Elbow and Sport

Luigi Adriano Pederzini
Denise Eygendaal • Matteo Denti
Editors

Elbow and Sport

Springer

ESSKA

Editors
Luigi Adriano Pederzini
Nuovo Ospedale di Sassuolo
Sassuolo
Italy

Denise Eygendaal
Department of Orthopedic Surgery
Amphia Hospital
Breda
The Netherlands

Matteo Denti
Istituto Clinico Humanitas
Rozzano
Milan
Italy

ISBN 978-3-662-48740-2 ISBN 978-3-662-48742-6 (eBook)
DOI 10.1007/978-3-662-48742-6

Library of Congress Control Number: 2016933454

Springer Heidelberg New York Dordrecht London

Printed on acid-free paper

Springer-Verlag GmbH Berlin Heidelberg is part of Springer Science+Business Media (www.springer.com)

Foreword

The editors of this informative and instructive *ESSKA* text, Luigi Pederzini, MD and Denise Eygendaal, MD, have invited my comments. This is a great honor, exhibiting their openness to commentary on their immense undertaking, together with numerous accomplished and respected authors and surgeons. Seeing the final product, I invite you into the pages and thoughts of surgeons who are inquisitive and creative, surgeons who can organize the complexities of orthopedic science to teach it with clarity, and surgeons who dare to break away from traditional elbow therapeutics with innovative insights and ideas.

It is a privilege to write this Foreword. Mine is a mature understanding of the upper extremity, mature but not fully grown. Maturity comes from age and experience, but as you will see in this text, there will always be new ideas and developments that further our knowledge of the upper extremity and of the elbow in particular. It was my good fortune to have been active, along with several others, during the pioneering stages of an upper extremity surgery revolution, a time when minimally invasive operative techniques proved more precise and advantageous to patients and to surgeons alike. That revolution is not over.

The various authors in this text are extensions of the main body of orthopedic surgical science. An elbow is where an extension – a river, stream, an arm, or an innovative surgeon – changes direction significantly or even radically. But the change permits a reach to a wholly new destination or to the same destination via a different route. These authors express their knowledge, opinions, and ideas which may subtly or radically change the direction of our understanding of the upper extremity in sports. The chapters in this book open new perspectives, new techniques, or nuances to upper extremity surgery.

Drs. Pederzini and Eygendaal have crafted a book not only *about* the elbow; it *is* the elbow in our thinking. It is current, cogent, comprehensive, and different; and it is organized into a very significant contribution to upper extremity surgical education.

Terry L. Whipple, MD

Contents

Clinical Relevant Anatomy of the Elbow

1

B. ten Brinke, A. Beumer, and D. Eygendaal

The elbow joint is a complex joint which combines a stable flexion and extension mechanism with a wide range of rotation and provides a stable position for a functional hand. To fulfill all these tasks, the elbow consists of three joints formed by the distal humerus, the proximal ulna, and the radial head: the radiohumeral joint (RHJ), the ulnohumeral joint (UHJ), and the proximal radioulnar joint (PRUJ). Knowledge of osteology and surrounding tissues such as ligaments, muscles, and neurovascular structures is crucial to understand the function of the elbow and the pathophysiology of elbow diseases.

1.1 Bones and Joints

The elbow plays a major role in the flexion-extension of the arm and supination-pronation of the forearm. There is also a slight medial and lateral mobility (abduction and adduction in frontal plane) and medial and lateral rotation (around the ulna in the transverse plane) [1]. The elbow is composed of three bones: the humerus, the ulna, and the radius (see Fig. 1.1a, b).

The shaft of the humerus ends in a lateral and medial ridge. Approximately 12 cm above the lateral ridge is a sulcus in which the radial nerve passes to the lateral side of the humerus. This is an important anatomical landmark in the surgical treatment of humeral fractures with plates or external fixators. Lateral and medial ridges end distally in the lateral and medial epicondyles (see Fig. 1.1a, b). The condyles of the humerus show a 30° anterior flexion in relation to the long axis, a 6–8° valgus tilt, and a 5° internal rotation in relation to the epicondylar line (see Fig. 1.1c–e).

To prevent anterior impingement during flexion of the elbow, the coronoid fossa and the radial fossa are located between the lateral and medial ridges on the anterior side of the distal humerus. On the posterior side, the olecranon fossa is located between the epicondyles to prevent posterior impingement during extension.

The trochlea is formed by the medial epicondyle, which forms the ulnohumeral joint with the olecranon of the ulna, which stabilizes the elbow during extension. The anterior side of the lateral epicondyle forms the capitellum. This convex structure articulates with the concave surface of the radial head. This is the radiohumeral joint, which plays a role in the stability of the elbow in flexion.

In the proximal ulna, the trochlear notch forms an angle of 30° with the ulna shaft, and there is also a slight 4° valgus angulation of the ulnar shaft (see Fig. 1.1f, g). The trochlear notch is divided into an anterior and a posterior part by the incisura trochlearis, a transverse portion composed of fatty tissue. This area of the olecranon can be used during an olecranon osteotomy to

B. ten Brinke • A. Beumer • D. Eygendaal (✉)
Department of Orthopaedic Surgery,
Amphia Hospital, Breda, The Netherlands
e-mail: denise@eygendaal.nl

L.A. Pederzini et al. (eds.), *Elbow and Sport*, DOI 10.1007/978-3-662-48742-6_1

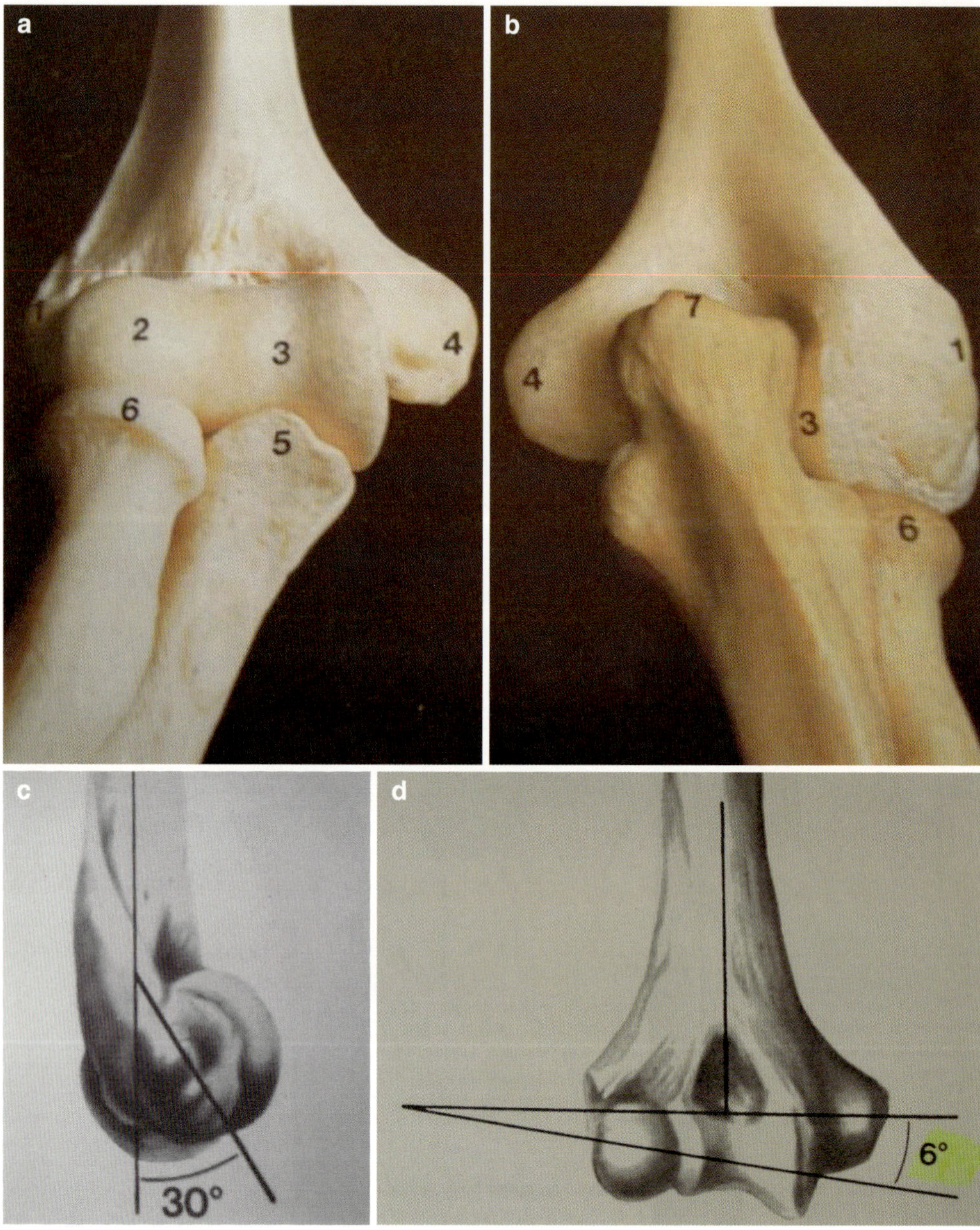

Fig. 1.1 (**a**) Anterior view: lateral epicondyle (*1*), capitellum (*2*), trochlea (*3*), medial epicondyle (*4*), coronoid process (*5*), and radial head (*6*). (**b**) Posterior view: olecranon (*7*). (**c–e**) The condyles of the humerus show a 30° anterior flexion in relation to the long axis, a 6–8° valgus tilt, and a 5° internal rotation in relation to the epicondylar line. (**f**, **g**) In the proximal ulna, the trochlear notch forms an angle of 30° with the ulna shaft, and there is also a slight 4° valgus angulation of the ulnar shaft. (**h–j**) The hyaline cartilage distribution of the proximal ulna varies and is often misinterpreted as osteochondral damage. (**k**) The radial head forms a 15° angle with the axis of the radial shaft

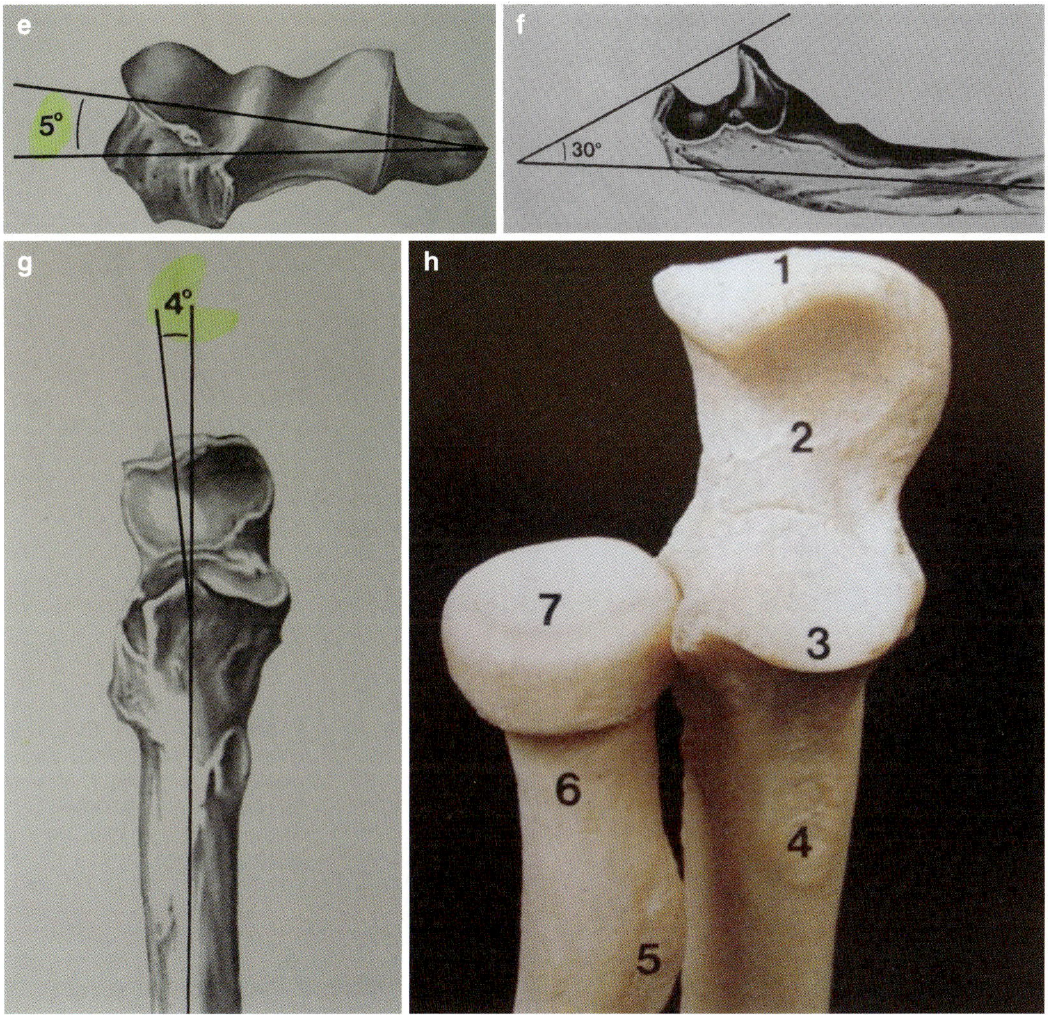

Fig. 1.1 (continued)

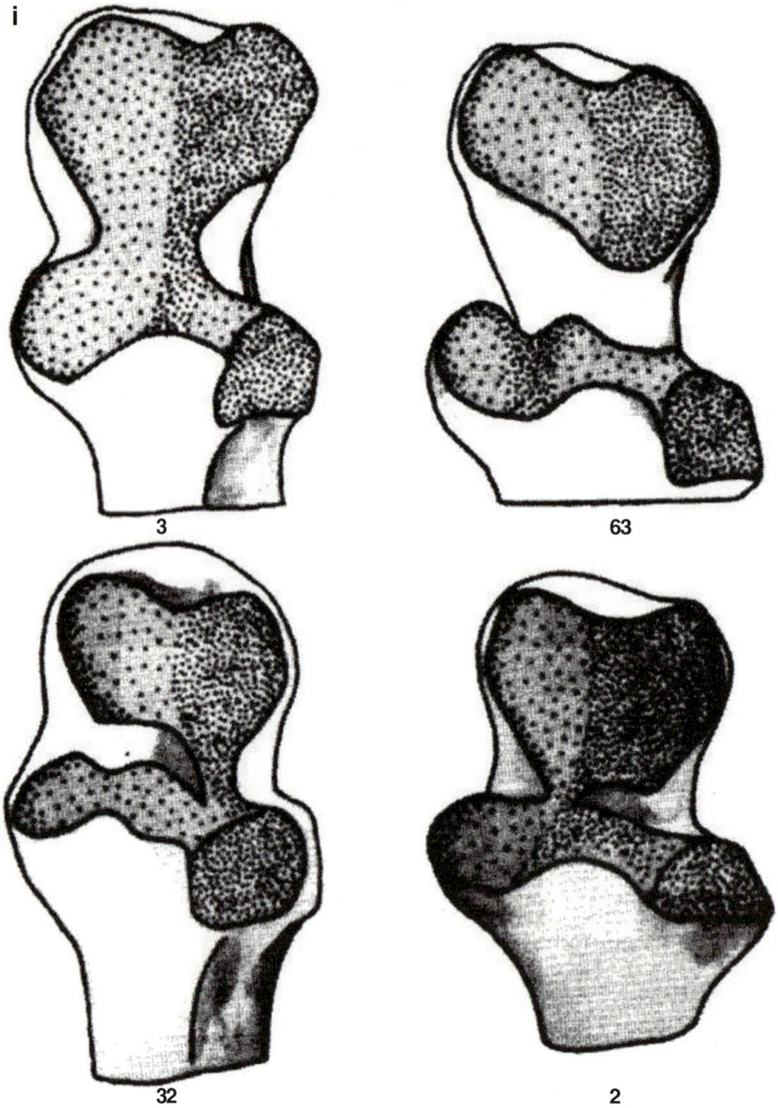

Fig. 1.1 (continued)

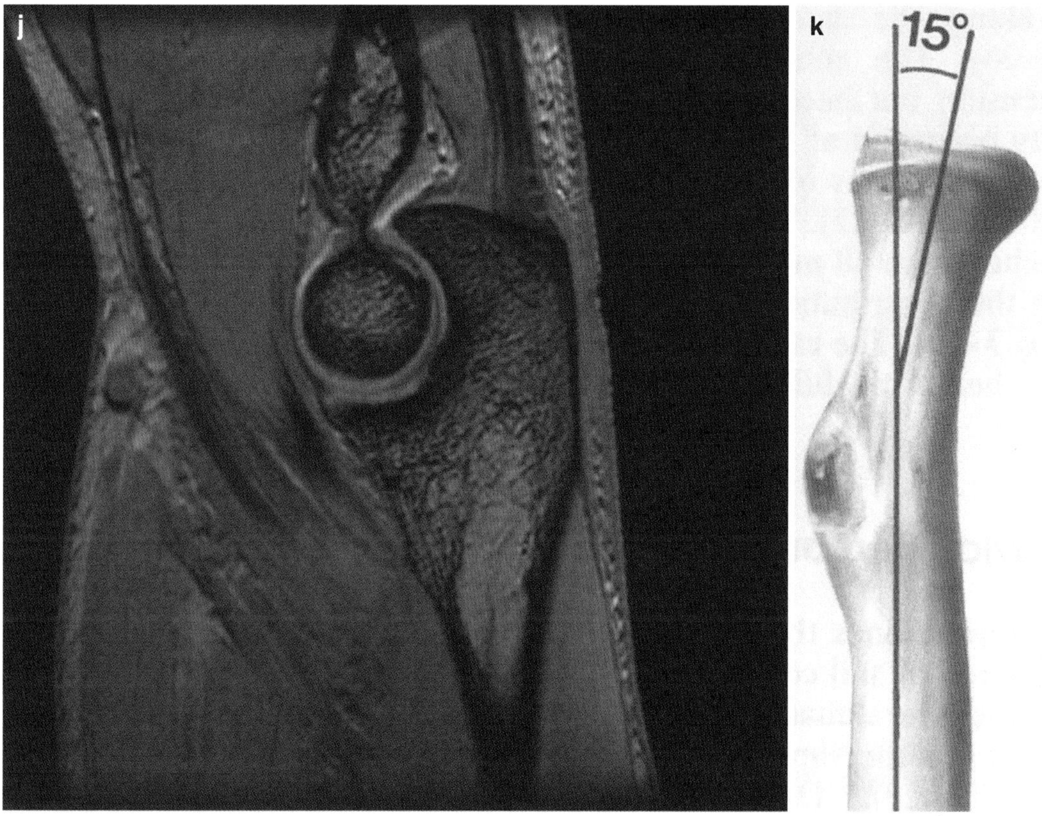

Fig. 1.1 (continued)

minimize cartilage damage. The hyaline cartilage distribution of the proximal ulna varies and is often misinterpreted as osteochondral damage (see Fig. 1.1h–j). The coronoid process, a protuberance of the ulna that demarcates the trochlear notch anteriorly, often fractures during dislocation of the elbow. Just distal and radial to the coronoid process, the radial notch of the ulna articulates with the radial head in the proximal radioulnar joint, contributing to pronation and supination of the forearm.

Since the radial head articulates with both the capitellum of the humerus and the radial notch of the ulna, it is covered with cartilage 280° around. The uncovered part of the radial head can be used for screw fixation in case of radial head fractures. The radial head forms a 15° angle with the axis of the radial shaft (see Fig. 1.1k).

There is a great amount of congruency between the articulating surfaces of the elbow. The tongue and groove-like fitting of the distal humerus on the ulna and radius make medial and lateral gliding almost impossible [2, 3].

The articular contact is influenced by the position of the elbow and the forearm. The radial head makes no contact with the cartilage of the capitellum during extension of the elbow. However, during flexion the radial head moves proximally resulting in an increased contact with the distal humerus. Supination of the forearm decreases the radiocapitellar contact, while pronation increases it. The knowledge of these positions is important during clinical examination of a degenerative elbow [4].

1.2 Joint Capsule and Ligaments

The three elbow joints are surrounded by a joint capsule. This capsule includes the olecranon, the coronoid fossa, and the radial fossa but not the humeral epicondyles. At the level of the radial head, distal from the radial annular ligament, the joint capsule forms a recess to preserve a good rotation of the radius (see Fig. 1.2a).

The joint capsule has a limited role in the stability of the elbow. To allow flexion and extension of the elbow, the capsule is loose on the anterior side and especially on the posterior. The volume of the capsule has been shown to average 23 ml. The capsule is most lax at 80° of flexion. Therefore patients with acute joint injury and inflammation combined with joint effusion find this position more comfortable. To prevent the capsule from sticking into the joints, small articular muscles radiate from the triceps brachii muscle and the brachial muscle. These muscles maintain sufficient tension on the capsule [5].

The collateral ligaments of the elbow are formed by thickenings of the capsule on the medial and lateral side. The medial collateral ligament consists of an anterior (AMCL) and a posterior (PMCL) bundle and a transversal ligament (also known as the Cooper ligament). The anterior and posterior bundles originate from the medial humeral epicondyle. The anterior bundle inserts the base of the coronoid process (sublime tubercle) of the ulna, and the posterior bundle inserts the medial part of the olecranon. The mean length of the AMCL is 27.1 mm and that of PMCL is 24.2 mm; the mean widths are about 4.7 mm and 5.3 mm, respectively. The function of these ligaments is to restrain valgus stress during extension (anterior bundle) and during flexion (posterior bundle) (see Fig. 1.2b) [6]. Studies reveal that the AMCL can be subdivided into three regions or bands according to their function [7, 8].

The lateral collateral ligament complex consists of three distinct bundles: the lateral ulnar collateral ligament (LUCL), the radial collateral ligament (RCL), and the annular ligament (AL) (see Fig. 1.2c). The LUCL and the RCL originate from the inferior part of the lateral epicondyle. The LUCL inserts into the crista supinatoris at the lateral side of the proximal ulna. The RCL extends to the AL. The AL encircles the radial head and originates and inserts on the ulna to maintain the radius to the ulna during rotations [3]. The function of the lateral collateral ligament complex is to provide stability during posterolateral directed forces on the elbow and during varus stress.

Similarly to the medial collateral ligament, various components of the lateral collateral ligament

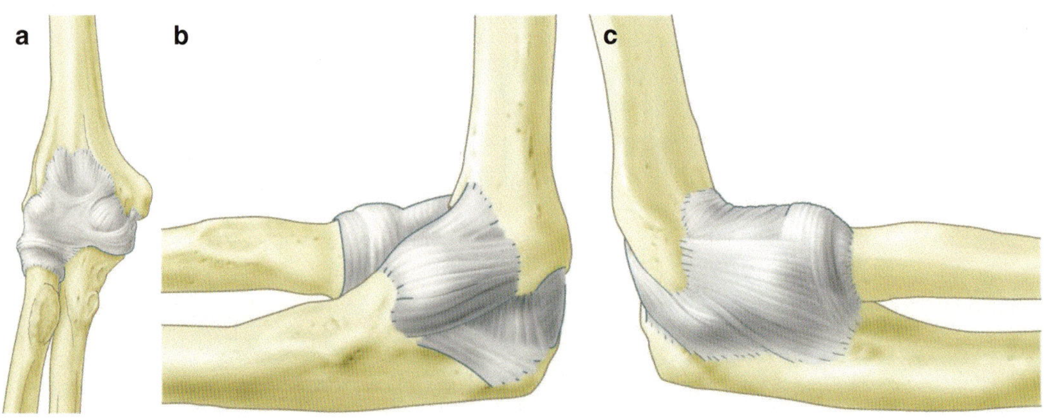

Fig. 1.2 (**a**) Anterior view of the joint capsule of the elbow. (**b**) Medial collateral ligement consisting of an anterior (AMCL) and posterior (PMCL) bundle and a transversal ligament. (**c**) Lateral collateral ligament complex consisting of the lateral ulnar collateral ligament (LUCL), the radial collateral ligament (RCL) and the annular ligament (AL)

play a different role in maintaining stability during varus stress. The anterior bundle of the RCL is tight during extension, while the posterior bundle is tightened during flexion. The middle part is taut in between extension and flexion. The LUCL is taut in extreme elbow flexion and tightens under varus stress.

The interosseous membrane (IOM) between the ulna and the radius prevents the displacement of the radius or ulna and regulates the acting forces on these two bones during closed chain activities [9].

1.3 Muscles

Three groups of muscles can be distinguished around the elbow: the extensor muscles of the elbow, the flexor muscles of the elbow, and the flexors/extensors of the wrist. Besides their role in all kinds of movements, muscles act as dynamic stabilizers as they compress the joint. Compression of the radial head and coronoid process in the articular surface of the distal humerus increases joint stability [10].

The most important extensor of the elbow is the triceps brachii muscle that originates from three proximal heads and inserts on the tip of the olecranon where it is palpable when the muscle is tensed against resistance. The anconeus muscle is a triangular muscle which originates from the lateral epicondyle and inserts posterolateral on the proximal ulna. The anconeus muscle is traditionally described as an extensor of the elbow, although its function is not fully understood. It mainly plays a stabilizing function on the elbow.

Primary flexors of the elbow are the brachialis, the biceps brachii, and the brachioradialis muscle.

The brachialis originates on both the humerus and the intermuscular septum and inserts on the anterior side of the proximal ulna. This muscle has the largest cross-sectional area of all flexors but suffers from a poor mechanical advantage because it crosses close to the axis of rotation. In addition, the brachialis seems to have an important role as a stabilizer against posterior subluxation [11]. The biceps brachii muscle has a two-headed origin. The short head originates from the coracoid process and inserts distally to the radial tuberosity and is a stronger flexor compared to the brachialis muscle. The long head originates from the superior glenoid aspect and inserts on the radial tuberosity and acts as a strong supinator. The brachioradialis muscle runs exclusively across the elbow. The muscle originates from the intermuscular septum and the lateral aspect of the distal humerus and inserts on the distal radius. It has the greatest mechanical advantage of any elbow flexor. Apart from its function as a flexor, it can contribute to pronation of the forearm when the arm is placed in supination.

The origin of the wrist extensor muscles is located at the lateral epicondyle. A common tendon is formed by the originating tendons of the extensor carpi radialis brevis, the extensor digitorum communis, the extensor digiti minimi, and the extensor carpi ulnaris. The supinator has a complex origin on the lateral epicondyle, the annular ligament, and the ulna. It inserts on the lateral proximal third of the radius. The extensor carpi radialis longus originates from the supracondylar bony ridge just below the origin of the brachioradialis.

At the medial epicondyle, the proximal insertion of the pronator teres, flexor carpi radialis, palmaris longus, flexor digitorum superficialis and profundus, and the flexor carpi ulnaris form the common flexor tendon. The palmaris longus is absent in approximately 15 % of normal individuals [12]. The pronator teres usually has a second site of origin on the medial part of the coronoid process, next to the second head of the flexor digitorum superficialis.

1.4 Neurovascular Structures

1.4.1 Nerves

The arm is innervated by three important nerves: the median nerve, the ulnar nerve, and the radial nerve (see Fig. 1.3a–c).

The median nerve is formed by the nerve roots from C6-T1 and first descends lateral to the brachial artery, anteriorly to the medial

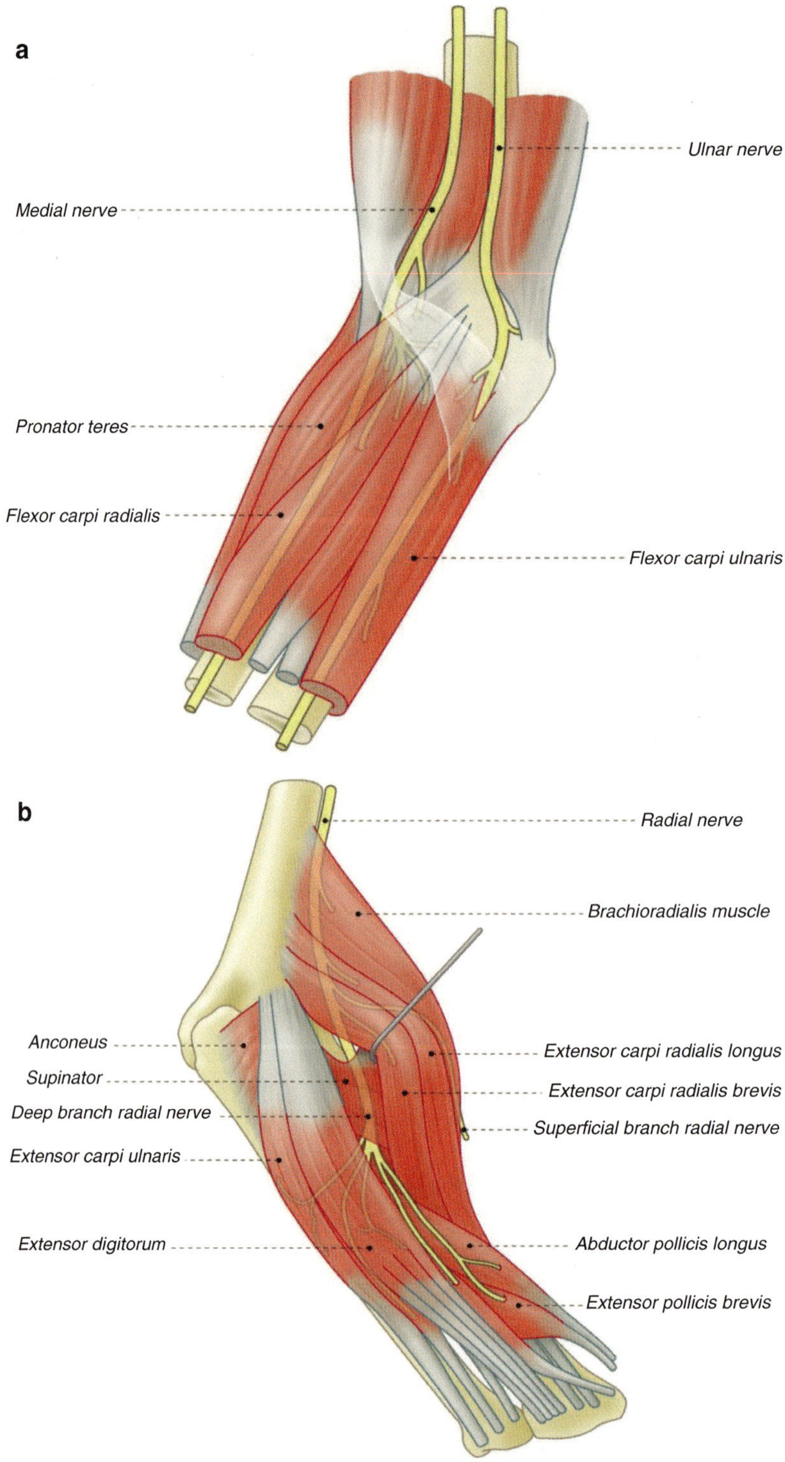

Fig. 1.3 (**a**) Anterior view of the medial and ulnar nerve. (**b**) Anterolateral view of the radial nerve and its branches. (**c**) Anterior view of the medial, radial and ulnar nerve. (**d**) Cuteneous innervation of the upper limb

c

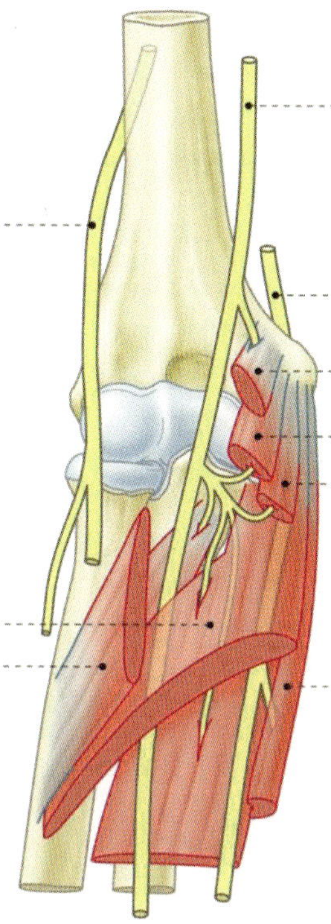

d

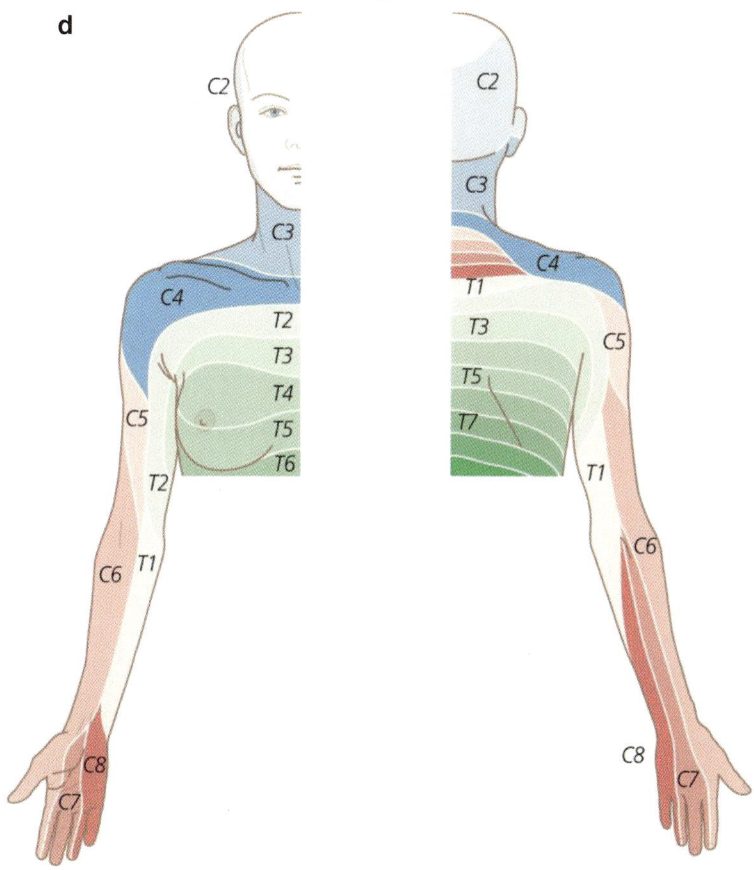

Fig. 1.3 (continued)

intermuscular septum. More distally, the median nerve crosses the brachial artery and continues medial to the artery. At the elbow, the median nerve lies in the cubital fossa, anterior to the brachioradialis muscle and posterior to the biceps tendon. Potential sites of entrapment are the ligament of Struthers (this is an anatomical variant where there is an accessory connection between a spur of bone and an accessory origin of the pronator teres muscle), under the biceps tendon, at the edge of the pronator teres muscle, and under the proximal free edge of the radial attachment of the flexor digitorum superficialis.

The ulnar nerve is derived from the nerve roots from C8-T1 and can be found medial to the brachial artery in the upper arm. The ulnar nerve enters the posterior compartment of the upper arm by crossing the medial intermuscular septum. At the elbow, the nerve lies in a shallow fibro-osseous sulcus at the posterior side of the medial epicondyle. It runs to the forearm between the two heads of the flexor carpi ulnaris muscle, where it can be compressed in the tunnel formed by the tendinous arch connecting these two heads to the humerus and the ulna.

The radial nerve originates from the nerve roots C8-T1 and initially runs dorsal to the humerus. It runs to the lateral aspect through the radial sulcus at the posterior side of the humeral shaft. The radial nerve runs deep between the brachialis and the brachioradial muscle proximally and the extensor carpi radialis longus distally. It divides into a motor, interosseous branch and a sensory, superficial branch. This sensory branch originates just before the radial tunnel, a tunnel between the anterior joint capsule and the proximal supinator muscle. Potential sites of radial nerve compression are fibrous bands of the radiocapitellar joint, the leash of Henry (where the radial nerve passes the recurrent radial artery), the medial edge of the extensor carpi radialis brevis, the proximal fascia of the supinator, and the distal edge of the supinator.

The cutaneous innervation of the elbow is variable; in general the proximal elbow is innervated by the lateral cutaneous (C5, C6) and medial cutaneous (C8, T1, T2) nerves. The skin of the distal elbow is innervated by the medial (C8, T1), lateral (C5, C6), and posterior (C6–C8) cutaneous nerves (see Fig. 1.3d).

1.4.2 Arteries

The subclavian artery forms the axillary artery that in turn forms the brachial artery. The first branches of the brachial artery are the profunda brachii artery, the superior collateral artery, and the inferior collateral ulnar artery. The brachial artery splits in a radial and ulnar artery at the anterior side of the elbow joint, close to the radial head. The radial recurrent artery is the first branch of the radial artery. This branch runs proximally to the brachioradialis muscle and the supinator and brachialis muscles to end in an anastomosis with the radial collateral branch of the profunda brachii artery. Further, the radial artery supplies the interosseous artery that is formed directly distal from the elbow.

The anterior and posterior ulnar recurrent arteries are the first two branches of the ulnar artery. The anterior branch runs through the anterior side of the medial epicondyle and forms an anastomosis with the inferior ulnar collateral artery. The posterior branch passes posterior to the medial epicondyle and makes an anastomosis with the inferior and superior ulnar collateral arteries.

1.4.3 Veins and Lymphatics

The deep venous structures are paired and run together with the arteries. The superficial veins are the basilic vein on the medial side and the cephalic vein on the lateral side of the elbow. These two veins are connected through the median cubital vein.

The elbow contains several lymph nodes that drain into the axillary lymphatic system. The most important lymph nodes are located supratrochlear, above the medial epicondyle.

1.5 Bursae

Around the elbow joint, several bursae have been described. Posteriorly, a superficial bursa is well known at the olecranon; a deep intratendinous bursa is present in the triceps tendon as it inserts at the tip of the olecranon. Bursae have also been described below the extensor carpi radialis brevis, deep in the anconeus muscle, on the medial and lateral aspect of the joint, and finally between the biceps tendon and the radial tuberosity.

References

1. Werner FW, An K-N. Biomechanics of the elbow and forearm. Hand Clin. 1994;10(3):357–73.
2. Van Glabbeek F. The effect of the length of the proximal part of the radial neck on the elbow function. Antwerp: Faculty of Medicine; University of Antwerp; 2005. p. 120.
3. Oatis CA. In: Wilkins WA, editor. The mechanics of human movement. Lippincott, Philadelphia; 2004.
4. McGinley JC, et al. Forearm and elbow injury: the influence of rotational position. J Bone Joint Surg Am. 2003;85-A(12):2403–9.
5. Platzer W. Atlas van de anatomie. 7th ed. SESAM, edition I (vol. 1). Baarn: Intro; 1999. p. 462.
6. Callaway GH, et al. Biomechanical evaluation of the medial collateral ligament of the elbow. J Bone Joint Surg Am. 1997;79(8):1223–31.
7. Regan WD, et al. Biomechanical study of ligaments around the elbow joint. Clin Orthop Relat Res. 1991; 271:170–9.
8. Tubbs RS, et al. The morphology and function of the quadrate ligament. Folia Morphol (Warsz). 2006; 65(3):225–7.
9. Pfaeffle HJ, et al. Reconstruction of the interosseous ligament restores normal forearm compressive load transfer in cadavers. J Hand Surg [Am]. 2005; 30(2):319–25.
10. Johnson JA, et al. Simulation of elbow and forearm motion in vitro using a load controlled testing apparatus. J Biomech. 2000;33(5):635–9.
11. King GJW, Morrey BF, An KN. Stabilizers of the elbow. J Shoulder Elbow Surg. 1993;2:165–74.
12. Sebastin SJ, et al. The prevalence of absence of the palmaris longus – a study in a Chinese population and a review of the literature. J Hand Surg [Br]. 2005; 30(5):525–7.

2 Biomechanics of the Elbow Joint in Overhead Athletes

Grzegorz Adamczyk

2.1 Introduction

The upper limb forms a kinematic chain, where all the elements are interrelated and functionally connected in order to optimalize its function. The basement is a shoulder girdle, the central part is an elbow, and the effector is the hand. These elements of the kinematic chain are strictly interconnected, and any elongation of the arm of the force by the sport attribute, for instance, tennis racquet, changes dramatically strains evoked at the level of the elbow joint. Majority of investigations of elbow biomechanics, used scales, concern daily living activities or are devoted to problems related to prosthetic design. The sport elbow function and athlete expectations are so complex that we should expect a new approach.

Sportsman needs a functional elbow "particularly fit" for a certain sport. One of my patients was a champion of Poland in Three-Day Event in horse riding, quite an extreme demanding sport competition, after a radial head removal, with a range of motion 30° of extension and 110° of flexion – he controls the horse mainly by relaxed wrist.

Athletes pose atypical strength, or speed, or precision of the joint motion. The role of proprioception cannot be overestimated. For instance, the biomechanical studies of the role of distal biceps rupture do concentrate on the loss of flexion strength, and the question is if reconstruction of distal biceps can allow to gain the flexion and supination. The matter of debate is when and how to suture it [14, 24]. I investigated three body builders, who lost their distal biceps and did not reconstruct it. Twenty-four weeks after trauma, they lost 20 % of the flexion strength, but 40 % of extension torque – probably due to proprioceptive problems with dynamic elbow stability (own unpublished data).

That's why we need always a complex, standardized biomechanical investigation of the whole limb – not only one joint, one movement study [17].

When one hits the tennis ball with a speed of 50 km/h, at the end of the racquet, in a backhand position and plays with a stiff wrist – taking under the consideration, that the wrist diameter is about 9 cm, the distance from the center of the grip to the ball 45 cm – the energy generated is such, that for the elbow it is an effort like lifting 25 kg. That's why the extensor mechanism then tears causing "tennis elbow" condition. So every technical mistake during the sport might have dramatical consequences on joint function, and meticulous knowledge of the elbow biomechanics in sport is crucial for the understanding of elbow diseases.

Grace to the shoulder girdle, in a trained person, upper limb rotates and covers more than the

G. Adamczyk
Gamma Medical Centre, Warsaw, Poland
e-mail: grzegorz.adamczyk@cmgamma.pl

L.A. Pederzini et al. (eds.), *Elbow and Sport*, DOI 10.1007/978-3-662-48742-6_2

hemisphere. That allows the hand to reach object located all around our body.

So, the complex anatomy of the elbow joint has to ensure both: the mobility and the stability of the whole construction. The main difference between the knee (central part of the lower limb concept) and the elbow is the key role of both: flexion-extension and prono-supination movements. On the other hand, it is absolutely untrue that because "people are not walking on hands," the elbow is shearing only limited forces. Bones of the upper limb are smaller in diameter, so the compression forces on square millimeter are relatively surprisingly high.

Elbow joint is composed from endings of three long bones: the distal humerus, proximal radius, and ulna. The articular surface of the distal humerus consists of the spool-shaped trochlea medially and the partially spherical capitellum laterally. From the strict lateral X-ray view, these articulations have approximately circular cross-sections, and these circles are nested concentrically together. That's why in the neutral position, elbow acts as a hinge joint and do not exist relative motions in between radius and ulna during flexion-extension.

To describe the type of possible motion of the elbow: flexion-extension and prono-supination one use expression – trochoginglymoid joint [2]. Elbow is composed of three interconnected articulations: the radio humeral, the ulno humeral and radioulnar one.

In majority of cases, the axis of flexion-extension activity is slightly valgus (male-female from 11° to 14°). One of possible reason for this difference is the width of the woman pelvis – for women is simply easier to carry heavy objects with upper limbs along their body when elbows are in valgus position [7]. This carrying angle in between the long axis of humerus and long axis of ulna is then approximately 6° with elbow extended and disappears with flexion.

Of course, meticulous video analysis showed that the elbow is not a pure hinge, due to obliquity of the trochlear groove, but helical pattern of these movements does not overpass 4–5°, so for the practical reason is better to see it as a pivot [2].

Axis of rotation is a line that passes through centers of curvatures of trochlear sulcus and capitellum.

When the carrying angle is 14°, the axis of flexion-extension movement is 7° from the base of coronoid process and the articular surface of radial head against the anterior surfaces of humeral fossae [4].

During the prono-supination, radius rotates around the ulna. Longitudinal axis of rotation passes from the center of concave surface of radial head to convex center of the ulnar distal head. Forearm rotation normally reaches 80° of pronation and 90° of supination [7]. The functional rotation of the object, like a pencil grasped in the hand, is much higher. Movement of the wrist and fingers, flexion of the fifth metacarpal bone in supination, adds another 30°. The axis of prono-supination is ulna. It's easy to check: when one positions the forearm on a table, with elbow, wrist, and fifth finger extended and keeps finger at its place, the ulna and radius are almost perfectly parallel. Supination of the forearm rotates then only the radius, and radial bone reaches a certain angle around the stable ulna. The anatomical axis of rotation passes from the center of the capitellum, through the center of the radial head proximally to the center of the ulnar head distally, then on toward the little finger.

Normally, the rotation axis passes along the long finger. Then pronation entails ulnar abduction, and supination causes ulnar adduction. If we then control the wrist motion with the opposite hand, the motion of the distal ulna can be noticed, it follows a rotary swing. This is not caused by the ulna rotating at the elbow; the shape of distal humerus and proximal ulna stable blocks such a possibility; however, it is circumduction. The curved path in space is accomplished by combinations of ulnar abduction and flexion during pronation and adduction and flexion during supination [4, 31].

Ray and James immobilized humerus by pins and took double-exposure radiographs in pronation and supination, and the humeroulnar varus-valgus motion of approximately 9° was documented [31].

Radial head is not perfectly circular, it is slightly elliptical and it allows sliding of the proximal radio-ulnar joint. This deviation from a circle gives support to the bearing surface against the ulna. Forearm rotation clearly involves rotational sliding motion between the concave end face of the radial head and the capitellum.

The proximal radioulnar joint is stabilized by the solid surrounding annular ligament that attaches strongly to the anterolateral corner of the coronoid and to the supinator ridge of the ulna. This structure prevents subluxation of the radial head during all activities and resists the anteriorly directed tension of the biceps tendon during elbow flexion.

For pronation and supination, the restraint is passive resistance of stretched muscles rather than the ligaments. The ROM of the intact cadaver arm is approximately 150°, whereas when muscles are excised 190° [2].

Meticulous knowledge of muscle attachments to the elbow forces generated by these muscles during different phases of sport activities is crucial factor for understanding the function of this joint. Growing expectation of the sportsmen, elongation of the limbs, and in consequence of arm forces, raising speed of well-trained arm and number of repetitions of some very particularly positioned upper limbs, causes the very new problems for our society.

2.2 Biomechanics of the Elbow

The forces around the joint must be in equilibrium, and their balance leads to zero resultant. Thus, the forces acting upward must be equal and opposite to those acting downward.

In this simplified analysis of elbow flexion, the muscle tension T is 200 N, and so the joint force JF is 180 N (Fig. 2.1). The lack of any muscle actions modeled along the forearm means that JF is predicted to act axially onto the distal humerus [26].

In normal circumstances, elbow flexion in man is from 0° to 150°, in woman from hyperextension 12–15° to 150°. The checking agent is an impact of the tip of olecranon to trochlear fossa – in full extension collateral ligaments are taut and stop the movement [26].

So, in example taken from book of Nordin and Frankel [26], the extension moment exerted by the load in the hand is 20 N times 0.35 m, or 7 Nm. This must be opposed by an equal and opposite flexion moment from the muscles. So, if the muscle exerts a moment of 7 N m at a moment arm of 35 mm (0.035 m), the muscle tension T must equal 7 Nm divided by 0.035 m, or 200 N. These calculations are of course simplification, treating elbow like pure hinge joint with all muscles acting parallel to long axis of humerus, like biceps and brachialis. Of course, in real situations, all other muscles (wrist and finger flexors) are clenched to stabilize the lifted object. The tensions in the finger flexor muscles compress the humeroulnar joint, due to flexor digitorum superficialis originating from the medial epicondyle and flex due to action of flexor digitorum profundus. We even sometimes use these muscles to restore elbow flexion in brachial plexus palsy (Steiner procedure). Clenched fist is stabilized as well by extensors – this pressure of the radial head against the humeral joint phenomenon might be illustrated by radial head migration after Monteggia fracture.

Generally, all actions that require a large force to be exerted cause all of the available muscles to contract, not just to produce a movement but also to stabilize the joints [23].

Basic works of Amis, Basmajian, and Long described the function of separate muscles using electromyography investigation. Lower limb carries the body weight during walking, so basic studies evaluate muscle function during gait phases, changing the position of the body. Studies of the upper limb are more difficult; we need to precise exactly, which action is of the interest: lifting heavy objects, stabilizing joints, operating peculiar machines, and ergonomics for industrial purposes.

2.2.1 Capacity and Contact Areas of the Elbow Joint

The capacity of the adult elbow joint is about 25 ml, reaching maximum at 80° of flexion – that's why stiff elbow most commonly is flexed [28]. The central depression of the radial head articulates with the dome of capitellum; medial triangular facet of TFCC is always in contact with the ulna. With the load of 10 N, about 9 %

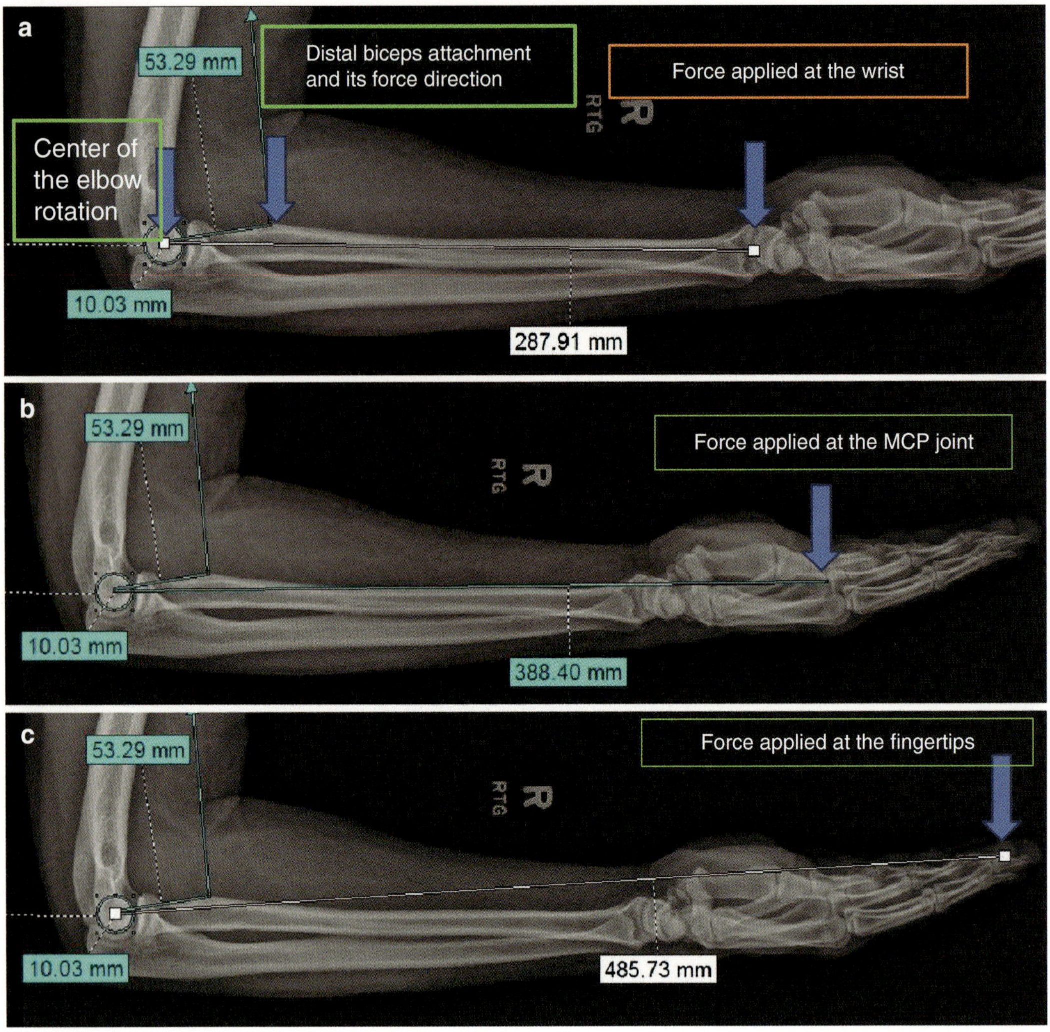

Fig. 2.1 Arm of the forces generated on the elbow joint, when the force is applied: (**a**) at the level of the wrist, (**b**) at the level of MCP joint, and (**c**) at the level of fingertips. Arc of rotation – center of capitellum, attachment of the distal biceps marked by green line on the radial tuberosity, distances in millimeters, my own forearm

contact of joint surfaces occurs, with the load of 120 N, it increases to almost 73 % [15].

2.2.2 Stabilization of the Elbow Joint

The elbow is one of the most congruent and stable joints of the human body.

Main reasons for that are almost parallel bony components of joint surfaces and very solid soft tissue stabilizers – lateral and medial collateral ligaments and anterior capsule. Lateral collateral ligament and anterior bundle of medial collateral ligament start from the endpoints of axis of rotation of the elbow joint [34, 35].

Medial collateral ligament has two components: the anterior bundle taut in extension but its posterior bundle is taut in flexion. Lateral collateral ligament assumes rather constant tension during all activities and functions with or without the radial head, central part of it called lateral collateral ulnar ligament that attaches to ulna, thus stabilizes the ulnar-humeral joint and controls the pivot-shift maneuver [27, 34, 35].

In extension, anterior capsule provides about 70 % of soft tissue restraint; in flexion main agent is a medial collateral ligament.

In extension, varus resistance is controlled equally by joint congruency, mainly olecranon in olecranon fossa and lateral collateral ligament; in flexion, joint congruency is responsible for 75 % of stability.

Valgus stress in extension is spread equally among the joint congruency, anterior capsule, and medial collateral ligament; in flexion in 74 %, the medial collateral ligament is responsible for resistance.

Varus and valgus laxity of the elbow depends on the forearm rotation [30]. Increased valgus/varus laxity in medially unstable joints puts, for instance, baseball pitchers in a risk of medial collateral ligament chronic injury due to permanent overload. So, one should clinically test the stability in sportsman in different ranges of prono-supination.

Bony eminences – like tip of olecranon, of coronoid process, and even partial excision of radial head – seem to play a crucial role in the elbow stability, and their restitution in traumatic setting is crucial for the athletes [10].

The role of muscles surrounding the elbow joint in its stabilization was postulated because of their course parallel to collateral ligaments. But in recent electromyographic studies, e.g., of flexor carpi ulnaris and extensor digitorum superficialis, muscles did not reveal their significant activity, when valgus or varus forces were applied [22]. Also baseball pitchers with medial collateral ligament insufficiency did not present any increased EMG activity of these muscles – so they probably do not support collaterals in their function [19].

2.2.3 Elbow Joint Load During Normal Activities

The size of the joint forces obviously relates to the external load. The elbow muscles work at a large mechanical disadvantage when comparing their small moment arms about the joint axis to the large moment arms of loads exerted on the lower limb. The radius of the curvature of joint surface, e.g., of capitellum and the length of the forearm, elongated by the hand and fingers, makes the articular forces surprisingly high.

The same muscles act differently in extension, neutral, and flexed position of the elbow.

In sagittal plane of motion, elbow is a hinge joint. Moments of forces applied at the hand are balanced by the muscles, tendons, ligaments, and contact forces on articular surfaces. In a single muscle, two-dimensional analysis basic equilibrium equation is used:

$$F = \frac{M}{P} = \cos\,\Psi \frac{d}{rf} + \sin\,\Psi \frac{rp}{rf}$$

$$\frac{R}{P} = \sqrt{f^2 + 2f\cos(\Theta + \Psi) + 1}$$

$$\phi = \tan^{-1} \frac{f\sin\,\Theta - \sin\,\Psi}{f\cos\,\Theta + \cos\,\Psi}$$

Where Ψ, Θ, and ϕ are the angles between the forearm axis and applied force, P, muscle pull, M, and resultant joint force, R, respectively [4, 7].

Classical works of Amis showed that when the elbow is near full extension, both the forearm muscles and the elbow flexors (principally biceps, brachialis, brachioradialis, and pronator teres) are pulling in similar directions. Their tensile forces then addict, resulting in very large forces acting onto the end of the humerus. This reaches a maximum of 5 kN at 30° flexion, for maximal isometric strength of a normal young male adult [4, 5]. Flexion starts from compressing the elbow joint and tearing radial head a little bit to the front, mainly by the biceps tendon.

In the bended elbow, flexors tend to distract the joint, in opposition to the forearm muscles that are always acting along the forearm. Thus, the elbow forces fall to their lowest values, 1 kN maximum.

Triceps is the primary elbow extensor; it is the strongest single muscle in the upper limb. The lateral head of the triceps does not insert into the tip of the olecranon and passes alongside it laterally and is attached to the fascia of the anconeus. Elbow extension causes large humeroulnar joint forces and that the triceps tension causes large tensile stresses in the olecranon. The joint force varies from 1.5 kN acting onto the distal aspect of the humerus at full extension, to 3.5 kN acting onto the anterodistal aspect at 120° flexion [7].

Pronator teres and pronator quadratus are the main pronators, while supination results primarily from actions in biceps and supinator. These muscles tend to cause forces acting transversely to the axis of the forearm, their action is reinforced by flexors and extensors of the wrist and fingers that pull the bones axially. The result is that the humeroradial and humeroulnar joints are loaded, while the proximal radioulnar joint is subjected to only small forces [4, 5, 11].

Pushing toward the centerline of the body with hand, when the elbow flexed, such as when pulling a mill or like they do in sumo, holding a large object causes torsion load on the humerus. This is in response to tensions in the anterior pectoral muscles causing internal rotation at the shoulder. The distal humerus has to be wide enough to resist the abduction action of the forearm. The load is resisted by a force couple: tension in the medial collateral ligament and compression in the humeroradial joint [4, 5].

When the force is directed along the centerline of the forearm (good technically boxer hit), then approximately 70 % of the load is transmitted by the radius directly to the capitellum [3]. When the force vector passes toward the lateral side of the elbow, in a slight varus position, then all of the load passes directly to the radius and the elbow is stable. If the force passes medially, in a slight valgus, the tenuous lateral collateral ligament structures do not maintain stability, but this situation is not normally encountered due to the carrying angle.

2.3 Interosseous Membrane

Pushing, or falling on extended hand, causes compressive forces to pass through the hand and wrist, then along the forearm to the elbow. One of the elements active in transmission of these forces is interosseous membrane. The exact role of an interosseous membrane is not fully known yet. The central part of the interosseous membrane includes strong interosseous ligament, and its resistance is estimated as similar to patellar tendon. This postulated structure links the radius and ulna, prevents proximal radius migration, and provides transverse stability in between forearm bones. In a fall, radius bears 80 % of the wrist load and 60 % of the elbow load. Interosseous ligament transfers load from hand to elbow and prevents radius and ulna from splaying.

The membrane has much lower stiffness than the radius, so it cannot transmit a significant load until it is stretched by a proximal migration of its radial attachment; this can only occur after radial head fracture.

Interosseous membrane loses when the forearm is pronated, the functional position when pushing or falling onto the outstretched hand. That also limits its role in transmission of forces.

An alternative hypothesis for the function of the interosseous membrane is that it is an extensive area for muscle attachment, and so it acts to transmit tensile force from the deep muscles to the radius, in equilibrium with the compressive force of the carpus loading the end of the radius.

In a fall forward onto the outstretched hand, the posture taken up automatically has the shoulder partly internally rotated, the elbow slightly flexed (approximately 15°), and the forearm semi-pronated, so that the palm faces the floor [12]. The flexed and elastic posture is important because after impact the elbow flexes and the shoulder extends, muscle stretching absorbs energy rather than bones. The landing posture places the lateral aspect of the elbow uppermost on impact. That's why the radius will be compressed and the medial collateral ligament tensed. Thus, 100 % of the impact force passes to the radial head and so it is the most common site of bone fracture at the elbow [8].

2.4 Distribution of Forces on the Articular Surfaces

When the elbow is extended and axially loaded, 40 % of force is transmitted across ulnohumeral joint and 60 % across radiohumeral [18]. In cadaveric studies, it has been noted that in severe valgus realignment, 12 % of load is transmitted through the distal ulna, in severe varus position 95 % [1].

When the elbow is flexed, internal rotation against resistance may lead to twice body weight transmission on medial collateral ligament and three times body weight on the radiohumeral joint [3].

The problem in analysis of these forces transmitted during activities is that it is extremely difficult to estimate them during sport or combat activities. Majority of investigation concerns daily living activities or is devoted to prosthetic design, very few studies concern sport or extreme possibilities of the human body.

2.5 Evaluation of the Elbow

Range of motion might be effectively investigated with the simple hand goniometer, and normal passive elbow flexion is from 0 to 140–150°, some elbow are hyperextended to 20°, pronation averages about 75°, and supination 85°. Some athletes, e.g., body builders and heavy weight lifters, with advancing age lose some range of motion due to overuse changes and muscle mass.

For majority of functions, the full ROM is not needed.

There are numerous methods to analyze three-dimensional joint motion: triaxial electrogoniometer, videotelemetry, miniature accelerometers, computer-simulated motions, and many others [17, 25].

One might distinguish three basic types of muscle contraction according to changes of length, force, and velocity of action.

If there's no change of length during contraction, the contracture is called isometric, when muscle lengthens while maintains tension, it's called eccentric, and while shortens, it's called concentric. The eccentric exercises are associated with muscle fiber tear, and it leads to muscle receptor damage that alters joint position sense [13, 25].

Isotonic contraction is the one when muscle produces a constant force and shortens, and when the angular speed of contraction is constant, the contraction is isokinetic.

In sport, rates of motion that reach 300° per second are common. For the training purposes, to build a power, isometric or slow motions are more effective than high-velocity exercises. Technique of measurement of isokinetic strength are mane, simple tensiometer, or accommodate resistance dynamometer is commonly sufficient. When evaluating strength, we define torque created around the joint or force generated by hand and forearm. Most of the torque is generated by brachialis, biceps, and brachioradialis.

There are many variables influencing the effect: motivation and the positive effect of repeating the measurement ("learning curve of instrument"). One should be very aware when motivating a sportsmen to do maximum effort – I've experienced several times even contusions with young athletes trying to obtain a maximum effect – we should pay extreme attention to warming, good preparation for testing.

2.6 Specific Sport Problems

Injuries to the elbow, forearm, and wrist account for approximately 25 % of all sport-related injuries. Specific elbow injury patterns can be so common to a specific sport that associated names have been applied to them such as tennis elbow, golfer's elbow, or little leaguer's elbow [29].

Nowadays, a useful tool becomes video recordings and even YouTube. Schreiber et al. [33] analyzing acute elbow dislocation from YouTube recordings available in net stated that acute elbow dislocations in vivo occur in relative extension irrespective of forearm position, a finding distinct from previous cadaveric studies. The most common mechanism appears to involve a valgus moment to an extended elbow, which suggests a requisite disruption of the medial collateral ligament, the known primary constraint to valgus force.

2.6.1 Chronic Elbow Injury

The biomechanics of the chronic elbow injury have been the most extensive examined during the baseball pitch, the football pass, the tennis serve, the javelin throw, and the underhand softball pitch – so-called overhead activities.

Because of location of many laboratories in US, primary emphasis has been placed on the baseball pitch. Professional pitcher might throw the ball up to 1200–1500 times a day, and each and every technical detail of this movement has to be carefully followed, to avoid elbow abuse. We all have in eyes picture of pitch divided into six phases [16]. They are windup, stride, arm cocking, arm acceleration, arm deceleration, and follow-through.

A maximum elbow angular velocity of 2,100° per second to 2,700° per second occurs at approximately halfway through the acceleration phase [16]. Roberts [32] reported that a pitcher with a paralyzed triceps because of a differential nerve block was able to throw a ball over 80 % of the speed attained before paralyzation. The triceps contraction does not generate all of the elbow extension velocity and that centrifugal force is a major factor.

Toyoshima et al. [37] compared "normal throwing" (using the entire body) with throwing using only the forearm to extend the elbow. It was stated that throwing only with the elbow contributed in less than 43 % to ball velocity and that a larger contribution percentage to ball velocity resulted from body rotation.

Fifty percent of pitchers have a flexion contracture averaging 5° of the dominant elbow, with 30 % demonstrating a cubitus valgus deformity [21].

2.6.1.1 Football

The motion in throwing a football is qualitatively similar to throwing a baseball [16]. During arm cocking, a quarterback showed greater elbow flexion than pitchers, with an average of 113°. Also during arm cocking, a maximum medial force of 280 N and a maximum varus torque of 54 nm are produced at the elbow. During arm acceleration, the elbow reaches a maximum extension velocity of 1,760° per second. To decelerate the elbow, a quarterback generates a flexion torque of 41 nm and a compressive force of 620 N. Slower elbow extension is probably responsible for less elbow injury in quarterbacks than pitchers.

2.6.1.2 Tennis

Elbow joint contributes 15 % of the force produced during the tennis serve [20]. As with the overhand throw, the tennis serve generates considerable angular velocity at the elbow. He stated that the angular velocity for elbow extension reaches 982° per second and pronation reaches 347° per second. Conflicting with these conclusions was a study by Sprigings [36] investigating the effectiveness of arm segment rotations in producing racquet-head speed. Forearm pronation had the fastest rotation of 1,375° per second.

Bibliography

1. An K. Biomechanics, basic relevant concepts. Section I – basic science. In: Morrey BF, editor. Joint replacement arthroplasty. New York: Churchill Livingstone; 1991. p. 7.
2. An K, Zobitz M, Morrey BF. Biomechanics of the elbow. In: Morrey BF, Sanchez-Sotelo J, editors. The elbow and its disorders. Philadelphia: Saunders-Elsevier; 2009. p. 39–63.
3. Amis A, Dowson D, Miller J, et al. Biomechanical aspects of the elbow: joint forces related to prosthesis design. IEEE Eng Med Biol Mag. 1981;10:65.
4. Amis AA, Dowson D, Unsworth A, et al. An examination of the elbow articulation with particular reference to variation of the carrying angle. Eng Med. 1977;6:76–80.
5. Amis A, Dowson D, Wright V. Muscle strengths and musculoskeletal geometry of the upper limb. Eng Med. 1977;8:41–56.
6. Amis AA, Dowson D, Wright V. Elbow joint force predictions for some strenuous isometric actions. J Biomech. 1979;13:765–75.
7. Amis AA, Miller JH. The elbow. Clin Rheum Dis. 1982;8:571–93.
8. Amis A, Miller J. The mechanisms of elbow fractures: an investigation using impact tests in vitro. Injury. 1995;26:163–8.
9. Amis A, Miller J, Dowson D, et al. Axial forces in the forearm. In: Stokes IAF, editor. Mechanical factors and the skeleton. London: Libbey; 1981. p. 29–37.
10. Askew L, An K, Morrey BF, et al. Isometric elbow strength in normal individuals. Clin Orthop. 1987;222: 261–71.
11. Basmajian J, DeLuca C. Muscles alive: their functions revealed by electromyography. Baltimore: Williams and Wilkins; 1985.
12. Carlsoo S, Johansson O. Stabilization of and load on the elbow joint in some protective movements. Acta Anatom Scand. 1962;48:224–31.
13. Chao EY. Experimental methods for biomechanical measurements of joint kinematics. In: Fenberg B,

Fleming D, editors. CRC handbook of engineering in medicine and biology; Section B: Instruments and measurements. West Palm Beach: CRC Press; 1978.
14. Chavan P, Duquin T, Bisson L. Repair of the ruptured distal biceps tendon: a systematic review. Am J Sports Med. 2008;36(8):1618–24.
15. Eckstein F, Lohe F, Muller-Gerbl M, et al. Stress distribution in the trochlear notch. A model of bicentric load transmission through joints. J Bone Joint Surg Br. 1994;76:647–80.
16. Fleisig G, Escamilla R. Biomechanics of the elbow in the throwing athlete. Oper Tech Sports Med. 1996;4(2):62–8.
17. Gribble P, Ostry D. Independent coactivation of shoulder and elbow muscles. Exp Brain Res. 1998; 125(3):355–68.
18. Halls A, Travill A. Transmission of pressures across the elbow joint. Anat Rec. 1964;150:245–52.
19. Hamilton C, Glousman R, Jobe F, et al. Dynamic stability of the elbow, electromyographic analyses of flexor pronator group and the extensor group in pitchers with valgus instability. J Shoulder Elbow Surg. 1996;5:547–62.
20. Kibler W. Clinical biomechanics of the elbow in tennis: implications for evaluation and diagnosis. Med Sci Sports Exerc. 1994;26:1203–6.
21. King J, Brelsford H, Tullos H. Analysis of the pitching arm of the professional baseball pitcher. Clin Orthop Relat Res. 1969;67:116–23.
22. Le Bozec S, Maton B, Cnockaert J. The synergy of elbow extensor muscles during dynamic work in man; Part 1. Elbow extension. Eur J Appl Physiol. 1980; 44:250–62.
23. Long C, Conrad P, Hall E, et al. Intrinsic-extrinsic muscle control of the hand in power group and precision handling. An electromyographic study. J Bone Joint Surg. 1970;53A:853–67.
24. Morrey BF. Injury of the flexors of the elbow. In: Morrey BF, editor. The elbow and it's disorders. Philadelphia: WB Saunders; 2000. p. 468–78.
25. Morrey B, An K. Functional evaluation of the elbow. In: Morrey B, Sanchez- Sotelo J, editors. The elbow and its disorders. Philadelphia: Saunders-Elsevier; 2009. p. 80–91.
26. Nordin M, Frankel V. Basic biomechanics of the musculoskeletal system. Philadelphia: Lea & Febiger; 1989.
27. O'Driscoll S, Bell D, Morrey BF. Posterolateral rotatory instability of the elbow. J Bone Joint Surg Am. 1991;73:440.
28. O'Driscoll S, Morrey BF, An K. Intraarticular pressure and capacity of the elbow. Arthroscopy. 1990;6: 100–6.
29. Plancher K, Minnich J. Sports-specific injuries. Clin Sports Med. 1996;15:207–8.
30. Pomianowski S, O'Driscoll S, Neale P, et al. The effect of forearm rotation on laxity and stability of the elbow. Clin Biomech (Bristol, Avon). 2001;16:401–12.
31. Ray R, Johnson R, Jameson R. Rotation of the forearm: an experimental study of pronation and supination. J Bone Joint Surg. 1951;33A:993–6.
32. Roberts T. Cinematography in biomechanical investigation. In: Selected topics on biomechanics: proceedings of the CIC symposium on biomechanics. Chicago: The Athletic Institute; 1971. p. 41–50
33. Schreiber J, Russell F, Hotchkiss R, et al. An online video investigation into the mechanism of elbow dislocation. J Hand Surg. 2013;38A:488–94.
34. Söbjerg J, Ovesen J, Gundorf C. The stability of the elbow following excision of the radial head and transection of the annular ligament. An experimental study. Arch Orthop Trauma Surg. 1987;106:248.
35. Söbjerg J, Ovesen J, Nielsen S. Experimental elbow instability after transection of medial collateral ligament. Clin Orthop. 1987;218:186.
36. Sprigings E, Marshall R, Elliott B, et al. A three-dimensional kinematic method for determining the effectiveness of arm segment rotations in producing racquet-head speed. J Biomech. 1994;27:245–54.
37. Toyoshima S, Hoshikawa T, Miyashita M. Contributions of the body parts of throwing performance. In: Nelson RC, Morehouse CA, editors. Biomechanics IV. Baltimore: University Park Press; 1974. p. 169–74.

Physical Examination of the Elbow 3

A. Van Tongel

The evaluation of elbow pain in the athlete can be challenging because of the complexity of the joint and its central location in the upper extremity. Although the elbow is not a weight bearing joint, it is subjected to significant loads, especially in overhead and throwing athletes.

To perform an adequate examination of the injured elbow, a good understanding of the anatomy of the elbow is required. The examination should be done in a systematic fashion using a step-by-step approach: (1) history, (2) inspection, (3) palpation, (4) passive motion, (5) active motion, (6) active motion against resistance, (7) a neurologic examination, and (8) a lidocaine test. These eight steps will allow a clinical diagnosis to be made in 90 % of athletes with elbow pathology.

3.1 History

Evaluation of elbow pathology begins with a thorough history, including comorbidities, hand dominance, and vocation. Evaluation of patient complaints with particular emphasis on pain, locking, stiffness, and paresthesia should allow the clinician to determine whether a single traumatic event or a series of repetitive traumatic episodes caused the symptoms.

Pain is the most common complaint. If the pain was first noted after a trauma, it is important to evaluate what, if anything, the athlete experienced just before and at the time of the injury. Also, it is important to ask about the presence and location of any swelling or bruising after the traumatic event and if there was a "pop." Any neurologic or vascular symptoms should also be identified.

If the pain started gradually, it is important to know the duration of the symptoms, during which activities the pain occurs, and any changes in the athlete's training or daily routine. This should include any changes in technique, equipment, and coaching [5]. A patient whose symptoms are related to throwing or to an occupational stress should be asked to reproduce the position that causes the symptoms.

The location and area of pain should be clearly identified because, for reasons that remain unclear, the posterior lateral ulnohumeral joint appears to be a "watershed" referral point for a spectrum of remote conditions. Dividing the elbow into four anatomic regions (i.e., lateral, medial, anterior, and posterior) helps to narrow the range of differential diagnoses (Tables 3.1 and 3.2).

Next, the evaluator should inquire about mechanical symptoms, such as clicking with motion, locking in extension, and catching, which can be caused by intra-articular pathology. Also loss of extension and/or flexion needs to be

A. Van Tongel
Department of Orthopaedic Surgery and Traumatology, Ghent University Hospital, De Pintelaan 185, B-9000 Gent, Belgium
e-mail: alexander.vantongel@uzgent.be

L.A. Pederzini et al. (eds.), *Elbow and Sport*, DOI 10.1007/978-3-662-48742-6_3

Table 3.1 Summary physical examination

1.	History	1. Co-morbidity		
		2. Etiology	Acute	
			Progressive	
		3. Symptoms	Pain	
			Stiffness	
			Locking	
			Paresthesia	
		4. Location		
2.	Inspection	1. Resting position		
		2. Localized swelling		
		3. Carrying angle		
		4. Anatomical areas		
		5. General inspection		
3.	Palpation	1. Lateral		
		2. Medial		
		3. Posterior		
		4. Anterior		
4.	Passive motion	1. Flexion – extension		
		2. Pronation – supination		
		3. Stability	Valgus	Valgus stress test
				Moving valgus test
				Milking maneuver
			Varus	Varus stress test
			Posterolateral	Lateral pivot shift
			Posteromedial	Medial pivot shift
5.	Active motion	1. Flexion – extension		
		2. Pronation – supination		
6.	Active motion against resistance	1. Brachialis		
		2. Biceps	Hooktest	
		3. Triceps		
		4. ECRB (tenniselbow)		
		5. FCR + pronator teres (golfer's elbow)		
		6. Stability	Posterolateral	Push-up test
				Chair test
7.	Neurologic examination	1. Ulnar nerve		
		2. Radial nerve		
		3. Median nerve		
8.	Lidocaine test			

Table 3.2 Anatomical area and differential diagnosis

Lateral	Medial	Anterior	Posterior
Radiocapitellaire artrose Osteochondrale loose body Radial head fracture Osteochondritis dissecans Tenniselbow	UCL lesion Ulnar neuritis Ulnar subluxation Golfer's elbow	Distal bicepstendon rupture Anterior capsule strain Coronoid osteophyte formation	Valgus extension overload Posterior osteophyte with impingement Tricepstendinitis Olecranon bursitis Olecranon stress fracture

identified and can occur progressively. Loss of range motion can be one of the first complaints in overhead athlete.

Patient reports of numbness and tingling distal to the elbow with specific attention to the ring finger and little finger need to be evaluated. Often, these symptoms come and go.

3.2 Inspection

Inspection and observation of the elbow begins as the patient walks into the examination room or as he or she comes off the field.

Inspection of the elbow should be carried out in a systematic fashion.

When starting the inspection of the elbow, it is important to visualize both arms for comparison. The examiner should note the resting position of the painful elbow. A patient with significant joint effusion will hold the elbow at 70–80° of flexion, as this corresponds to the position of maximum volume of the elbow joint [5].

Also localized swelling should be examined. For example, swelling over the olecranon can indicate olecranon bursitis from trauma or underlying inflammation.

Next, the carrying angle is evaluated (Fig. 3.1). The normal carrying angle in full extension is approximately 11–14° of valgus in adult men and 13–16 in adult women [11]. Variations in carrying angle may be due to previous trauma, developmental abnormality, injury, or adaptive changes. This angle is greatest in valgus at full extension, diminishing during flexion, and became varus at full flexion [8].

Regardless of the order of inspection, the clinician should make note of several important anatomic areas including the lateral recess, olecranon, medial epicondylar region, and antecubital fossa [5]. Also, differences seen in muscle mass may be due to injury or to hypertrophy in the dominant arm.

The clinician should complete the inspection by looking at the topographical landmarks of the entire upper extremity and trunk. Scapular winging or significant atrophy of the deltoid or

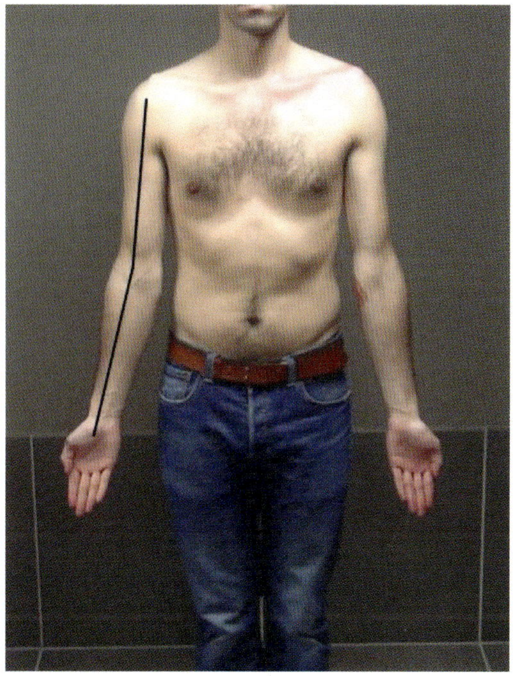

Fig. 3.1 Carrying angle

rotator cuff musculature may be the cause of abnormal mechanics that result in undue stresses across the elbow articulation. This determination will permit the clinician to prescribe appropriate treatment to correct the true pathology. Similarly, the distal aspect of the extremity should be inspected to assess for discoloration of the fingers and fingertips or bony deformity.

3.3 Palpation

Palpation of the elbow should be carried out in a systematic fashion and can also be subdivided into the four anatomic regions.

First, the lateral part of the elbow with the lateral epicondyle and the radial head are palpated. Pain directly at the lateral epicondyle can be due to trauma or LCL injury. Tenderness due to lateral epicondylitis is theoretically just anterior and distal to the epicondyle at the origin of the ECRB.

When palpating the radial head, there may be tenderness and associated clicking over the radial head with rotation seen in fractures, arthrosis, or a symptomatic posterolateral synovial plica. Next, palpation of the lateral recess, or soft spot, can easily identify an elbow effusion.

At the medial side, the medial epicondyle, medial collateral ligament (MCL), and the ulnar nerve can be palpated. The MCL is palpated with the elbow in 50–70° of flexion to move the overlying medial muscles anterior to the MCL.

The ulnar nerve can be palpated in the cubital tunnel. Percussion along the nerve may elicit the Tinel sign. Pain at the medial epicondyle or just distal can be seen in a patient with medial epicondylitis.

At the posterior side of the elbow, the olecranon fossa on either side of the triceps tendon can be felt by flexing the elbow. The clinician can also evaluate the olecranon bursa for swelling and fluctuation that indicate olecranon bursitis. Also, the proximal one-third medial subcutaneous border of the olecranon can be palpated because tenderness in this area can indicate a stress fracture. Next, the clinician evaluates the insertion of the triceps tendon. Finally, the clinician palpates the posterior, medial, and lateral aspects of the olecranon in varying degrees of flexion to detect osteophytes and loose bodies [2].

At last, the anterior structures can be palpated. The cubital fossa is bound laterally by the brachioradialis, the extensor carpi radialis longus, and the extensor carpi radialis brevis muscles, medially by the pronator teres muscle, and superiorly by the biceps muscle. The clinician can palpate the distal biceps tendon anteromedially in the antecubital fossa with the patient's forearm in supination and elbow in active flexion [1]. Tenderness in this area can indicate biceps tendinitis or a biceps tendon ruptures. Deep, poorly localized tenderness can result from anterior capsulitis or coronoid hypertrophy due to hyperextension injuries or repetitive hyperextension stress [3].

3.4 Passive Motion

Normal passive range of motion is approximately 0° of extension and 140 of flexion. Normally there is a hard stop in extension when the olecranon hits the olecranon fossa and a soft spot in flexion because flexion is limited due to the contact between the forearm and the upper arm. Full extension is often the first motion lost after injury.

Supination and pronation motion is approximately 80° in both directions. To determine pathologic differences, range of motion should always be compared with the contralateral side.

When evaluating the passive motion of the elbow, elbow stability can also be tested. Instability can occur around the frontal axis (valgus–varus) and around the longitudinal axis (posterolateral–posteromedial) of the elbow. Valgus stability is provided by the osseous anatomy of the olecranon and the humerus, the dynamic muscle forces, and the MCL complex. At less than 20° of extension, the interlocking bony anatomy of the olecranon with the olecranon fossa provides stability. If the elbow is bent more than 20°, the MCL is more important, and the majority of stress is placed on the anterior bundle of the MCL complex. Lesions of the MCL can be evaluated with the valgus stress test, the moving valgus stress test, and the milking maneuver.

The classic valgus stress test is performed in abduction and external rotation of the humerus. Next, the humerus is stabilized in 30° of flexion to unlock the bony restraint of the olecranon from the fossa and applying a valgus stress. The test has a positive result if the medial joint space opens and the patient reports pain.

Pseudovalgus instability, subtle posterolateral instability that can be present when the forearm is supinated, is eliminated as a confounding factor of possible medial laxity when the forearm is pronated (Fig. 3.2).

The moving valgus stress test is performed with the patient in an upright position and the shoulder abducted 90°. Starting with the elbow maximally flexed, a modest valgus torque is applied to the elbow until the shoulder reaches its limit of external rotation.

While a constant valgus torque is maintained, the elbow is quickly extended to about 30°. For an examination to be called positive, it must have two key components. First, the pain generated by the maneuver must reproduce the medial elbow pain at the MCL that the patient has with

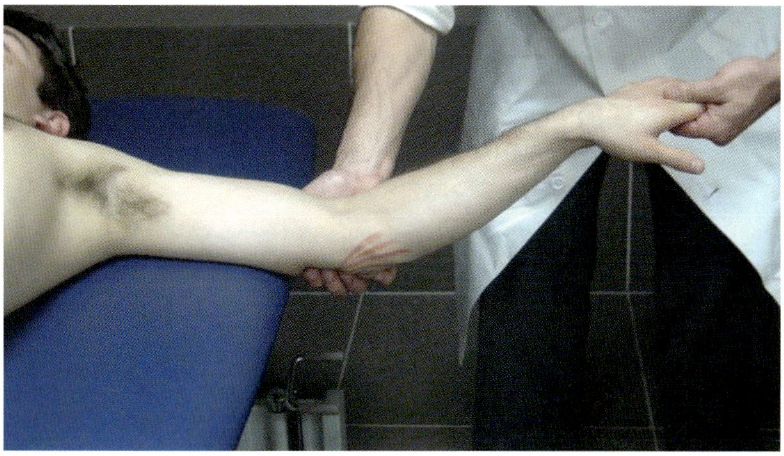

Fig. 3.2 Valgus stress test

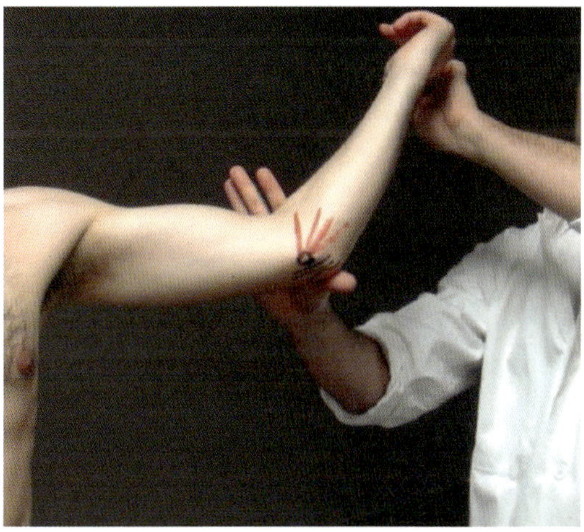

Fig. 3.3 Moving valgus stress

activities. Second, although the patient may experience pain throughout a range, the pain should be maximal between the position of late cocking (120°) and early acceleration (70°) as the elbow is extended [10] (Fig. 3.3).

During the "milking maneuver," the examiner grasps the thrower's thumb with the arm in the cocked position (90° shoulder abduction and 90° elbow flexion) and applies valgus stress by pulling down on the thumb [14]. This position is felt to be similar to pulling down on the teats when milking a cow (Fig. 3.4).

Varus stability is provided by the osseous anatomy of the olecranon and the humerus, also the dynamic muscle forces and the lateral collateral ligament (LCL) complex.

Varus instability is much less common. This reason can be found in the fact that a direct impact on the medial side causing varus of the elbow is difficult because the body protects the medial side most of the time.

During the varus stress test, the patient's arm is stabilized with one of the examiners hands at the medial distal humerus (elbow), and the other hand is placed above the patient's lateral distal radius (wrist) with the elbow flexed around 20°. An adduction or varus force is applied at the distal forearm by the examiner to test the radial collateral ligament. Varus stress is best applied with the humerus in full internal rotation.

During passive testing, posterolateral and posteromedial elbow instability can also be tested (active testing against resistance will be discussed below (Part 6)) [4].

Posterolateral instability is more common than posteromedial instability. The most common test for posterolateral instability is the passive lateral pivot-shift test described by O'Driscoll et al. [9]. During this test, the patient is supine with the affected limb overhead. With the forearm supinated, valgus and axial loading is applied, and the elbow is flexed from full extension. In posterolateral rotatory instability, as the elbow is flexed, the radial head subluxes/dislocates, seen as an osseous prominence posterolaterally. With flexion beyond 40°, the radial head suddenly reduces with a palpable and visible clunk. The test may also be done starting

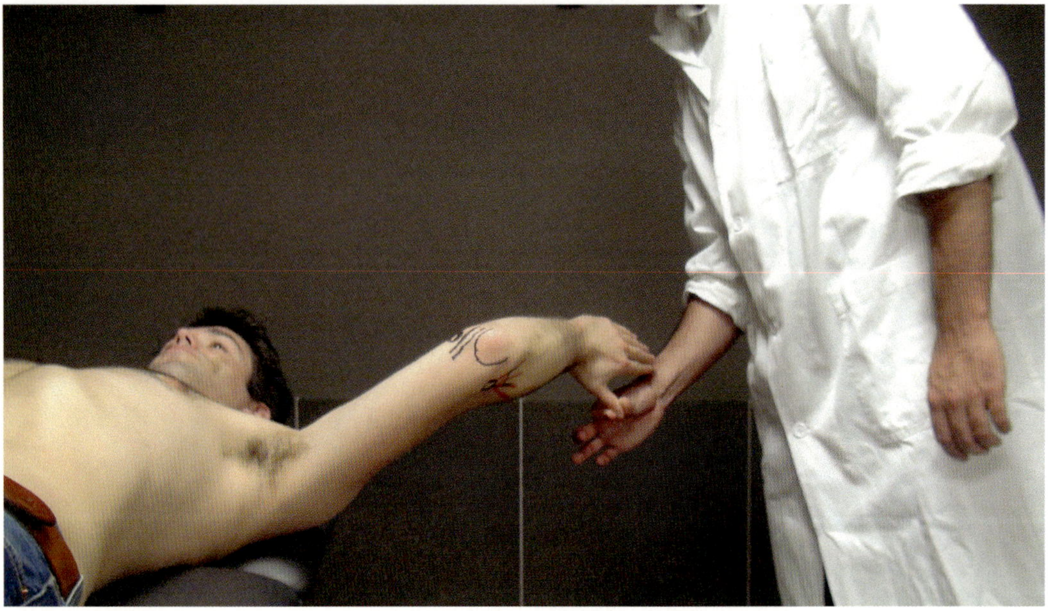

Fig. 3.4 Milking maneuver

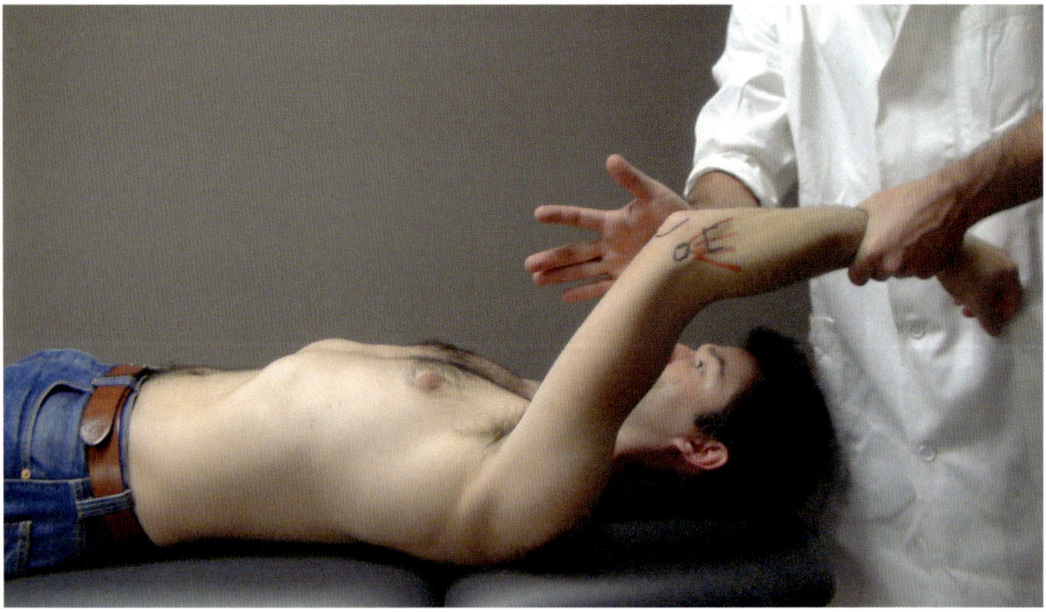

Fig. 3.5 Lateral pivot shift

with the elbow flexed and then extending, reversing the above sequence. The test is best done under general anesthesia for radial head dislocation and relocation to be seen (Fig. 3.5).

In posteromedial instability, theoretically, a subluxation can be obtained with the forearm pronated and varus and axial loading applied (medial pivot-shift test).

Because of the bony anatomy, this subluxation is only possible in the case of a coronoid fracture. This test cannot be performed in an awake patient.

3.5 Active Motion

As discussed during evaluation of passive ROM above, normal range of motion is approximately 0° of extension and 140 of flexion. Supination and pronation motion is approximately 80° in each direction. Loss of active motion can be seen in patients with tendon rupture and neurological problems. To evaluate active extension, it is important to exclude gravity and to ask the patient to actively extend the elbow while lying supine and with the shoulder flexed to 90°.

3.6 Active Motion against Resistance

Next several active tests against resistance can be performed to evaluate the strength and pain sensation of the different muscles.

The brachialis is tested with resisted flexion with the forearm in pronation, and this can be painful after a strain of the brachialis, as can be seen in climbers. The triceps is evaluated with resisted extension of the elbow while the patient is lying supine and the shoulder flexed 90°.

For evaluation of the biceps, a resisted flexion of the elbow is performed with the hand in supination. Also supination against resistance can be performed to evaluate the distal biceps. In patients with distal biceps tendinitis, these tests can be painful.

The hook test is a very sensitive and specific test for distal biceps ruptures. The patient abducts the shoulder, flexes the elbow to 90°, and actively fully supinates the forearm while the examiner attempts to hook his or her index finger laterally under the tendon. The test has a negative result if the finger can be inserted 1 cm beneath the tendon and a positive result if no cordlike structure can be hooked.

To evaluate the extensor carpi radialis brevis tendon, the primary structure involved in tennis elbow, dorsiflexion of the wrist against resistance can be performed. In patients with tennis elbow, this is more painful in extension of the elbow than in flexion.

Also, lifting a chair with pronated hands can induce pain at the lateral region. The flexor carpi radialis and the pronator teres are the primary structures involved in golfers' elbow and can be tested by palmar flexion of the wrist against resistance.

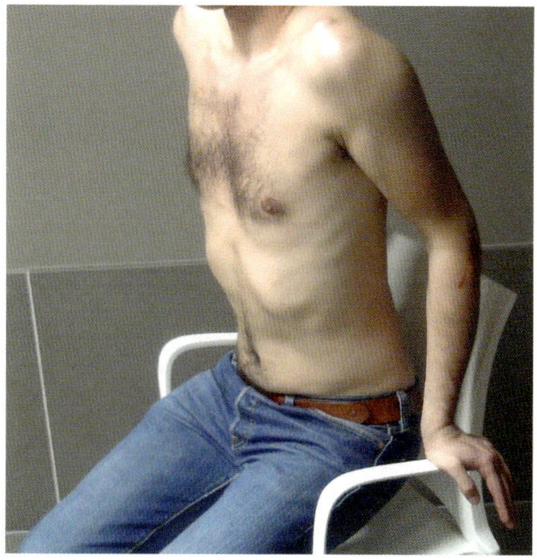

Fig. 3.6 Chair test

In golfer's elbow, it is also more painful with extension of the elbow than with flexion. It is also important to evaluate pain during pronation against resistance.

Also lifting a chair with supinated hands can induce pain at the medial region. When evaluating posterolateral instability of the elbow, in addition to passive testing, active tests are also conducted. The first is an active apprehension sign called the push-up test. The upper extremities are positioned with the elbow at 90° flexion, forearms supinated, and arms abducted to greater than shoulder width. The test is considered positive if apprehension occurs as the affected elbow is terminally extended from a flexed position together with voluntary and involuntary guarding [12].

A second active apprehension sign is the chair test. The technique consists of having the patient in a seated position with the elbows flexed 90°, the forearms supinated, and the arms abducted to greater than shoulder width. The test is considered positive if there is a reluctance to extend the elbow fully as the patient raises his or her body up from a chair using exclusively upper extremity force as a result of apprehension or with complete dislocation (Fig. 3.6). Regan et al. described that the chair test and push-up test are more sensitive than the pivot-shift sign in the awake patient and may be easily performed in the clinic environment [12].

3.7 Neurologic Examination

Determination of the sensory status of the extremity begins in the supraclavicular region and proceeds toward the axillary nerve distribution on the lateral aspect of the arm. Next, the posterior and medial aspect of the upper arm should be tested, followed by the antecubital fossa, which represents the sensory distribution of the musculocutaneous nerve. The volar, dorsal, radial, and ulnar aspects of the forearm should be tested, followed by a detailed sensory examination of the hand including each fingertip. The first dorsal web space (radial nerve), the pad of the index finger (median nerve), and the lateral border of the small digit (ulnar nerve) should be tested, as these are specific areas of sensory innervation with little overlap from contiguous sensory innervations.

Concerning the motor function of the three nerves passing the elbow, with five hand motions, the several nerves can be tested: (1) wrist extension (radial nerve), (2) thumb extension (posterior interosseus nerve), (3) opposition of thumb (median nerve), (4) OK sign (anterior interosseus nerve), and (5) abduction of fingers (ulnar nerve) (Fig. 3.7).

3.8 Lidocaine Test

The elbow is among the most common joints that is aspirated and/or injected. A common procedure is the aspiration of blood in patients with radial head fractures, although only very low-quality evidence suggests a beneficial effect of aspiration on pain relief immediately after aspiration [6].

When performing an aspiration and/or injection, the technique should be a convenient and

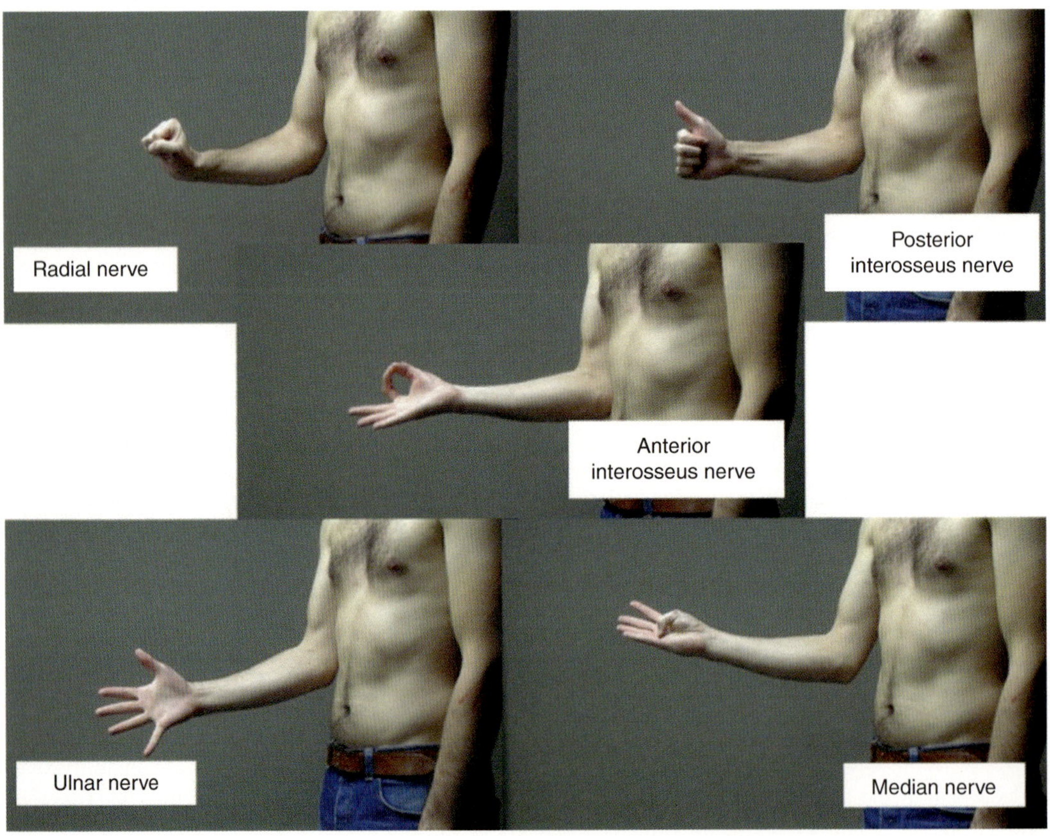

Fig. 3.7 Neurologic examination

safe procedure with minimal risk of complications. Several approaches to access the elbow joint have been outlined in the literature: the two most common locations are the soft spot and a posterior transtriceps approach [13].

Van Wagenberg et al. proposed a posterior transtriceps approach because this technique is easy to perform. It can also be used for arthrography because it avoids a diagnostic dilemma in presumed injuries to the lateral collateral ligament complex caused by contrast leakage using a radiocapitellar approach.

Accuracy is greater in the ultrasound-guided group [7]. No literature has described the importance of a positive lidocaine test in elbow pathology, but in my hands this technique is useful for confirmation of intra-articular pathology, objectivity of the complaints, and confirmation of the correct location when using intra-articular corticosteroids as treatment for intra-articular pathology.

Conclusion

A comprehensive history and physical examination of the elbow is the most important part of the evaluation of elbow disorders. This step-by step approach helps the clinician to examine the elbow thoroughly and in an orderly fashion.

Further diagnostic studies may be necessary to confirm the diagnosis or further narrow the scope of potential diagnoses.

Acknowledgement I want to thank Sheila McRae (PanAm clinic) for her linguistic support.

References

1. Andrews JR, Wilk KE, Satterwhite YE, Tedder JL. Physical examination of the thrower's elbow. J Orthop Sports Phys Ther. 1993;17:296–304.
2. Baker CL, Jones GL. History and physical examination of the elbow. In: Operative treatment of elbow injuries. Springer-Verslag New York, Inc; 2002. p. 41–54.
3. Barnes DA, Tullos HS. An analysis of 100 symptomatic baseball players. Am J Sports Med. 1978;6: 62–7.
4. Charalambous C, Stanley J. Posterolateral rotatory instability of the elbow. J Bone Joint Surg Br Vol. 2008;90:272–9.
5. Dugas JR, Andrews JR. Physical examination of the elbow. Athlete's elbow. Philadelphia: Lippincott Williams & Wilkins; 2001.
6. Foocharoen T, Foocharoen C, Laopaiboon M, Tiamklang T. Aspiration of the elbow joint for treating radial head fractures. Cochrane Database Syst Rev. 2014;11:CD009949. doi:10.1002/14651858.CD009949.pub2.
7. Gilliland CA, Salazar LD, Borchers JR. Ultrasound versus anatomic guidance for intra-articular and periarticular injection: a systematic review. Phys Sportsmed. 2011;39:121–31. doi:10.3810/psm.2011.09.1928.
8. Morrey BF, Chao EY. Passive motion of the elbow joint. J Bone Joint Surg Am. 1976;58:501–8.
9. O'driscoll S, Bell D, Morrey B. Posterolateral rotatory instability of the elbow. J Bone Joint Surg. 1991;73:440–6.
10. O'Driscoll SW, Lawton RL, Smith AM. The "moving valgus stress test" for medial collateral ligament tears of the elbow. Am J Sports Med. 2005;33: 231–9.
11. Paraskevas G, Papadopoulos A, Papaziogas B, Spanidou S, Argiriadou H, Gigis J. Study of the carrying angle of the human elbow joint in full extension: a morphometric analysis. Surg Radiol Anat: SRA. 2004;26:19–23. doi:10.1007/s00276-003-0185-z.
12. Regan W, Lapner PC. Prospective evaluation of two diagnostic apprehension signs for posterolateral instability of the elbow. J Shoulder Elbow Surg. 2006;15:344–6.
13. van Wagenberg JM, Turkenburg JL, Rahusen FT, Eygendaal D. The posterior transtriceps approach for intra-articular elbow diagnostics, definitely not forgotten. Skeletal Radiol. 2013;42:55–9. doi:10.1007/s00256-012-1430-5.
14. Veltri DM, O'Brien SJ, Field LD, Deutsch A, Altchek DW, Potter HG. The milking maneuver-a new test to evaluate the MCL of the elbow in the throwing athlete. J Shoulder Elbow Surg. 1995;4:S10.

4 Imaging of the Elbow in Overhead Athletes

R.L. van Steenkiste, J. Opperman, L.S. Kox, and M. Maas

4.1 Imaging of the Elbow in General

When it comes to imaging of the injured athlete's elbow, there is a vast array of image modalities to choose from, including conventional radiographs, ultrasound (US), computed tomography (CT), magnetic resonance imaging (MRI), and arthrography (CTA, MRA). Choosing the appropriate imaging technique is of vital importance for quick diagnosis and adequate treatment. This chapter will discuss the role of each image modality in the diagnostic workup for pathology around the elbow commonly encountered in overhead athletes. Specific conditions of the elbow will be discussed in detail with a focus on image findings.

4.1.1 Conventional Radiography

Radiography is the first choice in imaging of elbow injuries [1, 2]. It is common practice to depict at least two standard projections of the elbow: a lateral and an anteroposterior (AP) view.

R.L. van Steenkiste, MD • J. Opperman, BSc
L.S. Kox, MD • M. Maas, MD, PhD (✉)
Department of Radiology, Academic Medical Center, University of Amsterdam, Meibergdreef 9, 1106 AZ Amsterdam, The Netherlands
e-mail: denise@eygendaal.nl

The lateral view is obtained with the elbow flexed at 90° angle and the forearm in neutral position (thumb up). The anteroposterior view requires the elbow in full extension with the forearm supinated. In this position, the medial and lateral epicondyles are optimally visualized and the carrying angle can be estimated (normally slightly in valgus) [1, 2]. A radiocapitellar view can additionally be applied to optimally visualize the radiocapitellar joint. It resembles the lateral view with the elbow in 90° of flexion, yet the X-ray tube is angulated 45° anteriorly toward the joint. This view is particularly useful in the evaluation of osteochondral fractures of the capitellum or injuries to the radial head and neck [3, 4]. When evaluating the elbow on radiographic images, the following aspects should be assessed [1, 5]:

- Radiocapitellar line
  The radiocapitellar line is an imaginary line parallel to the long axis of the radial neck on a lateral view and should pass through the center of the capitellum [6]. If not, dislocation of the radius is implied [1, 7, 8]. However, in a *Monteggia* injury (see below), the radiocapitellar line may seem normal, even if the radial head is almost always dislocated. Careful evaluation of the total alignment of the elbow is therefore mandatory in all cases [5].
- Cortex of radial head and neck (in adults)
  The appearance of the cortex of the proximal radius is smooth on standard lateral and AP views in the normal situation. If injury is

L.A. Pederzini et al. (eds.), *Elbow and Sport*, DOI 10.1007/978-3-662-48742-6_4

present, the outlines of the cortex can display crinkles, steps, or irregularities due to (subtle) fracture lines [5].

– Anterior humeral line (in children)
  On a lateral view, the anterior humeral line can be drawn along the anterior cortex of the distal humeral shaft and should bisect the middle third of the capitellum [6]. If less than one third of the capitellum lies anterior to this line, a supracondylar fracture with posterior displacement is highly probable [5].
– Ossification centers
  Secondary ossification centers, also referred to as apophyses, serve as attachment sites for muscle-tendon units. Ossification centers are primarily composed of maturing chondrocytes which are biomechanically less resistant than musculotendinous structures. As a result, traction forces on an ossification center may result in an apophyseal avulsion injury [9]. During childhood, a total of six ossification centers develop in a set order: capitellum, radial head, medial epicondyle, trochlea, olecranon, and lateral epicondyle [10–12]. Being familiar with the pattern and appearance of these ossification centers is essential in differentiating normal anatomy from pathology on standard radiographs of the pediatrics elbow. Note that the exact timing of ossification shows great variability among young individuals [11, 12].
– Fat pads
  On a lateral view, the anterior fat pad is visible as a dark streak along the anterior side of the distal humerus. The posterior fat pad is never visible, unless intracapsular abnormalities are present. Joint effusion, for example, causes displacement of both the anterior and posterior fat pads, resulting in a positive *fat pad sign*. This makes the presence of a fracture more likely, but absence of a visible fat pad does not completely exclude a fracture [5]. The fat pad sign is specifically relevant in pediatric cases, as it can indicate fractures of the immature cartilaginous components of the elbow [1] (Table 4.1).

Table 4.1 Essential aspects of radiographic evaluation of the elbow joint

Children	Adults
1. Fat pads	1. Fat pads
2. Anterior humeral line	2. Cortex of radial head and neck
3. Radiocapitellar line	3. Radiocapitellar line
4. Ossification centers	

4.1.2 Magnetic Resonance Imaging and Magnetic Resonance Arthrography

Magnetic resonance imaging (MRI) is considered the next step in the imaging workup. Appropriate patient positioning, coil selection, and sequence technique are of vital importance in proper imaging of the elbow. The anatomical position with the patient lying supine, the elbow in full extension and the forearm in supination, is the most comfortable and a widely used position. Note that with this position, the elbow is located off-center of the scanner's magnetic field. This will reduce the signal-to-noise ratio and may introduce inhomogeneous fat suppression. For this reason, fat suppression by means of inversion recovery sequences is preferred over frequency-selective fat suppression techniques when the anatomical position is applied [13]. An alternative is the "superman position," where the patient lies prone with the elbow over the head and the forearm in pronation. This will bring the elbow closer to the center of the magnet which will increase overall image quality at the cost of markedly reduced patient comfort. In any case, a dedicated surface coil should be used for optimal imaging of the elbow [14]. Obtaining cross-sectional images in all three orthogonal planes will allow for adequate assessment of all relevant structures around the elbow.

T1-weighted (T1W) images are useful for illustrating anatomical detail, whereas fat-saturated T2-weighted (T2W) images or short-tau inversion recovery (STIR) images are suitable for detecting pathological changes manifesting as fluid or

Table 4.2 Characteristics of the elbow on MRI

	Appearance on:		
Tissue	T1-weighted images	T2-weighted images	T2-fat saturated images
Cortical bone	Hypointense	Hypointense	Hypointense
Medullary bone	Hyperintense	Hyperintense	Hypointense
Fibrous cartilage	Hypointense	Hypointense	Hypointense
Hyaline cartilage	Isointense	Isointense	Isointense
Bands and ligaments	Hypointense	Hypointense	Hypointense
Fluid	Hypointense	Hyperintense	Hyperintense
Fat	Hyperintense	Hyperintense	Hypointense
Muscle	Hypointense	Hyperintense	Hyperintense

edema. Furthermore, proton density-weighted (PDW) images can provide additional anatomical detail. Gradient-echo sequences are not routinely indicated but may enhance the visibility of intra-articular loose bodies [14, 15]. However, detecting loose bodies without intra-articular contrast remains difficult. Gadolinium is a contrast agent used in MR imaging that can be injected intravenously or directly into a joint, known as MR arthrography (MRA) (see below). Indirect MRA by means of *intravenous* administration of gadolinium may aid in the detection of post-traumatic disorders affecting the synovium. Direct MRA by means of *intra-articular* injection of gadolinium may provide superior visualization of disorders commonly encountered in throwing athletes, including partial capsular and ligamentous (ulnar collateral ligament) tears, intra- articular loose bodies, instability, and osteochondritis dissecans [16, 17].

For MRA, approximately 5–10 mL of gadolinium diluted in sterile saline (1:250) is injected with a 20- or 23-gauge needle into the elbow joint. The elbow joint space can be accessed via the standard lateral or posteromedial approach under fluoroscopy. For the lateral approach, the needle is inserted vertically at the superior third of the radiocapitellar joint line while the patient is lying prone with the elbow in 90° flexion and the forearm in supination. A disadvantage of this lateral approach is the possible extravasation of contrast agent around the radial collateral ligaments. For this reason, the alternative posteromedial approach can be employed with the patient lying supine on the fluoroscopic table, with the elbow over the head in 30° flexion and the forearm in pronation. The needle is then inserted between the olecranon and the medial epicondyle, approximately 1 cm lateral to the medial epicondyle to avoid damaging the ulnar nerve. Subsequently, the needle is advanced in anterolateral fashion into the olecranon fossa. Fat- saturated T1W and T2W sequences should be obtained immediately after contrast injection [18] (Table 4.2).

4.1.3 Computed Tomography and Computed Tomographic Arthrography

CT scans of the elbow are mainly used in the acute setting for assessing osseous abnormalities such as occult fractures and loose bodies, for further characterisation, and for support in preoperative planning [19, 20]. Current multi-detector CT scans allow for high-resolution images, multiplanar reconstruction, and fast scanning times. Typically, a section thickness of 1 mm is used with a matrix size of 512×512, and scanning is performed in the axial plane [21, 22]. The patient is scanned in the prone position with the elbow resting above the head at about 90° flexion [23–25].

In order to perform CTA, iodinated contrast agent is injected into the elbow joint. As in magnetic resonance arthrography (MRA), 5–10 mL of contrast agent is injected under fluoroscopic guidance through the lateral and, in some cases, the posteromedial approach. In addition to iodinated contrast agent, air can be injected into the elbow. This is defined as double-contrast arthrography. CT scans should be obtained within 30 min of contrast administration [26].

CTA is particularly useful in the evaluation of osteochondritis dissecans, osteochondral lesions, and loose bodies [27]. However, in the diagnostic workup of the athlete's injured elbow, MRA has essentially replaced the role of CTA. The main reasons for this are the absence of ionizing radiation in MRA and the fact that MRA is superior in the detection of concomitant soft tissue injury [18]. Nonetheless, CTA can be used as an alternative in patients with contraindications for MRA such as pacemakers, implanted devices, or gadolinium-based contrast allergies [28].

4.1.4 Ultrasound

The major advantage of ultrasound (US) is that it provides a low-cost, noninvasive, and dynamic evaluation of elbow structures, without ionizing radiation [29–31]. However, this imaging modality is highly operator-dependent and thus requires sufficient experience of the assessor. US can assist clinicians in the assessment of a wide variety of elbow injuries, including overuse syndromes, traumatic changes, inflammatory diseases, and neuropathies [31]. Transverse and longitudinal images of all four aspects (posterior, anterior, medial, and lateral) of the elbow in both flexion and extension are necessary for a complete examination [31].

Echogenicity is the characteristic ability of an elbow structure to return a signal in US examination; each tissue has its own characteristic appearance. A practical order of echogenicity in musculoskeletal ultrasound can be depicted as bone, ligament, tendon, nerve, and muscle [29]. In general, bone and gas-like substances are hyperechoic and fully reflect the sound waves, which is represented by a more intense appearance on US images. Muscles and fluids are less echogenic (hypoechoic) and are represented darker.

Ultrasound plays a major role in the examination of traumatic changes to ligaments and tendons of the elbow [29, 32]. Although these structures have a similar appearance, they can be distinguished because ligaments are slightly more echogenic than tendons. Moreover, the echogenicity of the fibrillar tendinous pattern increases when the tendon is being held under tension. Pathologic degeneration and partial tearing of a tendon are visualized as a structural hypoechoic gap. In case of a complete tear, the fibrillar pattern is completely absent. In addition, US may demonstrate intra-articular effusion due to a fracture even when the undisplaced fracture line is not detected on plain radiographs. Fractures can also be detected directly by US through depiction of irregularities or interruption of the hyperechoic bone cortex [31].

4.2 Osseous and Osteochondral Injury of the Elbow

4.2.1 Fractures of the Elbow

Elbow fractures in overhead athletes are most often caused by low energy trauma, such a fall onto an outstretched hand (FOOSH) and hyperextension or hyperflexion injuries [33]. Nontraumatic upper extremity fractures related to throwing are rare [34, 35]. However, stress fractures arising from repetitive microtrauma are not uncommon. In the following section, a description of fractures of the distal humerus, proximal ulna, and proximal radius, with associated characteristics on imaging, will be given.

4.2.1.1 Outline Pediatric Osseous Injury

In General

The immature skeleton contains growth plates, which appear as a radiolucency similar to cartilage on radiographs. Understanding of the developmental anatomy of the pediatric elbow is essential to distinguish normal ossification centers from a fracture fragment in radiography, since misinterpretation is not uncommon [36]. The mnemonic

CRITOE is a helpful tool in analyzing pediatric elbow injury. It represents the sequential order of appearance of the ossification centers of the elbow: capitellum, radial head, internal (medial) epicondyle, trochlea, olecranon, and external (lateral) epicondyle [1, 5]. This sequential order extends over the period from 1 year to 12 years of age [37].

Pediatric osseous injury differs in many aspects from adult osseous injury due to the differences in bone composition between children and adults [8, 38]. The thick periosteum of the immature skeleton, for example, inhibits displacement of a fracture. However, supracondylar fractures with posterior displacement occur frequently and are thus an exception to this rule. Finally, children's bones tend to be more flexible which can result in plastic bowing, torus, or greenstick fractures, mostly affecting the radius or ulna in FOOSH or hyperextension injury [5].

Physeal Injury

Since the cartilaginous physis is a more vulnerable structure than the surrounding ligaments and muscle tendons, injuries affecting the physis are common in childhood [2]. Fractures of the epiphysis and/or metaphysis are classified according to the Salter-Harris classification, which relates the radiographic appearance to the clinical importance of the fracture (see Table 4.3) [39]. Nevertheless, MRI is considered superior for evaluating fractures of the cartilaginous epiphysis in children [40].

4.2.1.2 Fractures of the Distal Humerus

Fractures of the distal humerus can broadly be categorized into supracondylar, transcondylar, or intercondylar fractures (above the olecranon fossa, through the olecranon fossa, or between the condyles, respectively) [41, 42]. More specific and commonly used is the AO classification system, in which type A describes an extra-articular fracture, type B an intra-articular fracture of a single column, and type C an intra-articular fracture of both columns with no portion of the joint contiguous with the shaft (see Table 4.4) [41]. Each type is subdivided into three subtypes to classify the degree of comminution, with subtype 3 being the highest degree of comminution. Anteroposterior, lateral, and oblique views in plain radiography can be used to confirm the presence and location of distal humeral fractures [42].

Supracondylar (type A) fractures are common and account for more than half of all elbow fractures in children, but are relatively uncommon in

Table 4.3 Salter-Harris classification for physeal fractures [39]

Type	Mnemonic	Description of fracture
I	"Slipped"	Through the physis without involvement of bone, epiphysis, or metaphysis
II	"Above"	Involving part of the metaphysis and extending to the physis
III	"Lower"	Involving the epiphysis and extending to the physis
IV	"Through"	Involving epiphysis and metaphysis and extending to the physis
V	"Rammed"	Involving compression of the physis

Table 4.4 AO/OTA classification of distal humerus fractures

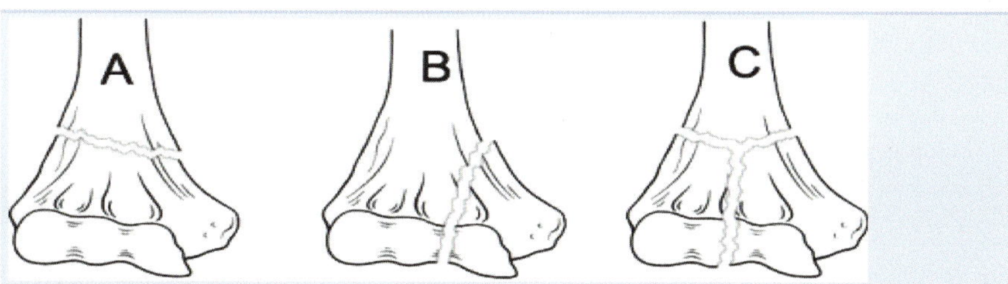

Type A	Extra-articular	Supracondylar
Type B	Intra-articular, single column	Partial articular-isolated condylar, coronal shear, epicondyle
Type C	Intra-articular, both columns	Complete articular

adults [6]. Pediatric supracondylar fractures are classified according to the classification of Gartland [43]. Type I fractures are non-displaced, type II fractures are partially displaced (with intact posterior cortex) and type III fractures are completely displaced. The anterior humeral line in particular can be used to assess the direction of the displacement, which is commonly posterior [5]. A rare, but important complication of pediatric supracondylar fractures is the *fishtail deformity* (see Sect. 4.2.2) [44, 45].

Transcondylar (type B) fractures include fractures of the lateral and medial humeral condyle. Fractures of the lateral condyle are the most common fractures in children under the age of 7 years [5]. When only the cartilaginous part of the distal humeral epiphysis is involved, this fracture equals a Salter-Harris type IV epiphyseal fracture. A specific type of transcondylar fractures of the capitellum and trochlea are *coronal shear fractures*. These fractures occur when the radial head impacts into the anterior articular cortex of the distal humerus and both the capitellum and the lateral ridge of the trochlea are sheared off. Indicative for this injury is the *double-arc sign* on lateral view radiographs [46, 47]. This sign represents an increased radiographic density due to overprojection of the subchondral bone of the displaced capitellum and the lateral trochlear ridge. Coronal shear fractures can also be visualized with a radial head-capitellum view [48].

Regarding other imaging modalities, two- and three-dimensional CT images have been shown to be of particular benefit in preoperative decision making and planning of the operative treatment [49]. Nonoperative treatment (i.e., immobilization and bracing) is only recommended in case of non-displaced fractures. Patients with displaced, comminuted, or highly unstable distal humeral fractures should be referred to an orthopedic surgeon, since surgical intervention is the standard treatment [41, 42].

4.2.1.3 Fractures of the Proximal Ulna

Olecranon process fractures can be the result of a direct trauma to the elbow, for example a fall on the elbow with the arm flexed. As a consequence, the olecranon collides with the distal humerus and is often comminuted [50]. These fractures occur more frequently in adults than in children, as the immature olecranon is relatively stronger than the distal humerus (which also explains the higher occurrence of supracondylar fractures in children). Indirect forces are mostly due to a FOOSH injury together with forceful contraction of the triceps which may show transverse or short oblique fractures on plain radiographs [50, 51]. Undisplaced, simple fractures are easily assessed on plain radiographs. Displaced or comminuted fractures require two- and three-dimensional CT imaging in support of surgery [52].

In addition to traumatic injury, the olecranon process is the most common location for stress fractures in throwers [2]. During throwing, repetitive forces in valgus load are applied through excessive pulling of the triceps on the olecranon, which may result in posteromedial osseous stress syndrome. This comprises trabecular collapse and transverse or short oblique stress fractures. Since plain radiographs may not show significant alterations in the appearance of the proximal ulna, accurate assessment is justified [53, 54]; progression of small stress fractures to a complete and displaced fracture is possible. Either a hairline fracture or a lucent region surrounded by a sclerotic margin (indicating nonunion and periosteal new bone formation) can be seen. These features can also be detected with CT [2]. However, MR imaging is the most sensitive method for identifying early changes consistent with osseous stress injury, like bone marrow edema and hyperemia [53]. These changes on T1-weighted images consist of poorly defined, patchy areas of low signal intensity in the affected bone.

Fractures of the coronoid process rarely occur isolated. Since the coronoid is responsible for resisting posterior displacement of the ulna, these fractures are often associated with other elbow injuries that increase joint instability. In the O'Driscoll classification, three major traumatic injury patterns are linked to coronoid fractures [55]. This classification can aid in predicting associated injuries of coronoid fractures [56]. Type I includes a small transverse fracture of the coronoid tip. This fracture accounts for one of the three distinct injuries in the *terrible triad*, the others being a fracture of the radial head and a posterior elbow dislocation [57]. If external rotation forces and valgus stress are loaded axially in a FOOSH injury, the lateral collateral ligament (LCL) is typically torn as well. Type II fractures of the anteromedial facet are often seen with varus posteromedial rotatory instability pattern injuries, occurring after an elbow subluxation. Associated injury includes an LCL avulsion from the lateral epicondyle. Varus stress radiographs often reveal radiocapitellar widening and ulnohumeral narrowing. Type III includes relatively large fractures of the coronoid process, associated with transolecranon fracture-dislocations (anterior or posterior).

4.2.1.4 Fractures of the Proximal Radius

Radial head fractures are the most common type of elbow fracture in athletes and represent 50 % of all elbow fractures in adults [33]. In children, the radial neck is more commonly involved (leading to Salter-Harris II fracture). Based on results of 100 cases of radial head fractures, Mason established a classification system to guide treatment based on the injury pattern [58]. Type I fractures include non-displaced or peripheral fractures of the rim, type II includes displaced fractures of the rim, and type III fractures are comminuted and displaced fractures of the entire radial head. Johnston added a fourth type to this classification, which denotes a fracture of the radial head with associated dislocation [59]. Initially, type I fractures are treated nonoperatively, type II may be treated either nonoperatively or operatively, while types III and IV require surgical management. However, although these guidelines of the Mason-Johnston classification are widely used, there is a paucity of data confirming the outcomes of surgical management [60].

Isolated radial head fractures resulting from a fall with the elbow extended and the forearm pronated occur rarely. Investigation of radial head fractures with MR imaging showed that radial head fractures in three-quarters of cases are associated with soft tissue injuries [61, 62]. Common injuries occurring in association with these fractures are posterior dislocation of the elbow, medial collateral ligament rupture, capitellar fracture, terrible triad injuries, and Monteggia injuries [63]. If a radial head fracture is suspected, anteroposterior and lateral radiographs of the elbow should be obtained. A radiocapitellar view may help delineate the fracture. In addition, computed tomography can identify fractures not visualized in plain radiographs. CT may help in identifying the fracture pattern, the degree of comminution (if present), possible associated injuries and in planning surgical treatment [63, 64].

4.2.2 OCD and Avascular Necrosis Around the Elbow

4.2.2.1 Osteochondritis Dissecans of the Capitellum

Osteochondritis dissecans (OCD) is an idiopathic disorder of the subchondral bone with dissection of the articular surface and underlying bone of the immature skeleton. OCD is commonly localized in the capitellum of the dominant elbow but can also occur in the trochlea, radial head, and olecranon [65]. It typically affects young, competitive athletes in overhead sports such as baseball or weight-bearing sports like gymnastics, in which repetitive valgus stress is placed on the elbow joint [66, 67]. Patients, most commonly adolescent boys, present with lateral elbow pain, swelling, tenderness, stiffness, and locking of the joint. Although the etiology remains unclear, it is believed that the underlying pathogenesis involves repetitive microtrauma due to compression and shear forces, leading to overuse injury of the vulnerable and relatively hypovascular epiphyseal cartilage [65].

Although prevention is the best treatment for OCD, early detection and classification of the lesion are necessary to protect athletes from developing irreversible damage [68, 69]. The International Cartilage Repair Society (ICRS) divides OCD lesions into four categories. To determine the best treatment option for capitellar OCD in young athletes, it is important to differentiate between stable and unstable lesions: ICRS I and II are classified as stable and ICRS III and IV as unstable [69–72]. However, the major drawback of this classification is that it is based on intraoperative findings. To assess the stability of the OCD lesion in a noninvasive way, the use of ultrasound, radiographs, MRI, or CT is recommended [72]. The characteristics of each imaging modality will be discussed in the following section (Table 4.5).

Ultrasound is useful in the initial examination of cartilaginous changes in capitellar OCD [74]. US can visualize the subchondral bone and overlying articular cartilage simultaneously in one dynamic image [75]. The image should be obtained in both an anterior and a posterior longitudinal view to display the whole capitellum. The normal capitellum is shown as a highly echogenic band with the overlying cartilage as an overlying hypoechoic band. Subchondral bone flattening causes the highly echogenic band to narrow. Moreover, non-displaced or (slightly) displaced bony fragments, marrow gap formation, or complete osteochondral defects can be seen on ultrasound imaging [74]. It is advised to compare findings on ultrasound with MRI and/or radiographic assessment to identify both cartilaginous and bone changes, so the lesion can be more accurately classified [74, 76].

Table 4.5 International cartilage repair society – OCD classification for lesion stability [73]

Type	Description
I	Stable lesions with a continuous but softened area covered by intact cartilage
II	Lesions with partial discontinuity that are stable when probed
III	Lesions with a complete discontinuity that are not yet dislocated but are unstable when probed (dead in situ)
IV	Empty defects as well as defects with a dislocated fragment or a loose fragment within the bed

Routine AP radiographic examination of the elbow for detecting capitellar OCD and intra-articular loose bodies has limited sensitivity [77]. However, radiographic images of the capitellum on radiocapitellar view or AP view with the elbow 45° flexed can show the following:

Grade I. Localized flattening or subchondral radiolucency
Grade II. Non-displaced bone fragment(s)
Grade III. Displaced or detached fragment(s)

Takahara et al. [71] proposed a guideline for treatment, based on findings at initial presentation of the patient, supplemented with radiographic findings (Table 4.6) [71]. In stable OCD, an immature capitellum with open growth plate is present with flattening or radiolucency of the subchondral bone (Grade I), but with normal elbow motion. The preferred treatment is conservative; elbow rest and analgesics are recommended. In unstable OCD, the capitellum is mature (the growth plates have closed) and fragments (Grade II or III) may occur. The fragments or loose bodies can lead to restricted elbow motion due to narrowing of the articular space. In this case, surgical treatment is indispensable to prevent further damage. The advantage of this classification system is that it directly links radiographic findings with the ICRS classification and thus is useful in the choice for treatment [78].

Magnetic resonance imaging has been approved as the most sensitive and reliable means

Table 4.6 Classification and preferred treatment of OCD lesions [71]

Classification of lesion	Capitellar growth plate	Radiographic grade	Range of motion	ICRS classification	Preferred treatment
Stable	Open	I	Normal	I	Elbow rest
Unstable	Closed	II or III	Restricted	II	Fixation and bone-peg graft
				III	Fixation and bone-peg or iliac bone graft
				IV	Fragment removal and reconstruction for large defect

ICRS International Cartilage Repair Society

for the assessment of osteochondritis dissecans [74, 79]. MRI provides information about size, location, presence of joint effusion, bone marrow change, and loss of continuity or cartilage over the OCD lesion [79]. Cartilage changes in early disease may not be obvious radiographically, but can be visualized with MRI [68]. These early changes of osteochondral defects are detectable on T1-weighted images and appear normal on T2 images [67]. Advanced changes are detectable in both T1 and T2 images. T2-weighted images may show high-signal intensity interfaces between fragments and their beds or reflect the interposition of synovial fluid interposed through the articular cartilage. Focal articular defects may be seen as well [69, 72]. The MRI staging system developed by Itsubo et al. [79] provides evidence regarding the instability of the OCD and the corresponding stages of the ICRS classification, but has not yet been validated in other studies [79].

It should be noted that the literature on imaging of capitellar OCD by computed tomography (CT) is limited. The general consensus on the advantages of CT over radiography or MRI is that CT can aid in defining the subchondral bone condition and that it is often used to determine the extent of the osseous lesion and the presence of ossified loose bodies [80]. However, CT should not be used to detect cartilaginous change at the lesion; for this purpose, computed tomographic arthrography (CTA) is more suitable. CTA favors examination of the overlying cartilage and can confirm the intra-articular position of calcified loose bodies, yet this can also be achieved with MRI [73, 81].

4.2.2.2 Panner's Disease

It is important to distinguish Panner's disease from OCD of the capitellum. Although the presentation and clinical features may be similar, Panner's disease is a self-limiting condition of the epiphysis and will resolve with rest and conservative treatment [65]. In general, it affects a younger age group (mainly boys under the age of 10 years) and it is not necessarily related to sports. The characteristic appearance of Panner's disease on radiographs is the initially subchondral rarefaction, which is in a later stage followed by translucency and fragmentation of the entire capitellum. Magnetic resonance imaging shows low T1 signal and high T2 signal of the entire capitellum. Loose bodies are seldom seen [65].

4.2.2.3 Hegemann's Disease

In the continuum of disorders of endochondral ossification like OCD and Panner's disease, in 1951 Hegemann described a total of 15 cases of avascular osteonecrosis of the humeral trochlea [82]. Since then, reports on this disease have been limited. This condition seems to affect predominantly preadolescent boys and is seldom accompanied by pain. Swelling and decreased range of motion are more often described [83]. In contrast to OCD, there is no locking of the joint and radiography shows rarefaction of the entire epiphyseal center of the trochlea (instead of the subchondral bone only) [84]. Another condition that strongly resembles Hegemann's disease is the *fishtail deformity* of the trochlea, a late complication of pediatric supracondylar fractures [45]. Claessen et al. [85] provided an overview of the most recent knowledge on the etiology, radiographic findings, and treatment options of both these rare conditions [85].

4.2.3 Apophysitis and Apophysiolysis: Little Leaguer's Elbow

The apophysis is a secondary ossification center located outside the joint surface. Injury of the medial epicondylar apophysis occurs almost exclusively in young athletes performing overhead sports and is referred to as the clinical diagnosis *Little Leaguer's elbow* [86–88]. The medial epicondyle is relatively weak compared to the increasing muscle strength in adolescents. Therefore, apophysiolysis or apophyseal avulsion fractures are often the consequence of sustained valgus stress forces with traction of the common origins of the flexor muscles at the apophysis, due to repetitive overhead throwing [5, 89, 90]. Moreover, avulsion fractures can also be the consequence of an acute traumatic event such as a dislocation due to FOOSH injury [91].

AP and lateral radiographic images with comparative views of the unaffected side should be used in the initial evaluation [1]. Although these images appear normal in 85 % of cases, they may reveal a hypertrophic medial epicondyle with bony fragmentations and apophyseal widening or complete avulsion from the underlying humerus, with possible entrapment of the fragment in the joint [87, 89].

MRI is not warranted in the initial imaging workup, but can be justified to outline the surrounding structures [92]. MR images in such cases may show bone marrow edema in the apophysis (or distal in the humerus) and tendinopathy of the common flexor tendon. Contrary to previous literature, there is a growing consensus that the ulnar collateral ligament (UCL) is not involved in the pathology of the Little Leaguer's elbow, but solely associated with valgus extension overload in adult patients (see Sect. 4.3.1) [92].

4.2.4 Degeneration, Osteophytosis, and Loose Bodies

While traumatic injury may precipitate secondary degenerative arthritis in the elbow, primary degeneration is not associated with acute elbow trauma or rheumatologic disease. Primary degenerative arthritis of the elbow is a relatively rare condition, but occurs to a greater extent in overhead athletes at whom excessive stress on the elbow joint is placed [93, 94]. The pathologic changes that occur in both the radiohumeral and ulnohumeral compartments of the elbow can be divided in three stages [95]. The first stage involves loss and fragmentation of the cartilage due to repetitive impaction of the coronoid process and the tip of the olecranon against the olecranon fossa membrane. As a response to this erosion, hypertrophic bone and cartilage formation results in so-called osteophytes and loose bodies. Osteophytes or bone spurs reduce the amount of joint space needed for a full, pain-free range of motion, giving rise to symptoms as pain, locking, or reduced elbow motion. In the final stage, the impingement caused by these small protuberances (particularly in the olecranon fossa) leads to distortion and in most severe cases to contracture of the elbow joint. Arthroscopic intervention with removal of the eroded bone and its fragments is the best treatment option to prevent further degeneration of the elbow [96]. Plain radiography and computed tomography are the modalities of choice when assessing the condition of the elbow.

Two views in plain radiography are usually sufficient for the initial evaluation of primary osteoarthritis. Standard lateral radiographs allow identification of the most frequent features of the osteoarthritic elbow (i.e., osteophytes of all involved bony structures, thickening of the olecranon fossa membrane, and joint space narrowing). The anteroposterior view in addition enables the assessment of the olecranon fossa membrane [97].

In preoperative planning, computed tomography (CT) is favorable when heterotopic ossification or intra-articular loose bodies are suspected [93]. More advanced three-dimensional CT scans can specifically determine the size, location, and bony architecture of the hypertrophic bone spurs and loose bodies [97, 98].

4.2.5 Goalkeeper's Elbow

Shot blocking of a ball with the forearm fully extended induces repeated hyperextension trauma of the elbow, mostly seen in goalkeepers of handball and soccer [99]. The injury pattern resembles elbow lesions in overhead athletes: repeated impaction of the posteromedial olecranon leads to arthritic changes with cartilage damage, osteophyte formation, and intra-articular loose bodies [100]. The presence of these pathological alterations can be confirmed by radiological evaluation. Soft tissue lesions can be visualized by US or MRI and may comprise bilateral thickening of the medial collateral ligament, flexor-pronator tendon, triceps tendon, and ulnar nerve [100].

4.3 Ligamentous Injury of the Elbow

Various osseous and soft tissue constraints provide static and dynamic stability to the elbow joint, respectively. Primary stabilization is provided by the ulnohumeral articulation as well as by the medial (ulnar) and lateral (radial) collateral ligament complexes. The medial ulnar collateral ligament (MCL/UCL) complex comprises anterior, posterior, and transverse bundles, of which the anterior bundle is the primary restraint against valgus stress. The lateral ligament complex includes the radial collateral ligament, the lateral collateral ligament (LCL), and the annular ligament, of which the LCL provides both varus- and posterolateral stability [101]. The radiocapitellar articulation, the common extensor tendon, the flexor-pronator tendon, and the joint capsule all contribute to secondary stabilization [102].

Ligamentous injury of the elbow in athletes can be caused by repetitive overhead activities or by an acute traumatic event like an elbow dislocation. Timely recognition of injuries to these structures is very important; disruption of the ligaments may threaten elbow stability and can possibly be career ending for an athlete [102, 103]. MR imaging is indispensable in the assessment of the ligaments, since it provides superior soft tissue contrast and allows for simultaneous evaluation of bony structures in a single examination [104]. In the following section, an overview of elbow ligament injuries and their appearance on various imaging methods are provided.

4.3.1 Ulnar Collateral Ligament Injury and Valgus Extension Overload

Valgus extension overload is a spectrum of symptoms that are commonly seen in competitive overhead athletes [105]. Large valgus and extension forces in the acceleration phase of throwing lead to major tensile stress on medial structures, compressive forces on the lateral structures (see Sect. 4.2.2), and shear forces posteriorly (see Sect. 4.2.4). These chronic tensile forces lead to inflammation, microtearing, and laxity of the ligament, which may progress into disruption of the UCL. Less commonly, the UCL may be injured after traumatic elbow dislocation [105].

Plain radiographs may not provide any direct information on ligamentous injuries, but can be indirectly supportive if focal calcifications of the UCL are present [106, 107]. When compared to the normal appearance of the UCL on US, UCL sprains show thickening, decreased echogenicity, and hyperechoic areas demonstrating local calcifications [31, 107]. A completely ruptured UCL appears as a hypoechoic band surrounded by fluid.

On normal axial MR images, the anterior band of the UCL has uniform low signal intensity on T1W and T2W images. However, a completely normal UCL on MRI in a competitive throwing athlete is rarely seen [108]. Adaptations in response to forces in throwing include thickening of the anterior band of the UCL and posteromedial subchondral sclerosis of the trochlea. Therefore, MRI ought to be used to differentiate between acute versus chronic injury and to observe the degree of remodeling of the chronic ligament deformity [109]. Ruptures, sprains, laxity, or other irregularities manifest as a discontinuity with hyperintense fluid filling the hiatus on both T1W and T2W images [14, 104]. Avulsion fracture of the medial epicondyle may be present.

MR arthrography may be of particular benefit when partial-thickness tearing is suspected, since it improves the sensitivity of detecting such tears [18]. In case of a partial-thickness tear, the so-called T-sign may demonstrate increased signal intensity at the distal insertion near the sublime tubercle [14, 110].

4.3.2 Dislocation of the Elbow Joint

Dislocation of the elbow is the most common dislocation in children and the second most common dislocation in adults (after dislocation of the shoulder) [111]. The elbow owes its stability to the osseous architecture of the ulnohumeral joint, which provides the most stability in the anteroposterior direction. The surrounding capsuloligamentous and musculotendinous aspects (including the collateral ligaments, joint capsule, and adjacent muscles) provide further stability. If these components are disrupted by trauma, elbow dislocation may result.

Dislocations of the elbow can either be simple or complex depending on the absence or presence of associated bony injury, respectively. Simple dislocations are described by the direction of the dislocated ulna relative to the humerus. Posterior displacement occurs in over 90 % of cases, with posterolateral dislocation as its most common subtype [112]. The injury mechanism is considered to be a combination of axial compression, supination, and valgus stress, often seen in FOOSH-type injuries [103]. Lateral and anterior displacements are rare and may result from a direct posterior blow to a flexed elbow [113]. Bony injuries of the olecranon and avulsion of the medial and lateral condyles and epicondyles can be present. Complex dislocations with combined fractures of the radial head or neck and the coronoid process are referred to as the *terrible triad* (see Sect. 4.2.1) [57, 102].

Accompanying ligamentous and capsular disruption can be described according to the Horii circle [103]. Stage 1 involves disruption of the LUCL with posterolateral rotatory subluxation of the ulna. In stage 2, the coronoid places on the trochlea (i.e., incomplete dislocation) and the other adjacent lateral ligaments are torn, including anterior and posterior aspects of the joint capsule. Finally in stage 3, the elbow is completely dislocated with the coronoid located posteriorly to the humerus. The MCL may be disrupted only posteriorly (stage 3A) or completely (stage 3B). Thus, elbow dislocation is the result of a posterolateral rotatory subluxation followed by a total disruption of the surrounding soft tissue from the lateral to the medial side [102].

Posterolateral dislocation can lead to permanent valgus instability that correlates with a worse overall clinical and radiographic result. All treatment options are therefore primarily aimed at restoring functional elbow stability [102]. Simple dislocations may be treated nonoperatively after reduction under adequate muscular relaxation and appropriate analgesia. To prevent joint contractures, definitive management involves limited mobilization and early active range of motion [114]. Complex fracture-dislocations require operative management with fixation of fractures and repair of damaged surrounding soft tissues. Damage to the brachial artery or median and ulnar nerve must be ruled out, although neurovascular injury is uncommon in the setting of a FOOSH injury [103].

Anteroposterior, lateral, and oblique radiographs should be obtained to determine the direction of the dislocation and the potential presence of associated fractures. An intact radiocapitellar line should be evident on all views, since this is no longer aligned in posterior elbow dislocations [8]. Post-reduction radiographs are required to ensure correct positioning of the elbow.

Concerning preoperative planning after complex elbow dislocation, CT can be used to delineate fractures, and MR imaging is helpful to visualize the extent of the soft tissue disruption [57, 115, 116].

4.3.3 Chronic Insufficiency of the LCL: Posterolateral Rotatory Instability

Elbow dislocation from a FOOSH trauma poses a substantial risk for recurrent elbow instability, since the stabilizing architecture of the surrounding ligaments, the radial head, and the coronoid process can be significantly disrupted. This condition has also been reported following coronoid insufficiency, radial head excision, or steroid injections for lateral epicondylitis [18].

Several criteria are used to classify the degree of the instability: the articulation(s) involved, the direction of the displacement (valgus, varus, anterior or posterolateral), the degree of displacement (subluxation or dislocation), the timing of displacement (acute, chronic or recurrent), and the presence or absence of associated fractures [103]. The most common type of chronic elbow instability is posterolateral rotatory instability (PLRI) [117]. PLRI implies a dislocation by which external rotation of the radius and the ulna relative to the distal humerus results in posterior displacement of the radial head relative to the capitellum. Contrary to isolated dislocation of the radial head, the radioulnar joint does not dislocate because the annular ligament is not affected [118].

The lateral ligament complex limits external rotation of the radius and ulna relative to the humerus and is therefore considered the weakest link in the pathogenesis of PLRI [102]. However, the medial collateral ligament may contribute as well [119, 120].

The diagnosis is made clinically based on the patient's history and physical examination. Patients with PLRI often have a history of ulnohumeral dislocation; recurrent symptoms of lateral pain, locking, clicking, snapping, or popping can be present. The feeling of instability mostly occurs when the elbow is actively brought from flexion into extension with the forearm in supination. Several specific apprehension tests are available to provoke these symptoms [118, 121]. During the lateral pivot-shift maneuver, the elbow is in supine position and mild valgus stress is applied while the elbow is flexed. The test is positive if apprehension or frank subluxation of the radius and the ulna (rotating away from the humerus) occurs [122]. The posterolateral rotatory drawer test involves overhead placement of the elbow in 40° of flexion. Subsequent application of an anteroposterior force on the ulna and the radius (with the forearm in external rotation) will subluxate the forearm away from the humerus on the lateral side, pivoting on the intact medial ligaments [122]. A more adequate evaluation of instability by these tests may be performed with the patient under anesthesia. The radial head then visibly subluxates posteriorly, whereas apprehension occurs when the patient is awake.

The primary treatment goal in patients with PLRI is to restore elbow stability. Nonoperative measures are applied in the first days after reduction. These measures include both splinting of the arm as well as rehabilitation to strengthen the surrounding musculature [123]. If unsatisfactory results are yielded by conservative management, surgical treatment may be considered. The majority of surgically treated patients encounter satisfactory outcomes regarding elbow stability [118]. Surgical management aimed at the reconstruction of ligaments can be performed either open or arthroscopically [123]. Deficiency of the radial head or coronoid may require bony reconstructions. In that case, computed tomography is of particular use to delineate complex fracture patterns and to assist in surgical planning [115].

Plain radiographs are used to demonstrate changes in the alignment of the elbow by reviewing the integrity of the radial head, coronoid process, and capitellum. The *drop sign*, indicative for PRLI, represents ulnohumeral separation on lateral radiographs [124]. Posterior displacement of the radial head in relation to the capitellum may be visible as well.

Although MRI has been well established as an effective method for the assessment of ligamentous injury to the LCL, the role of MRI in the diagnosis of PLRI remains questionable [121, 125]. However, examination through MR arthrography is advantageous if uncertainty about the diagnosis remains even though PLRI is suspected [123]. Arthrography reveals laxity of the LCL, widening of the lateral joint space, and osteochondral lesions at the radiocapitellar joint [18, 118].

4.3.4 Monteggia Injury of the Forearm

The ulna and the radius act as a single functional unit through binding via the interosseous membrane and ligaments in the forearm. As a consequence, hyper-pronation injury with fracture of the ulna is often accompanied by a dislocation of the proximal radioulnar joint. This combination of injuries was first described by Monteggia in 1814 and further classified by Bado [126]. Depending on the location of displacement of the radial head, four types can be distinguished (see Table 4.7).

Since the long-term range of motion of the elbow is seriously threatened in Monteggia injury, early recognition is important [127]. Pediatric patients may sustain injuries slightly different to Monteggia injury, including plastic deformation, incomplete or greenstick fractures, and ulnar metaphyseal fractures [127]. Although conservative management can be successful in the younger population, operative treatment is warranted for the majority of adults [127, 128].

Table 4.7 Bado classification of Monteggia injury [126]

Type	Description
I	Anterior dislocation of the radial head and fracture of the ulnar shaft with anterior angulation
II	Posterior dislocation of the radial head and fracture of the ulnar shaft with posterior angulation
III	Lateral dislocation of the radial head and fracture of the ulnar metaphysis
IV	Anterior dislocation of the radial head, fracture of the proximal third of the radius and ulna

The treatment goal is to restore the cooperative functioning of the radius, ulna, and their associated articulations.

Radiographic examination should comprise AP, lateral, and oblique views of both the forearm and the wrist. The distal forearm should be evaluated for displacement of the ulna relative to the radius. The radiocapitellar line must accurately be assessed in the proximal forearm, since it may seem normal due to concurrent displacement of the ulnar shaft [5].

4.3.5 Isolated Dislocation of the Radial Head

Isolated dislocation of the proximal radius, also termed *nursemaid's elbow* or *pulled elbow*, is the result of a sudden pull on the arm. This longitudinal traction force with the forearm in pronation and extension pulls the radial head trough the annular ligament. Due to relative laxity of the annular ligament, this injury is common in children aged 0–5 years [129]. After the age of 5 years, the annular ligament is stronger and less likely to tear or be displaced. Generally, the diagnosis is based on the clinical presentation. The injured child is likely to not use the affected arm and holds it in pronation, mild flexion, and abduction against the body. Radiography (AP view) should be considered if the diagnosis is equivocal, if the mechanism of injury other than a pull is suspected, or if reduction attempts are unsuccessful [130].

4.4 Musculotendinous Injury of the Elbow

4.4.1 Epicondylitis

4.4.1.1 Lateral Epicondylitis

Lateral epicondylitis, also known as tennis elbow, is the most common cause of lateral elbow pain [131]. Any sport or occupation that demands repetitive wrist extension can result in this type of injury. Lateral epicondylitis most commonly occurs in the fourth and fifth decades of life, with both sexes affected equally [132]. The common extensor tendon (CET) originates from the anterior aspect of the lateral epicondyle of the elbow and consists of the three conjoining tendons of the extensor carpi radialis brevis (ECRB), the extensor digitorum communis (EDC), and the extensor carpi ulnaris (ECU) muscles [133]. Lateral epicondylitis represents a condition where repetitive contractions of the ECRB, and to a lesser extent the EDC and ECU, lead to microtearing with subsequent degeneration, immature repair, and tendinosis [131, 134]. Tendinopathy or tearing of the ECRB tendon is invariably seen in lateral epicondylitis [132]. Physical examination typically reveals tenderness at the origin of the ECRB tendon and pain exacerbating with active wrist extension [135, 136]. The clinical picture is often sufficient for making the diagnosis. However, when symptoms are atypical or patients do not respond to therapy, imaging may be performed.

In case of suspected lateral epicondylitis, elbow radiographs may show some calcification along the lateral epicondyle. Nevertheless, radiographs are often false-negative and the routine use of plain films does not seem justified in the diagnostic process [137]. Both magnetic resonance imaging (MRI) and ultrasound (US) are useful tools in diagnosing lateral epicondylitis. US provides an inexpensive and fast imaging method, whereas MRI is more expensive and time-consuming. Presently, MRI is considered the golden standard with a diagnostic sensitivity ranging between 90 % and 100 %. The sensitivity for US ranges between 60 % and 80 % [138]. Additional US techniques have no extra benefit over standard gray-scale ultrasonography in detecting abnormal musculoskeletal findings in painful elbows [138].

The CET origin in individuals with lateral epicondylitis shows increased signal intensity on T2-weighted fat-suppressed MR images within the substance of the tendon, most commonly the ECRB, with or without tendon thickening [138–140]. However, CET thickening and increased signal intensity on T2-weighted images have also been observed in asymptomatic high-performance athletes [140]. MRI can be used to categorize epicondylitis into several grades of severity. In mild epicondylitis, the CET is thickened with increased internal signal intensity. In moderate epicondylitis, there is a partial-thickness tear with thinning and focal disruption that does not extend across the full thickness of the tendon. Severe epicondylitis consists of a near-complete or complete tear, characterized as a fluid-filled gap separating the tendon from its origin at the lateral epicondyle [132]. This grading system has a significant role in surgical planning [139].

4.4.1.2 Medial Epicondylitis

Medial epicondylitis, also known as golfer's elbow, is another common cause of elbow pain among athletes and workers in occupations that demand repetitive flexion of the wrist. In throwing athletes, medial epicondylitis may result from repetitive stress to the flexor-pronator mass, consisting of the pronator teres and flexor carpi radialis muscles [141]. The tendon origin of the flexor-pronator mass attaches to the anterior aspect of the medial epicondyle of the humerus and is most commonly affected in medial epicondylitis [133, 142]. This condition has the same pathogenesis as lateral epicondylitis, repetitive microtrauma at the tendinous insertion of the flexor-pronator mass leading to degeneration, tendinosis, and ultimately tearing [143–145]. Patients most often report a history of activities involving wrist flexion and forearm pronation, as is the case in golf, racket sports, and overhead throwing [142, 146]. Examination typically reveals painful flexion and pronation against resistance, decreased grip strength, and tenderness over the origin of the flexor-pronator mass at the medial epicondyle [147].

When clinical signs are confounding, the diagnosis of medial epicondylitis can be further explored using both US and MRI. Plain radiographs may show calcification or traction osteophytes at the flexor-pronator mass origin, but these findings have overall low sensitivity [148]. US may demonstrate focal hypoechoic or anechoic areas in the tendon, cortical irregularity at the tendinous insertion, tendon thickening, and calcification. Most abnormalities occur in the tendons of the flexor carpi radialis and pronator teres but changes may also be seen inside the tendon of the palmaris longus and flexor digitorum superficialis [30]. MRI is considered more sensitive than US and may demonstrate findings similar to those described in lateral epicondylitis: focal thickening and increased signal intensity within the flexor-pronator tendons accompanied by surrounding soft tissue edema best seen on T2-weighted fat-suppressed MR image series. In both lateral and medial epicondylitis however, clinical evaluation remains the mainstay of the diagnosis and the role of imaging is primarily to confirm the presence of suspected tendon pathology [135].

4.4.2 Tendon Pathology

4.4.2.1 Distal Biceps Tendon

Distal biceps tendon (DBT) pathology is a relatively rare cause of anterior elbow pain and ranges from tendinopathy to partial tearing and complete tears of the DBT. A complete tear of the DBT is the most common entity, followed by partial tearing, with isolated tendinopathy being exceedingly rare [135]. Complete ruptures of the DBT typically occur in male weightlifters and athletes between 40 and 60 years of age [149, 150]. Risk factors include smoking, anabolic steroid use, and a history of previous DBT rupture [151].

Rupture of the DBT is classically an acute injury occurring when a strong eccentric force is applied on the contracted biceps with the elbow in 90° flexion, leading to tear at the insertion site of the DBT into the radial tuberosity [135]. In the case of a full DBT rupture, physical examination often shows a palpable defect within the antecubital fossa and proximal bulging of the biceps muscle due to retraction of the ruptured tendon. Pain over the antecubital fossa and weakness of forearm supination and elbow flexion can be observed in both partial and complete tears [135].

Imaging has an important role in distinguishing partial from complete tears [152–154]. Plain radiographs are not indicated unless concomitant injury of the elbow is suspected [148]. A complete tear can be diagnosed on US as a complete absence of the DBT that is retracted proximally, often more than 10 cm from the insertion at the radial tuberosity [155]. In addition to diagnosing complete tears, MRI is useful for visualizing partial tears of the DBT. A partial rupture of the distal biceps tendon is characterized by the presence of increased signal intensity within the tendon [156, 157]. Secondary MRI findings of partial tears may include the presence of bone marrow edema within the radial tuberosity, indicative of a micro-avulsion at the DBT's insertion site. Differentiating partial tears from tendinopathy proves to be challenging both clinically and radiologically [158]. As such, MRI is indicated when the presence of a complete versus a partial rupture is uncertain. This distinction is clinically important as complete tears need to be repaired surgically. This is in contrast with partial tears and tendinopathy of the DBT, where conservative treatment is often adequate [148].

4.4.2.2 Distal Triceps Tendon

Tendinosis and rupture of the distal triceps tendon constitute the least common type of elbow tendinopathy [159]. Males are affected twice as often as females and triceps injuries have been reported in professional football players, soccer players, softball players, skiers, and weightlifters [160–162]. In contrast to biceps tendon injuries, triceps injuries are exclusively seen at the distal insertion of the triceps tendon onto the olecranon. Presently, no proximal tendon avulsion of the triceps has been described in the English literature [163]. Several risk factors for triceps tendon pathology have been explored, including chronic renal failure, endocrine disorders, metabolic bone disease, and steroid use [164–166]. The most common mechanism of injury is a fall on an outstretched hand in which a deceleration load is applied to the triceps while it is actively contracting [167]. In case of a complete triceps rupture, the most universal finding on physical examination is the inability to extend the elbow against gravity [168].

Tendinosis and partial tears of the triceps can be more difficult to diagnose on physical examination and this is where imaging comes into play. Plain radiographs often show osseous flakes, also termed the *flake sign*, which is considered pathognomonic for avulsion injuries of the triceps [169]. Radiographs are indicated in traumatic settings to rule out concomitant injuries of the elbow. Both US and MRI can differentiate between either a partial or full tear of the distal triceps tendon. Moreover, the degree of tearing is of major value in deciding whether surgical repair or conservative treatment is indicated [167]. US may diagnose all types of triceps tendon injury ranging from tendinosis to complete tears along with retraction of the tendon. However, data on sensitivity and specificity have not been documented [170]. MRI is an acknowledged imaging modality for confirming the presence of complete tendon tears and staging partial tears. The triceps tendon is best visualized on sagittal images. Partial ruptures of the triceps tendon are characterized by a small fluid-filled defect within the distal triceps tendon with edema in the surrounding subcutaneous tissue of the posterior elbow. Complete rupture of the triceps tendon is characterized by a large fluid-filled gap between the distal triceps tendon and the olecranon process with a large amount of edema in the adjacent subcutaneous tissue. The distal edges of the torn triceps tendon are frayed and show heterogeneous signal intensity. A variable amount of retraction of the distal triceps tendon is usually present [135, 171].

4.4.2.3 Snapping Medial Head of the Triceps with Subluxating Ulnar Nerve

The medial head of the triceps originates just inferior to the radial sulcus of the humerus, traverses posterior to the medial epicondyle, and inserts into the olecranon process of the ulna. During flexion of the elbow, a portion of the medial head of the triceps may dislocate or "snap" anteriorly over the medial epicondyle [172]. The ulnar nerve is in close relationship with the medial head of the triceps and may also dislocate during flexion. This condition often presents as a combination of medial elbow pain, a single- or double-snapping sensation during flexion of the elbow, and additional symptoms of ulnar nerve irritation [172]. A symptomatic dislocating medial head of the triceps muscle is frequently associated with overhead activities in throwing athletes and with weightlifting in bodybuilders. Predisposing factors include hypertrophy of the triceps musculature, post-traumatic alteration of bone alignment, and congenital predisposition owing to anatomical variations of the triceps [173]. Snapping of the medial head of the triceps is relatively easily observable during physical examination compared to snapping of the ulnar nerve [172].

Because the snapping syndrome is a dynamic and intermittent condition, MRI and CT are unfavorable for confirming the diagnosis. Nonetheless, axial imaging with CT or MRI may demonstrate the structures that dislocate with the elbow positioned in different degrees of flexion [174]. US is the modality of choice and can provide a dynamic assessment of the structures involved during a snapping sensation. With an isolated dislocating ulnar nerve, the nerve and medial triceps will often appear to separate during flexion of the elbow, whereas with a dislocating medial triceps, the ulnar nerve and triceps appear to travel as one unit over the medial epicondyle in the anterior direction [175]. Differentiating between these two entities is of clinical importance as it aids in deciding which type of surgery is indicated [176].

4.4.2.4 Bursitis of the Elbow

Two main bursae can be found in the elbow joint. Anteriorly, the bicipitoradial bursa fills the antecubital fossa. Posteriorly, the olecranon bursa is located just below the skin. The bicipitoradial bursa encases the distal biceps tendon and reduces friction between this tendon and the radial tuberosity during joint movement [177]. Repeated supination and pronation of the forearm is believed to be a possible cause of chronic bicipitoradial bursitis [178]. Due to its close relationship with the distal biceps tendon, bicipitoradial bursitis may be accompanied by tendinopathy of the biceps [179]. In contrast with the bicipitoradial bursa, the olecranon bursa is located more superficially and therefore prone to direct trauma leading to acute, post-traumatic bursitis. Traumatic olecranon bursitis has been reported in athletes who train and play on hard surfaces [180]. In general, bursitis of the elbow in athletes is an aseptic condition [181].

Although the diagnosis of bursitis is mainly clinical, the affected bursa can be excellently visualized on US. Imaging signs include bursal wall distension with presence of local hypoechoic or anechoic intra-bursal material [182]. Power Doppler is able to demonstrate the presence of pathological signal enhancement in case of active inflammation [170]. An added benefit of US is the possibility to guide the needle into the bursa for direct aspiration and injection of corticosteroids. In case of bicipitoradial bursitis, US can provide information about concomitant radial nerve injury [183]. Both bicipitoradial and olecranon bursitis can be further evaluated on MRI, especially in more severe cases where extensive damage of surrounding structures is suspected and preoperative planning. MRI aspects of olecranon bursitis include hypointensity on T1-weighted images and variable signal intensity in T2-weighted sequences over the olecranon, with adjacent soft tissue edema and contrast enhancement of the bursal margins [184]. MRI aspects of bicipitoradial bursitis include increased signal intensity within the lesion on T2-weighted images suggestive of a fluid collection. Furthermore, hypointense septal structures may be observed. A biceps tendon with low signal intensity on both T1- and T2-weighted images can be detected at the anterior edge of the bursa [185].

4.5 Neurological Injury of the Elbow

4.5.1 Cubital Tunnel Syndrome

Next to dislocation of the ulnar nerve, as described in a snapping medial head of the triceps, the ulnar nerve may also become compressed at the cubital tunnel of the elbow. Compression of the ulnar nerve, also known as cubital tunnel syndrome, is the second most common compression neuropathy in the upper limp, following carpal tunnel syndrome [186]. In most instances, the ulnar nerve can become entrapped at the entrance of the cubital tunnel due to a thickened aponeurosis connecting the two heads of the flexor carpi ulnaris muscle [187]. This may lead to ulnar neuropathy with clinical symptoms of paresthesia and weakness of the intrinsic musculature around the fourth and fifth digits and the hypothenar region of the hand [188]. The diagnosis is confirmed with electromyography (EMG), showing a decrease in compound muscle action potential amplitude (CMAP) and slowing of focal conduction along the elbow segment [189]. EMG however is a rather uncomfortable procedure and several other diagnostic approaches have therefore been investigated, including high-resolution ultrasound (HRU) and magnetic resonance imaging (MRI) [190–192].

Qualitatively, US findings suggestive of ulnar neuropathy include abnormal enlargement of the nerve with an abrupt caliber change or loss of the normal fascicular pattern [193]. Numerous quantitative US findings have been investigated, including the ulnar nerve cross-sectional area (UNCSA), nerve diameter, and swelling ratio. The UNCSA measured at the site of greatest enlargement is a useful parameter for diagnosing cubital tunnel syndrome [194]. With the elbow in full extension and supination, the UNCSA measured at the cubital tunnel is significantly elevated in case of suspected cubital tunnel syndrome [195]. HRU may also demonstrate signs of ulnar nerve dedifferentiation consisting of edematous infiltration with a homogeneous hypoechoic aspect of the nerve. These HRU findings correspond well with cubital tunnel syndrome as diagnosed on EMG [195]. In addition, HRU can assess ulnar nerve instability during active flexion and extension of the elbow, one of the causes for ulnar neuropathy [193].

A universal MRI finding of neuropathy involves a hyperintense signal on short-tau inversion recovery (STIR) sequences. However, this finding has low specificity and is occasionally seen in healthy nerves [196]. Diffusion weighted imaging (DWI) is useful for imaging tissues with an organized microstructure such as the peripheral nerves, and the diagnostic value of DWI in median nerve entrapment neuropathy proves to be high [197]. When the ulnar nerve is entrapped, DWI is able to highlight diffusion restriction appreciable as an increase in signal intensity. Contrary to STIR sequences, an increased signal intensity of the ulnar nerve on DWI images is only visible in case of cubital tunnel syndrome as diagnosed with EMG [198].

4.5.2 Median Nerve Entrapment Syndromes

Pronator syndrome (PS) is a rare and controversial diagnosis that was originally coined to describe a compression syndrome of the median nerve between the humeral and ulnar heads of the pronator teres (PT) muscle [199]. Despite its name, compression of the median nerve can occur at several other, less common sites as it travels through the antecubital region into the forearm. Proximally, the median nerve may become entrapped as it dives under the ligament of Struthers, a ligament present in 2–3 % of the population connecting a residual supracondylar process with the medial epicondyle of the humerus [200–202].

The nerve then runs across the antecubital fossa and enters the forearm deep to the bicipital aponeurosis, another potential site of median nerve compression around the elbow. Distal to the elbow, the nerve travels between the two heads of PT muscle and passes beneath the proximal arch of the flexor digitorum superficialis (FDS) muscle [203]. PS is characterized by proximal, volar forearm pain with paresthesias of the first three digits and radial half of the fourth digit but has varying clinical manifestations due to the multiple potential sites of nerve entrapment [204]. Furthermore, the median nerve gives off a branch deep to the FDS muscle which may also become entrapped, resulting in another compression syndrome called the anterior interosseous nerve (AIN) syndrome [203].

Diagnosing median nerve entrapment around the elbow may be challenging and EMG studies are often inconclusive [205]. Conventional elbow radiographs are considered an initial step in the imaging workup and can show a residual supracondylar process of the distal humerus indicative of a Struthers' ligament [206]. To date, no studies concerning the diagnostic efficacy of MRI and US have been published. However, both MRI and US are useful for ruling out secondary causes of median nerve compression such as ganglion cysts of nerve (sheath) tumors. Moreover, MRI can demonstrate the presence of denervation edema resulting from compression neuropathy when AIN syndrome is suspected. Denervation edema is visible in the muscles enervated by the AIN, mostly the pronator quadratus (PQ) muscle, and presents as a hyperintense signal within the affected muscles on fat-saturated T2-weighted images [207, 208].

Fatty atrophy of the affected muscles, presenting as hyperechogenicity on US, is another characteristic of chronic median nerve entrapment syndromes. However, US and MRI findings of fatty atrophy correlate poorly [209].

4.5.3 Radial Nerve Compression Syndromes

Next to ulnar and median nerve compression neuropathies in the elbow, the radial nerve is the least involved in compression injury with an annual incidence of 0.003 % for radial nerve compression syndromes [210]. As the radial nerve continues along the antecubital fossa, it branches into the motor posterior interosseous nerve (PIN) and sensory superficial radial nerve (SRN). The SRN is a subcutaneous sensory branch of the radial nerve and compression of this nerve is exceedingly rare [211]. More common is entrapment of the PIN as it courses through the radial tunnel and gives rise to either PIN syndrome or radial tunnel syndrome (RTS). Remarkably, RTS and PIN syndrome are both the result of entrapment of the same deep branch of the radial nerve, or PIN, but symptoms of both compression neuropathies show considerable diversity among patients. PIN syndrome is dominated by loss of motor function of the innervated musculature, whereas RTS is dominated by posterolateral forearm pain. This discrepancy in symptoms may be explained by the degree and duration of nerve compression [203].

There are at least five anatomical landmarks responsible for entrapment of the deep branch of the radial nerve along the radial tunnel: fibrous bands between the brachialis and brachioradialis muscles at the level of the radiocapitellar joint; the anastomosing vessels of the radial recurrent artery at the level of the radial neck, also referred to as the *leash of Henry*; the proximal edge of the extensor carpi radialis brevis (ECRB) muscle; the proximal edge of the supinator muscle, also referred to as the *arcade of Fröhse*; and the distal edge of the supinator muscle [203]. The arcade of Fröhse or proximal edge of the supinator muscle may undergo tendinous thickening due to repetitive pronosupination and is the most common site for PIN compression, hence its alternative name *supinator syndrome* [212, 213].

Because motor function is commonly affected in PIN syndrome, nerve conduction studies often reveal abnormal findings and are thus a useful tool for the diagnosis in addition to physical examination. Imaging studies are not routinely indicated in PIN syndrome, but MRI may reveal soft tissue masses responsible for nerve compression. Moreover, reported MRI findings in patients with suspected PIN syndrome include denervation edema of the supinator muscle, marked by an increased signal intensity of the muscle as seen on fluid-sensitive sequences with fat suppression [214]. Ultrasound may show hypoechogenicity, increased diameter of the radial deep branches, and hyperemia of the nerve on power Doppler in

PIN syndrome as compared to healthy individuals [215]. However, standardized cutoff values have yet to be developed and sensitivity is relatively poor. Consequently, the role of imaging studies is limited and may be used to further strengthen the diagnosis of suspected PIN syndrome or rule out other pathology. In contrast with PIN syndrome, electrodiagnostic studies are often normal in RTS, which add to the difficulty and controversy of this diagnosis [203]. Symptoms of RTS may mimic those of lateral epicondylitis and this is where ultrasound can be used to rule out epicondylitis [211]. This distinction can usually be made during physical examination, where lateral epicondylitis presents with focal tenderness at the insertion of the ECRB, whereas RTS presents with pain starting a few centimeters more distally from the lateral epicondyle radiating into the forearm [216].

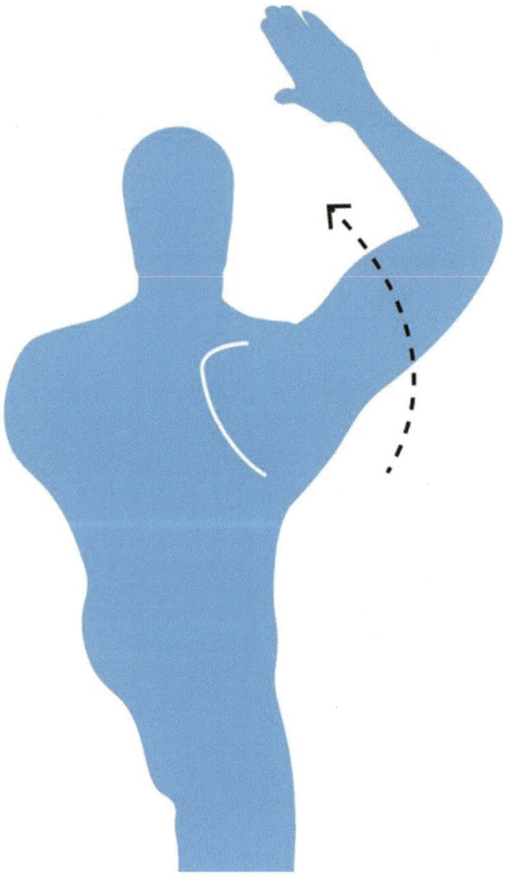

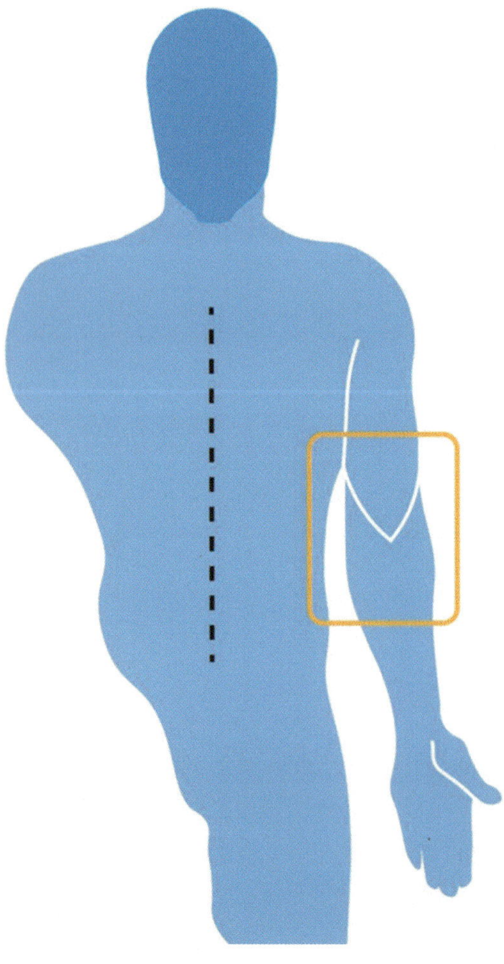

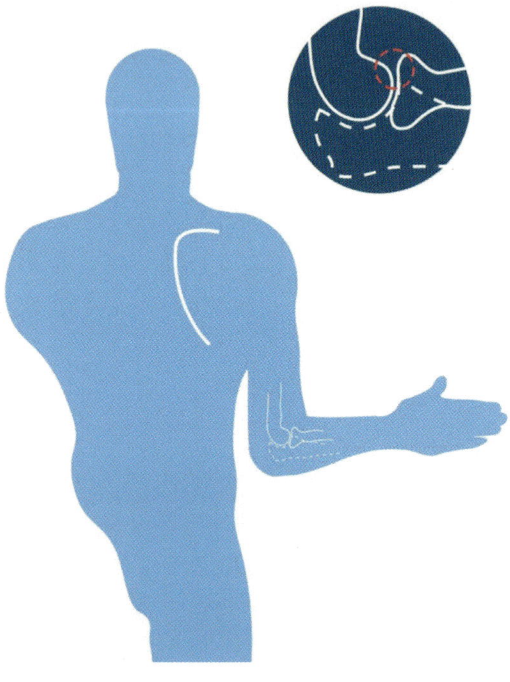

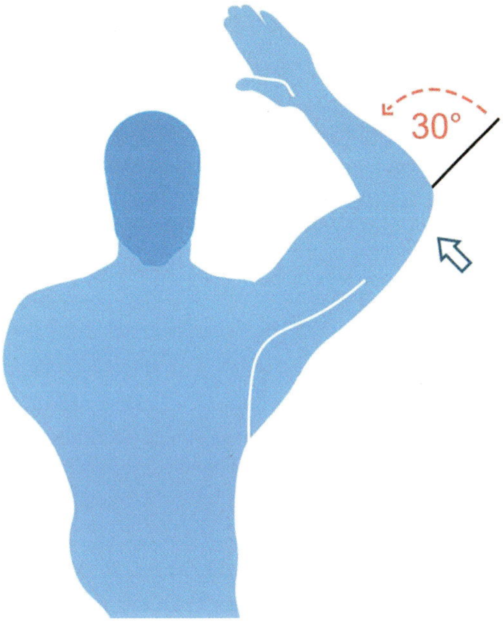

References

1. Grayson D. The elbow: radiographic imaging pearls and pitfalls. Semin Roentgenol. 2005;40(3):223–47.
2. Cain E, Dugas J, Wolf R, Andrews J. Elbow injuries in throwing athletes: a current concepts review. Am J Sports Med. 2003;31(4):621–35.
3. Chen A, Youm T, Ong B, Rafii M, Rokito A. Imaging of the elbow in the overhead throwing athlete. Am J Sports Med. 2003;31(3):466–73.
4. Greenspan A, Norman A, Rosen H. Radial head-capitellum view in elbow trauma: clinical application and radiographic-anatomic correlation. Am J Roentgenol. 1984;143(2):355–9. doi:10.2214/ajr.143.2.355.
5. Raby N, Berman L, De Lacey G. Accident and emergency radiology. 3rd ed. London: Bailliere Tindall; 2005.
6. Rogers L, Malave SJ, White H, Tachdjian M. Plastic bowing, torus and greenstick supracondylar fractures of the humerus: radiographic clues to obscure fractures of the elbow in children. Radiology. 1978;128(1):145–50. doi:10.1148/128.1.145.
7. Frick M. Imaging of the elbow: a review of imaging findings in acute and chronic traumatic disorders of the elbow. J Hand Ther. 2006;19(2):98–113. doi:10.1197/j.jht.2006.02.007.
8. Iyer R, Thapa M, Khanna P, Chew F. Pediatric bone imaging: imaging elbow trauma in children. A review of acute and chronic injuries. Am J Roentgenol. 2012;198(5):1053–68. doi:10.2214/AJR.10.7314.
9. LaBella CR. Common acute sports-related lower extremity injuries in children and adolescents. Clin Pediatr Emerg Med. 2007;8(1):31–42.
10. Shrader MW. Pediatric supracondylar fractures and pediatric physeal elbow fractures. Orthop Clin N Am. 2008;39(2):163–71. doi:10.1016/j.ocl.2007.12.005. v.
11. Patel B, Reed M, Patel S. Gender-specific pattern differences of the ossification centers in the pediatric elbow. Pediatr Radiol. 2009;39(3):226–31. doi:10.1007/s00247-008-1078-4.
12. Cheng JC, Wing-Man K, Shen WY, Yurianto H, Xia G, Lau JT, Cheung AY. A new look at the sequential development of elbow-ossification centers in children. J Pediatr Orthop. 1998;18(2):161–7.
13. Hayter C, Giuffre B. Overuse and traumatic injuries of the elbow. Magn Reson Imaging Clin N Am. 2009;17(4):617–38. doi:10.1016/j.mric.2009.06.004.
14. Sampath S, Sampath S, Bredella M. Magnetic resonance imaging of the elbow: a structured approach. Sports Health. 2013;5(1):34–49. doi:10.1177/1941738112467941.
15. Brunton L, Anderson M, Pannunzio M, Khanna A, Chhabra B. Magnetic resonance imaging of the elbow: update on current techniques and indications. J Hand Surg [Am]. 2006;31(6):1001–11. doi:10.1016/j.jhsa.2006.04.006.
16. Ouellette H, Bredella M, Labis J, Palmer W, Torriani M. MR imaging of the elbow in baseball pitchers. Skelet Radiol. 2008;37(2):115–21. doi:10.1007/s00256-007-0364-9.
17. Schwartz M, Al-Zahrani S, Morwessel R, Andrews J. Ulnar collateral ligament injury in the throwing athlete: evaluation with saline-enhanced MR arthrography. Radiology. 1995;197(1):297–9. doi:10.1148/radiology.197.1.7568841.
18. Delport A, Zoga A. MR and CT arthrography of the elbow. Semin Musculoskelet Radiol. 2012;16(1):15–26. doi:10.1055/s-0032-1304298.
19. Bohndorf K, Kilcoyne R. Traumatic injuries: imaging of peripheral musculoskeletal injuries. Eur Radiol. 2002;12(7):1605–16. doi:10.1007/s00330-002-1461-8.
20. Rosas H, Lee K. Imaging acute trauma of the elbow. Semin Musculoskelet Radiol. 2010;14(4):394–411. doi:10.1055/s-0030-1263255.
21. Zubler V, Saupe N, Jost B, Pfirrmann C, Hodler J, Zanetti M. Elbow stiffness: effectiveness of conventional radiography and CT to explain osseous causes. Am J Roentgenol. 2010;194(6):515–20. doi:10.2214/ajr.09.3741.
22. Schaeffeler C, Waldt S, Woertler K. Traumatic instability of the elbow – anatomy, pathomechanisms and presentation on imaging. Eur Radiol. 2013;23(9):2582–93. doi:10.1007/s00330- 013-2855-5.
23. Sauser D, Thordarson S, Fahr L. Imaging of the elbow. Radiol Clin N Am. 1990;28(5):923–40.
24. Franklin P, Dunlop R, Whitelaw G, Jacques EJ, Blickman J, Shapiro J. Computed tomography of the normal and traumatized elbow. J Comput Assist Tomogr. 1988;12(5):817–23.

25. Frahm R, Wimmer B. The search for joint loose bodies in the elbow joint – conventional or CT arthrography? Radiologe. 1990;30(3):113–5.
26. Steinbach L, Schwartz M. Elbow arthrography. Radiol Clin N Am. 1998;36(4):635–49.
27. Waldt S, Bruegel M, Ganter K, Kuhn V, Link T, Rummeny E, Woertler K. Comparison of multislice CT arthrography and MR arthrography for the detection of articular cartilage lesions of the elbow. Eur Radiol. 2005;15(4):784–91. doi:10.1007/s00330-004-2585-9.
28. Hodge J. Musculoskeletal procedures: diagnostic and therapeutic. Austin: Landes Bioscience; 2003.
29. Nofsinger C, Konin J. Diagnostic ultrasound in sports medicine: current concepts and advances. Sports Med Arthrosc. 2009;17(1):25–30. doi:10.1097/JSA.0b013e3181982add.
30. Martinoli C, Bianchi S, Giovagnorio F, Pugliese F. Ultrasound of the elbow. Skelet Radiol. 2001;30(11):605–14. doi:10.1007/s002560100410.
31. Draghi F, Danesino G, de Gautard R, Bianchi S. Ultrasound of the elbow: examination techniques and US appearance of the normal and pathologic joint. J Ultrasound. 2007;10(2):76–84. doi:10.1016/j.jus.2007.04.005.
32. Lee KS, Rosas HG, Craig JG. Musculoskeletal ultrasound: elbow imaging and procedures. Semin Musculoskelet Radiol. 2010;14(4):449–60. doi:10.1055/s-0030-1263260.
33. Badia A, Stennett C. Sports-related injuries of the elbow. J Hand Ther. 2006;19(2):206–27. doi:10.1197/j.jht.2006.02.006.
34. Miller A, Dodson C, Ilyas A. Thrower's fracture of the humerus. Orthop Clin N Am. 2014;45(4):565–9. doi:10.1016/j.ocl.2014.06.011.
35. Curtin P, Taylor C, Rice J. Thrower's fracture of the humerus with radial nerve palsy: an unfamiliar softball injury. Br J Sports Med. 2005;39(11):40. doi:10.1136/bjsm.2004.016345.
36. Sofka C, Potter H. Imaging of elbow injuries in the child and adult athlete. Radiol Clin N Am. 2002;40(2):251–65. doi:10.1016/S0033-8389(02)00011-8.
37. Little K. Elbow fractures and dislocations. Orthop Clin N Am. 2014;45(3):327–40. doi:10.1016/j.ocl.2014.03.004.
38. Merkel D, Molony J. Recognition and management of traumatic sports injuries in the skeletally immature athlete. Int J Sports Phys Ther. 2012;7(6):691–704.
39. Salter R, Harris R. Injuries involving the epiphyseal plate. J Bone Joint Surg Am. 1963;45(3):587–622.
40. Beltran J, Rosenberg Z, Kawelblum M, Montes L, Bergman A, Strongwater A. Pediatric elbow fractures: MRI evaluation. Skelet Radiol. 1994;23(4):277–81.
41. Seth A, Baratz M. Fractures of the elbow. In: Trumble T, Budoff J, Cornwall R, editors. Hand, elbow, shoulder. Philadelphia: Mosby; 2006. p. 522–31.
42. Wong A, Baratz M. Elbow fractures: distal humerus. J Hand Surg Am. 2009;34(1):176–90. doi:10.1016/j.jhsa.2008.10.023.
43. Gartland J. Management of supracondylar fractures of the humerus in children. Surg Gynecol Obstet. 1959;109(2):145–54.
44. Kim H, Song M, Conjares J, Yoo C. Trochlear deformity occurring after distal humeral fractures: magnetic resonance imaging and its natural progression. J Pediatr Orthop. 2002;22(2):188–93.
45. Narayanan S, Shailam R, Grottkau B, Nimkin K. Fishtail deformity – a delayed complication of distal humeral fractures in children. Pediatr Radiol. 2014. doi:10.1007/s00247-014-3249-9.
46. Guitton T, Doornberg J, Raaymakers E, Ring D, Kloen P. Fractures of the capitellum and trochlea. J Bone Joint Surg Am. 2009;91(2):390–7. doi:10.2106/jbjs.g.01660.
47. Lee J, Lawton J. Coronal shear fractures of the distal humerus. J Hand Surg [Am]. 2012;37(11):2412–7. doi:10.1016/j.jhsa.2012.09.001.
48. Sen R, Tripahty S, Goyal T, Aggarwal S. Coronal shear fracture of the humeral trochlea. J Orthop Surg (Hong Kong). 2013;21(1):82–6.
49. Doornberg J, Lindenhovius A, Kloen P, van Dijk C, Zurakowski D, Ring D. Two and three- dimensional computed tomography for the classification and management of distal humeral fractures. Evaluation of reliability and diagnostic accuracy. J Bone Joint Surg Am. 2006;88(8):1795–801. doi:10.2106/jbjs.e.00944.
50. Newman S, Mauffrey C, Krikler S. Olecranon fractures. Injury. 2009;40(6):575–81. doi:10.1016/j.injury.2008.12.013.
51. Sahajpal D, Wright T. Proximal ulna fractures. J Hand Surg Am. 2009;34(2):357–62. doi:10.1016/j.jhsa.2008.12.022.
52. Baecher N, Edwards S. Olecranon fractures. J Hand Surg Am. 2013;38(3):593–604. doi:10.1016/j.jhsa.2012.12.036.
53. Schickendantz M, Ho C, Koh J. Stress injury of the proximal ulna in professional baseball players. Am J Sports Med. 2002;30(5):737–41.
54. Stephenson D, Love S, Garcia G, Mair S. Recurrence of an olecranon stress fracture in an elite pitcher after percutaneous internal fixation: a case report. Am J Sports Med. 2012;40(1):218–21. doi:10.1177/0363546511422796.
55. O'Driscoll S, Jupiter J, Cohen M, Ring D, McKee M. Difficult elbow fractures: pearls and pitfalls. Instr Course Lect. 2003;52:113–34.
56. Doornberg J, Ring D. Coronoid fracture patterns. J Hand Surg [Am]. 2006;31(1):45–52. doi:10.1016/j.jhsa.2005.08.014.
57. Ring D, Jupiter J, Zilberfarb J. Posterior dislocation of the elbow with fractures of the radial head and coronoid. J Bone Joint Surg Am. 2002;84(4):547–51.
58. Mason M. Some observations on fractures of the head of the radius with a review of one hundred cases. Br J Surg. 1954;42(172):123–32. doi:10.1002/bjs.18004217203.
59. Johnston G. A follow-up of one hundred cases of fracture of the head of the radius with a review of the literature. Ulster Med J. 1962;31(1):51–6.
60. Struijs P, Smit G, Steller E. Radial head fractures: effectiveness of conservative treatment versus surgical intervention. A systematic review. Arch Orthop

Trauma Surg. 2007;127(2):125–30. doi:10.1007/s00402-006-0240-4.
61. Kaas L, Turkenburg J, van Riet R, Vroemen J, Eygendaal D. Magnetic resonance imaging findings in 46 elbows with a radial head fracture. Acta Orthop. 2010;81(3):373–6. doi:10.3109/17453674.2010.483988.
62. Itamura J, Roidis N, Mirzayan R, Vaishnav S, Learch T, Shean C. Radial head fractures: MRI evaluation of associated injuries. J Should Elb Surg. 2005;14(4):421–4. doi:10.1016/j.jse.2004.11.003.
63. Kumar V, Wallace W. Radial head fractures – update on classification and management. Orthop Traumatol. 2012;26(2):124–31. doi:10.1016/j.mporth.2012.04.002.
64. Pike J, Athwal G, Faber K, King G. Radial head fractures – an update. J Hand Surg Am. 2009;34(3):557–65. doi:10.1016/j.jhsa.2008.12.024.
65. Baker 3rd C, Romeo A, Baker CJ. Osteochondritis dissecans of the capitellum. Am J Sports Med. 2010;38(9):1917–28.doi:10.1177/0363546509354969.
66. Ruchelsman D, Hall M, Youm T. Osteochondritis dissecans of the capitellum: current concepts. J Am Acad Orthop Surg. 2010;18(9):557–67.
67. Kijowski R, De Smet A. MRI findings of osteochondritis dissecans of the capitellum with surgical correlation. Am J Roentgenol. 2005;185(6):1453–9. doi:10.2214/AJR.04.1570.
68. Bradley J, Petrie R. Osteochondritis dissecans of the humeral capitellum. Diagnosis and treatment. Clin Sports Med. 2001;20(3):565–90.
69. Takahara M, Ogino T, Takagi M, Tsuchida H, Orui H, Nambu T. Natural progression of osteochondritis dissecans of the humeral capitellum: initial observations. Radiology. 2000;216(1):207–12. doi:10.1148/radiology.216.1.r00jl29207.
70. van den Ende K, McIntosh A, Adams J, Steinmann S. Osteochondritis dissecans of the capitellum: a review of the literature and a distal ulnar portal. Arthroscopy. 2011;27(1):122–8. doi:10.1016/j.arthro.2010.08.008.
71. Takahara M, Mura N, Sasaki J, Harada M, Ogino T. Classification, treatment, and outcome of osteochondritis dissecans of the humeral capitellum. J Bone Joint Surg Am. 2007;89(6):1205–14. doi:10.2106/jbjs.f.00622.
72. Satake H, Takahara M, Harada M, Maruyama M. Preoperative imaging criteria for unstable osteochondritis dissecans of the capitellum. Clin Orthop Relat Res. 2013;471(4):1137–43. doi:10.1007/s11999-012-2462-9.
73. Brittberg M, Winalski C. Evaluation of cartilage injuries and repair. J Bone Joint Surg Am. 2003;85:58–69.
74. Takahara M, Ogino T, Tsuchida H, Takagi M, Kashiwa H, Nambu T. Sonographic assessment of osteochondritis dissecans of the humeral capitellum. Am J Roentgenol. 2000;174(2):411–5. doi:10.2214/ajr.174.2.1740411.
75. Takenaga T, Goto H, Nozaki M, Yoshida M, Nishiyama T, Otsuka T. Ultrasound imaging of the humeral capitellum: a cadaveric study. J Orthop Sci. 2014;19(6):907–12. doi:10.1007/s00776-014- 0637-9.
76. Harada M, Takahara M, Sasaki J, Mura N, Ito T, Ogino T. Using sonography for the early detection ofelbow injuries among young baseball players. Am J Roentgenol. 2006;187(6):1436–41. doi:10.2214/AJR.05.1086.
77. Kijowski R, De Smet A. Radiography of the elbow for evaluation of patients with osteochondritis dissecans of the capitellum. Skelet Radiol. 2005;34(5):266–71. doi:10.1007/s00256-005- 0899-6.
78. Smith M, Bedi A, Chen N. Surgical treatment for osteochondritis dissecans of the capitellum. Sports Health. 2012;4(5):425–32. doi:10.1177/1941738112444707.
79. Itsubo T, Murakami N, Uemura K, Nakamura K, Hayashi M, Uchiyama S, Kato H. Magnetic resonance imaging staging to evaluate the stability of capitellar osteochondritis dissecans lesions. Am J Sports Med. 2014;42(8):1972–7. doi:10.1177/0363546514532604.
80. Holland P, Davies A, Cassar-Pullicino V.Computed tomographic arthrography in the assessment of osteochondritis dissecans of the elbow. Clin Radiol. 1994;49(4):231–5. doi:10.1016/S0009-9260(05)81846-X.
81. Jans L, Ditchfield M, Anna G, Jaremko J, Verstraete K. MR imaging findings and MR criteria for instability in osteochondritis dissecans of the elbow in children. Eur J Radiol. 2012;81(6):1306–10. doi:10.1016/j.ejrad.2011.01.007.
82. Hegemann G. [Spontaneous aseptic bone necrosis of the elbow] (Die "spontanen" aseptischen Knochennekrosen des Ellenbogengelenkes). Fortschr Geb Rontgenstr. 1951;75(1):89–92.
83. Beyer W, Heppt P, Gluckert K, Willauschus W. Aseptic osteonecrosis of the humeral trochlea (Hegemann's disease). Arch Orthop Trauma Surg. 1990;110(1):45–8.
84. Patel N, Weiner S. Osteochondritis dissecans involving the trochlea: report of two patients (three elbows) and review of the literature. J Pediatr Orthop. 2002;22(1):48–51.
85. Claessen F, Louwerens J, Doornberg J, van Dijk C, van den Bekerom M, Eygendaal D. Hegemann's disease and fishtail deformity: aetiopathogenesis, radiographic appearance and clinical outcome. J Child Orthop. 2015. doi:10.1007/s11832-014-0630-z.
86. Brogdon B, Crow N. Little leaguer's elbow. Am J Roentgenol Radium Ther Nucl Med. 1960;83:671–5.
87. Zellner B, May M. Elbow injuries in the young athlete – an orthopedic perspective. Pediatr Radiol. 2013;43 Suppl 1:S129–34. doi:10.1007/s00247-012-2593-x.
88. Banks KP, Ly JQ, Beall DP, Grayson DE, Bancroft LW, Tall MA. Overuse injuries of the upper extremity in the competitive athlete: magnetic resonance imaging findings associated with repetitive trauma. Curr Probl Diagn Radiol. 2005;34(4):127–42.
89. Hang D, Chao C, Hang Y. A clinical and roentgenographic study of Little League elbow. Am J Sports Med. 2004;32(1):79–84.
90. Frush T, Lindenfeld T. Peri-epiphyseal and overuse injuries in adolescent athletes. Sports Health. 2009;1(3):201–11.doi:10.1177/1941738109334214.
91. Davis K. Imaging pediatric sports injuries: upper extremity. Radiol Clin N Am. 2010;48(6):1199–211. doi:10.1016/j.rcl.2010.07.020.

92. Wei A, Khana S, Limpisvasti O, Crues J, Podesta L, Yocum L. Clinical and magnetic resonance imaging findings associated with Little League elbow. J Pediatr Orthop. 2010;30(7):715–9. doi:10.1097/BPO.0b013e3181edba46.
93. Biswas D, Wysocki R, Cohen M. Primary and post-traumatic arthritis of the elbow. Arthritis. 2013;2013:1–6. doi:10.1155/2013/473259.
94. Lim Y, van Riet R, Mittal R, Bain G. Pattern of osteophyte distribution in primary osteoarthritis of the elbow. J Should Elb Surg. 2008;17(6):963–6. doi:10.1016/j.jse.2008.03.012.
95. Suvarna S, Stanley D. The histologic changes of the olecranon fossa membrane in primary osteoarthritis of the elbow. J Should Elb Surg. 2004;13(5):555–7. doi:10.1016/j.jse.2004.02.014.
96. Savoie Iii F, Nunley P, Field L. Arthroscopic management of the arthritic elbow: indications, technique, and results. J Should Elb Surg. 1999;8(3):214–9. doi:10.1016/S1058-2746(99)90131-3.
97. Dalal S, Bull M, Stanley D. Radiographic changes at the elbow in primary osteoarthritis: a comparison with normal aging of the elbow joint. J Should Elb Surg. 2007;16(3):358–61. doi:10.1016/j.jse.2006.08.005.
98. Nishiwaki M, Willing R, Johnson J, King G, Athwal G. Identifying the location and volume of bony impingement in elbow osteoarthritis by 3-dimensional computational modeling. J Hand Surg [Am]. 2013;38(7):1370–6. doi:10.1016/j.jhsa.2013.03.035.
99. Tyrdal S, Finnanger A. Osseous manifestations of 'handball goalie's elbow'. Scand J Med Sci Sports. 1999;9(2):92–7.
100. Popovic N, Lemaire R. Hyperextension trauma to the elbow: radiological and ultrasonographic evaluation in handball goalkeepers. Br J Sports Med. 2002;36(6):452–6. doi:10.1136/bjsm.36.6.452.
101. Bryce C, Armstrong A. Anatomy and biomechanics of the elbow. Orthop Clin N Am. 2008;39(2):141–54. doi:10.1016/j.ocl.2007.12.001.
102. O'Driscoll S, Jupiter J, King G, Hotchkiss R, Morrey B. The unstable elbow. J Bone Joint Surg Am. 2000;82(5):724.
103. O'Driscoll S, Morrey B, Korinek S, An K. Elbow subluxation and dislocation. A spectrum of instability. Clin Orthop Relat Res. 1992;(280):186–97.
104. Kaplan L, Potter H. MR imaging of ligament injuries to the elbow. Magn Reson Imaging Clin N Am. 2004;12(2):221–32. doi:10.1016/j.mric.2004.02.006.
105. Dugas J, Chronister J, Cain EJ, Andrews J. Ulnar collateral ligament in the overhead athlete: a current review. Sports Med Artrosc Rev. 2014;22(3):169–82. doi:10.1097/jsa.0000000000000033.
106. Cain EJ, Andrews J, Dugas J, Wilk K, McMichael C, 2nd Walter J, Riley R, Arthur S. Outcome of ulnar collateral ligament reconstruction of the elbow in 1281 athletes: results in 743 athletes with minimum 2-year follow-up. Am J Sports Med. 2010;38(12):2426–34. doi:10.1177/0363546510378100.
107. Hariri S, Safran M. Ulnar collateral ligament injury in the overhead athlete. Clin Sports Med. 2010;29(4):619–44. doi:10.1016/j.csm.2010.06.007.
108. Hurd W, Eby S, Kaufman K, Murthy N. Magnetic resonance imaging of the throwing elbow in the uninjured, high school-aged baseball pitcher. Am J Sports Med. 2011;39(4):722–8. doi:10.1177/0363546510390185.
109. Potter H, Sofka C. Imaging of the athlete's elbow. In: Altchek D, Andrews J, editors. The athlete's elbow. Philadelphia: Lippincott-Raven; 2001. p. 59–80.
110. Timmerman L, Schwartz M, Andrews J. Preoperative evaluation of the ulnar collateral ligament by magnetic resonance imaging and computed tomography arthrography: evaluation in 25 baseball players with surgical confirmation. Am J Sports Med. 1994;22(1):26–32. doi:10.1177/036354659402200105.
111. Parsons B, Ramsey M. Acute elbow dislocations in athletes. Clin Sports Med. 2010;29(4):599–609. doi:10.1016/j.csm.2010.06.005.
112. Kuhn M, Ross G. Acute elbow dislocations. Orthop Clin N Am. 2008;39(2):155–61. doi:10.1016/j.ocl.2007.12.004.
113. Taylor F, Sims M, Theis J, Herbison G. Interventions for treating acute elbow dislocations in adults. Cochrane Database Syst Rev. 2012;4:Cd007908. doi:10.1002/14651858.CD007908.pub2.
114. McCabe M, Savoie Iii F. Simple elbow dislocations: evaluation, management, and outcomes. Physicians. 2012;40(1):62–71. doi:10.3810/psm.2012.02.1952.
115. Tarassoli P, McCann P, Amirfeyz R. Complex instability of the elbow. Injury. 2013. doi:10.1016/j.injury.2013.09.032.
116. Potter H, Schachar J, Jawetz S. Imaging of the elbow. Oper Tech Orthop. 2009;19(4):199–208. doi:10.1053/j.oto.2009.09.002.
117. O'Driscoll S. Classification and evaluation of recurrent instability of the elbow. Clin Orthop Relat Res. 2000;370:34–43.
118. Charalambous C, Stanley J. Posterolateral rotatory instability of the elbow. J Bone Joint Surg (Br). 2008;90(3):272–9. doi:10.1302/0301-620x.90b3.19868.
119. Schreiber J, Potter H, Warren R, Hotchkiss R, Daluiski A. Magnetic resonance imaging findings in acute elbow dislocation: insight into mechanism. J Hand Surg Am. 2014;39(2):199–205. doi:10.1016/j.jhsa.2013.11.031.
120. Eygendaal D, Verdegaal S, Obermann W, van Vugt A, Poll R, Rozing P. Posterolateral dislocation of the elbow joint. Relationship to medial instability. J Bone Joint Surg Am. 2000;82(4):555–60.
121. Anakwenze O, Kancherla V, Iyengar J, Ahmad C, Levine W. Posterolateral rotatory instability of the elbow. Am J Sports Med. 2014;42(2):485–91. doi:10.1177/0363546513494579.
122. O'Driscoll S, Bell D, Morrey B. Posterolateral rotatory instability of the elbow. J Bone Joint Surg Am. 1991;73(3):440–6.
123. Savoie III F, Field L, Ramsey J. Posterolateral rotatory instability of the elbow: diagnosis and management. Oper Tech Sports Med. 2006;14(2):81–5. doi:10.1053/j.otsm.2006.03.001.
124. Coonrad R, Roush T, Major N, Basamania C. The drop sign, a radiographic warning sign of elbow

instability. J Should Elb Surg. 2005;14(3):312–7. doi:10.1016/j.jse.2004.09.002.

125. Grafe M, McAdams T, Beaulieu C, Ladd A. Magnetic resonance imaging in diagnosis of chronic posterolateral rotatory instability of the elbow. Am J Orthop. 2003;32(10):501–4.
126. Bado J. The Monteggia lesion. Clin Orthop Relat Res. 1967;50:71–86.
127. Beutel B. Monteggia fractures in pediatric and adult populations. Orthopedics. 2012;35(2):138–44. doi:10.3928/01477447-20120123-32.
128. Dahmoush H, Pollock A. Monteggia fracture-dislocation. Pediatr Emerg Care. 2013;29(3):406–7. doi:10.1097/PEC.0b013e318286495e.
129. Browner E. Nursemaid's elbow (annular ligament displacement. Pediatr Rev. 2013;34(8):366–7. doi:10.1542/pir.34-8-366.
130. Krul M, van der Wouden J, van Suijlekom-Smit L, Koes B. Manipulative interventions for reducing pulled elbow in young children. Cochrane Database Syst Rev. 2012;1:Cd007759. doi:10.1002/14651858.CD007759.pub3.
131. Faro F, Wolf J. Lateral epicondylitis: review and current concepts. J Hand Surg Am. 2007;32(8):1271–9. doi:10.1016/j.jhsa.2007.07.019.
132. Walz D, Newman J, Konin G, Ross G. Epicondylitis: pathogenesis, imaging, and treatment. Radiographics. 2010;30(1):167–84. doi:10.1148/rg.301095078.
133. Blease S, Stoller D, Safran M, Li A, Fritz R. The elbow. In: Stoller D, editor. Magnetic resonance imaging in orthopaedics and sports medicine. 3rd ed. Philadelphia: Lippincott, Williams & Wilkins; 2007. p. 1463–625.
134. Bunata R, Brown D, Capelo R. Anatomic factors related to the cause of tennis elbow. J Bone Joint Surg Am. 2007;89(9):1955–63. doi:10.2106/jbjs.f.00727.
135. Kijowski R, Tuite M, Sanford M. Magnetic resonance imaging of the elbow. Part II: abnormalities of the ligaments, tendons, and nerves. Skelet Radiol. 2005;34(1):1–18. doi:10.1007/s00256-004-0854-y.
136. Wessely M, Grenier J. Elbow MRI: part 2: the imaging of common disorders affecting the elbow region. Clin Chiropr. 2007;10(1):43–9. doi:10.1016/j.clch.2006.12.001.
137. Pomerance J. Radiographic analysis of lateral epicondylitis. J Should Elb Surg. 2002;11(2):156–7.
138. Miller T, Shapiro M, Schultz E, Kalish P. Comparison of sonography and MRI for diagnosing epicondylitis. J Clin Ultrasound. 2002;30(4):193–202. doi:10.1002/jcu.10063.
139. Potter H, Hannafin J, Morwessel R, DiCarlo E, O'Brien S, Altchek D. Lateral epicondylitis: correlation of MR imaging, surgical, and histopathologic findings. Radiology. 1995;196(1):43–6. doi:10.1148/radiology.196.1.7784585.
140. Martin C, Schweitzer M. MR imaging of epicondylitis. Skelet Radiol. 1998;27(3):133–8.
141. Grana W. Medial epicondylitis and cubital tunnel syndrome in the throwing athlete. Clin Sports Med. 2001;20(3):541–8.
142. Ciccotti M, Schwartz M, Ciccotti M. Diagnosis and treatment of medial epicondylitis of the elbow. Clin Sports Med. 2004;23(4):693–705. doi:10.1016/j.csm.2004.04.011.
143. Nirschl R, Pettrone F. Tennis elbow. The surgical treatment of lateral epicondylitis. J Bone Joint Surg Am. 1979;61(6):832–9.
144. Nirschl R, Pettrone F. Lateral and medial epicondylitis. Master techniques in orthopedic surgery: the elbow. New York: Raven Press; 1994.
145. Nirschl R. Prevention and treatment of elbow and shoulder injuries in the tennis player. Clin Sports Med. 1988;7(2):289–308.
146. Bernard F, Regan W. Elbow and forearm. In: DeLee JC, editor. DeLee and Drez's orthopaedic sports medicine. 2nd ed. Philadelphia: Saunders; 2003.
147. Pienimaki T, Siira P, Vanharanta H. Chronic medial and lateral epicondylitis: a comparison of pain, disability, and function. Arch Phys Med Rehabil. 2002;83(3):317–21.
148. Taylor S, Hannafin J. Evaluation and management of elbow tendinopathy. Sports Health. 2012;4(5):384–93. doi:10.1177/1941738112454651.
149. Morrey B, Askew L, An K, Dobyns J. Rupture of the distal tendon of the biceps brachii. A biomechanical study. J Bone Joint Surg Am. 1985;67(3):418–21.
150. Thompson K. Rupture of the distal biceps tendon in a collegiate football player: a case report. J Athl Train. 1998;33(1):62–4.
151. Safran M, Graham S. Distal biceps tendon ruptures: incidence, demographics, and the effect of smoking. Clin Orthop Relat Res. 2002;404:275–83.
152. RaAntanen J, Orava S. Rupture of the distal biceps tendon. A report of 19 patients treated with anatomic reinsertion, and a meta-analysis of 147 cases found in the literature. Am J Sports Med. 1999;27(2):128–32.
153. Aldridge J, Bruno R, Strauch R, Rosenwasser M. Management of acute and chronic biceps tendon rupture. Hand Clin. 2000;16(3):497–503.
154. Ramsey M. Distal biceps tendon injuries: diagnosis and management. J Am Acad Orthop Surg. 1999;7(3):199–207.
155. Tran N, Chow K. Ultrasonography of the elbow. Semin Musculoskelet Radiol. 2007;11(2):105–16. doi:10.1055/s-2007-1001876.
156. Fitzgerald S, Curry D, Erickson S, Quinn S, Friedman H. Distal biceps tendon injury: MR imaging diagnosis. Radiology. 1994;191(1):203–6. doi:10.1148/radiology.191.1.8134571.
157. Falchook F, Zlatkin M, Erbacher G, Moulton J, Bisset G, Murphy B. Rupture of the distal biceps tendon: evaluation with MR imaging. Radiology. 1994;190(3):659–63. doi:10.1148/radiology.190.3.8115606.
158. Williams B, Schweitzer M, Weishaupt D, Lerman J, Rubenstein D, Miller L, Rosenberg Z. Partial tears of the distal biceps tendon: MR appearance and associated clinical findings. Skelet Radiol. 2001;30(10):560–4. doi:10.1007/s002560100397.
159. Anzel S, Covey K, Weiner A, Lipscomb P. Disruption of muscles and tendons; an analysis of 1.014 cases. Surgery. 1959;45(3):406–14.

160. Sierra R, Weiss N, Shrader M, Steinmann S. Acute triceps ruptures: case report and retrospective chart review. J Should Elb Surg. 2006;15(1):130–4. doi:10.1016/j.jse.2005.01.004.
161. Mair S, Isbell W, Gill T, Schlegel T, Hawkins R. Triceps tendon ruptures in professional football players. Am J Sports Med. 2004;32(2):431–4.
162. Sollender J, Rayan G, Barden G. Triceps tendon rupture in weight lifters. J Should Elb Surg. 1998;7(2): 151–3.
163. Blackmore S, Jander R, Culp R. Management of distal biceps and triceps ruptures. J Hand Ther. 2006;19(2):154–68. doi:10.1197/j.jht.2006.02.001.
164. Johnson D, Allen A. Biceps and triceps tendon injury. In: Altchek D, Andrews J, editors. The athlete's elbow. Philadelphia: Lippincott Williams & Wilkins; 2001. p. 105–20.
165. Stannard J, Bucknell A. Rupture of the triceps tendon associated with steroid injections. Am J Sports Med. 1993;21(3):482–5.
166. Bach BJ, Warren R, Wickiewicz W. Triceps rupture. A case report and literature review. Am J Sports Med. 1987;15(3):285–9.
167. Stucken C, Ciccotti M. Distal biceps and triceps injuries in athletes. Sports Med Arthrosc. 2014;22(3):153–63. doi:10.1097/jsa.0000000000000030.
168. van Riet R, Morrey B, Ho E, O'Driscoll S. Surgical treatment of distal triceps ruptures. J Bone Joint Surg Am. 2003;85(10):1961–7.
169. Pina A, Garcia I, Sabater M. Traumatic avulsion of the triceps brachii. J Orthop Trauma. 2002;16(4): 273–6.
170. Radunovic G, Vlad V, Micu M, Nestorova R, Petranova T, Porta F, Iagnocco A. Ultrasound assessment of the elbow. Med Ultrason. 2012;14(2): 141–6.
171. Gaines S, Durbin R, Marsalka D. The use of magnetic resonance imaging in the diagnosis of triceps tendon ruptures. Contemp Orthop. 1990;20(6):607–11.
172. Spinner R, Goldner R. Snapping of the medial head of the triceps: diagnosis and treatment. Tech Hand Upper Extrem Surg. 2002;6(2):91–7.
173. Spinner R, Goldner R. Snapping of the medial head of the triceps and recurrent dislocation of the ulnar nerve. Anatomical and dynamic factors. J Bone Joint Surg Am. 1998;80(2):239–47.
174. Spinner R, Hayden FJ, Hipps C, Goldner R. Imaging the snapping triceps. Am J Roentgenol. 1996;167(6): 1550–1. doi:10.2214/ajr.167.6.8956595.
175. Jacobson J, Jebson P, Jeffers A, Fessell D, Hayes C. Ulnar nerve dislocation and snapping triceps syndrome: diagnosis with dynamic sonography – report of three cases. Radiology. 2001;220(3):601–5. doi:10.1148/radiol.2202001723.
176. Spinner R, O'Driscoll S, Jupiter J, Goldner R. Unrecognized dislocation of the medial portion of the triceps: another cause of failed ulnar nerve transposition. J Neurosurg. 2000;92(1):52–7. doi:10.3171/jns.2000.92.1.0052.
177. Wenzke D. MR imaging of the elbow in the injured athlete. Radiol Clin N Am. 2013;51(2):195–213. doi:10.1016/j.rcl.2012.09.013.
178. Bak B. Bicipitoradial bursitis. Ugeskr Laeger. 2008;170(40):3123–4.
179. Bond J, Sundaram M, Beckenbaugh R. Radiologic case study. Partial tear of the distal biceps tendon with mass-like bicipitoradial bursitis and associated hyperostosis of the radial tuberosity. Orthopedics. 2003;26(4):448–50.
180. Larson R, Osternig L. Traumatic bursitis and artificial turf. J Sports Med. 1974;2(4):183–8.
181. Del Buono A, Franceschi F, Palumbo A, Denaro V, Maffulli N. Diagnosis and management of olecranon bursitis. Surgeon. 2012;10(5):297–300. doi:10.1016/j.surge.2012.02.002.
182. Blankstein A, Ganel A, Givon U, Mirovski Y, Chechick A. Ultrasonographic findings in patients with olecranon bursitis. Ultraschall Med. 2006;27(6):568–71. doi:10.1055/s-2006-926569.
183. Draghi F, Gregoli B, Sileo C. Sonography of the bicipitoradial bursa: a short pictorial essay. J Ultrasound. 2012;15(1):39–41. doi:10.1016/j.jus.2012.02.003.
184. Floemer F, Morrison W, Bongartz G, Ledermann H. MRI characteristics of olecranon bursitis. Am J Roentgenol. 2004;183(1):29–34. doi:10.2214/ajr.183.1.1830029.
185. Hoi T, Lui T. Bicipitoradial bursitis: a review of clinical presentation and treatment. JOTR. 2013;8(1):7–11. doi:10.1016/j.jotr.2013.12.009.
186. Aliandro P, La Torre G, Padua R, Giannini F, Padua L. Treatment for ulnar neuropathy at the elbow. Cochrane Database Syst Rev. 2012;7:Cd006839. doi:10.1002/14651858.CD006839.pub3.
187. Tewart J, Shantz S. Perioperative ulnar neuropathies: a medicolegal review. Can J Neurol Sci. 2003; 30(1):15–9.
188. Bordalo-Rodrigues M, Rosenberg Z. MR imaging of entrapment neuropathies at the elbow. Magn Reson Imaging Clin N Am. 2004;12(2):247–63. doi:10.1016/j.mric.2004.02.002.
189. Zrieli Y, Weimer L, Lovelace R, Gooch C. The utility of segmental nerve conduction studies in ulnar mononeuropathy at the elbow. Muscle Nerve. 2003;27(1):46–50. doi:10.1002/mus.10293.
190. Aumer P, Dombert T, Staub F, Kaestel T, Bartsch A, Heiland S, Bendszus M, Pham M. Ulnar neuropathy at the elbow: MR neurography – nerve T2 signal increase and caliber. Radiology. 2011;260(1):199–206. doi:10.1148/radiol.11102357.
191. Eekman R, Schoemaker M, Van Der Plas J, Van Den Berg L, Franssen H, Wokke J, Uitdehaag B, Visser L. Diagnostic value of high-resolution sonography in ulnar neuropathy at the elbow. Neurology. 2004; 62(5):767–73.
192. Yromlou H, Tarzamni M, Daghighi M, Pezeshki M, Yazdchi M, Sadeghi-Hokmabadi E, Sharifipour E, Ghabili K. Diagnostic value of ultrasonography and

magnetic resonance imaging in ulnar neuropathy at the elbow. ISRN Neurol. 2012. doi:10.5402/2012/491892.
193. Bojniewicz A. US for diagnosis of musculoskeletal conditions in the young athlete: emphasis on dynamic assessment. Radiographics. 2014;34(5):1145–62. doi:10.1148/rg.345130151.
194. Eekman R, Visser L, Verhagen W. Ultrasonography in ulnar neuropathy at the elbow: a critical review. Muscle Nerve. 2011;43(5):627–35. doi:10.1002/mus.22019.
195. Abusiaux D, Laulan J, Bouilleau L, Martin A, Adrien C, Aubertin A, Rabarin F. Contribution of static and dynamic ultrasound in cubital tunnel syndrome. Orthop Traumatol Surg Res. 2014;100(4 Suppl):S209–12. doi:10.1016/j.otsr.2014.03.008.
196. Jarvik J, Yuen E. Diagnosis of carpal tunnel syndrome: electrodiagnostic and magnetic resonance imaging evaluation. Neurosurg Clin N Am. 2001;12(2):241–53.
197. Ba K, Wada T, Tamakawa M, Aoki M, Yamashita T. Diffusion-weighted magnetic resonance imaging of the ulnar nerve in cubital tunnel syndrome. Hand Surg. 2010;15(1):11–5. doi:10.1142/s0218810410000445x.
198. Ltun Y, Aygun M, Cevik M, Acar A, Varol S, Arikanoglu A, Onder H, Uzar E. Relation between electrophysiological findings and diffusion weighted magnetic resonance imaging in ulnar neuropathy at the elbow. J Neuroradiol. 2013;40(4):260–6. doi:10.1016/j.neurad.2012.08.004.
199. Eyffarth H. Primary myoses in the M. pronator teres as cause of lesion of the N. medianus (the pronator syndrome). Acta Psychiatr Neurol Scand Suppl. 1951;74:251–4.
200. Newman A. The supracondylar process and its fracture. Am J Roentgenol Radium Ther Nucl Med. 1969;105(4):844–9.
201. Truthers J. On hereditary supracondyloid process in man. Lancet. 1873;1:231–2.
202. Lonsdale H. A sketch of his life and writings of Robert Knox, the anatomist. London: Macmillan; 1870.
203. Ang A, Rodner C. Unusual compression neuropathies of the forearm, part I: radial nerve. J Hand Surg Am. 2009;34(10):1906–14. doi:10.1016/j.jhsa.2009.10.016.
204. Johnson R, Spinner M, Shrewsbury M. Median nerve entrapment syndrome in the proximal forearm. J Hand Surg Am. 1979;4(1):48–51.
205. Pinner M, Linscheid R. Nerve entrapment syndromes. In: Morrey B, editor. The elbow and its disorders. 2nd ed. Philadelphia: Saunders; 1993. p. 813–32.
206. Arnard L, McCoy S. The supra condyloid process of the humerus. J Bone Joint Surg Am. 1946;28(4):845–50.
207. L-Qattan M. Gantzer's muscle. An anatomical study of the accessory head of the flexor pollicis longus muscle. J Hand Surg (Br). 1996;21(2):269–70.
208. Rainger A, Campbell R, Stothard J. Anterior interosseous nerve syndrome: appearance at MR imaging in three cases. Radiology. 1998;208(2):381–4. doi:10.1148/radiology.208.2.9680563.
209. Iller T, Reinus W. Nerve entrapment syndromes of the elbow, forearm, and wrist. Am J Roentgenol. 2010;195(3):585–94. doi:10.2214/ajr.10.4817.
210. Atinovic R, Gulliford M, Hughes R. Incidence of common compressive neuropathies in primary care. J Neurol Neurosurg Psychiatry. 2006;77(2):263–5. doi:10.1136/jnnp.2005.066696.
211. Sai P, Steinberg D. Median and radial nerve compression about the elbow. Instr Course Lect. 2008;57:177–85.
212. Lavert P, Lutz J, Adam P, Wolfram-Gabel R, Liverneaux P, Kahn J. Frohse's arcade is not the exclusive compression site of the radial nerve in its tunnel. Orthop Traumatol Surg Res. 2009;95(2):114–8. doi:10.1016/j.otsr.2008.11.001.
213. Uillain G, Courtellemont R. Role of the supinator in radial nerve paralysis: pathogenesis of a partial radial nerve paralysis in an orchestra conductor. Presse Med. 1905;7:50–2.
214. Erdinand B, Rosenberg Z, Schweitzer M, Stuchin S, Jazrawi L, Lenzo S, Meislin R, Kiprovski K. MR imaging features of radial tunnel syndrome: initial experience. Radiology. 2006;240(1):161–8. doi:10.1148/radiol.2401050028.
215. Bodner G, Harpf C, Meirer R, Gardetto A, Kovacs P, Gruber H. Ultrasonographic appearance of supinator syndrome. J Ultrasound Med. 2002;21(11):1289–93.
216. Roles N, Maudsley R. Radial tunnel syndrome: resistant tennis elbow as a nerve entrapment. J Bone Joint Surg Br. 1972;54(3):499–508.

Medial-Sided Elbow Pain

5

Alan H. Lee and Marc R. Safran

In baseball pitchers, tennis players, water polo competitors, volleyball players, and javelin throwers, overhead athletes place high strain on the medial aspect of the elbow, specifically the ulnar collateral ligament (UCL), flexor-pronator mass, and ulnar nerve.

5.1 Throwing Mechanics and Pathophysiology of the Thrower's Elbow

Repeated valgus stress to the elbow during overhead throwing in athletes leads to (1) traction forces on the medial structures (i.e., UCL, ulnar nerve, flexor-pronator mass), (2) compression on the lateral side of the elbow, and (3) medially directed posterior shear forces on the posteromedial olecranon.

The medial structures of the elbow are most susceptible to tensile forces, with the UCL at particular risk. When the UCL is compromised, the tensile forces are then transferred to the other structures in the medial elbow, specifically the flexor-pronator mass and the ulnar nerve. The UCL is the most important static stabilizer to valgus stress between 30 and 120° of elbow flexion [1, 2] and thus is at increased risk for injury (including microscopic tearing leading to attenuation as well as rupture) from repeated valgus force sustained during throwing activities. The primary dynamic stabilizers to valgus stress include the FCU and FDS [3, 4] and, when fatigued, may result in increasing stress to the UCL. Concomitantly, rupture or laxity of the UCL exposes the medial dynamic stabilizers to additional stress, and there are reports of avulsion of the flexor-pronator mass found association with UCL tears [5, 6].

Chronic traction to the UCL may also lead to thickening of the ligament or marginal osteophytes. An incompetent UCL may exacerbate traction neuritis of the ulnar nerve, as it is stretched beyond its normal course. When the elbow is flexed and the wrist extended (as in late cocking and early acceleration), the pressure within the ulnar nerve has been found to be three times that of normal [7]. With further elbow flexion, wrist extension, and shoulder abduction, the pressure can increase to up to sixfold normal [7]. Many baseball and tennis players have increased cubitus valgus and a fixed flexion contracture of the elbow [8, 9], which may further exacerbate ulnar nerve pathology. The ultimate result of excessive traction is fibrosis from direct injury and possibly ischemia of the nerve due to prolonged or repeated elevation of pressures and stretching injury [10–13].

A.H. Lee, MD
Orthopaedic Surgery, Stanford University, Redwood City, CA, USA

M.R. Safran, MD (✉)
Orthopaedic Surgery, Sports Medicine, Stanford University, Redwood City, CA, USA
e-mail: msafran@stanford.edu

L.A. Pederzini et al. (eds.), *Elbow and Sport*, DOI 10.1007/978-3-662-48742-6_5

Valgus extension overload from chronic UCL laxity results from repetitive impaction of the posteromedial olecranon into the olecranon fossa. This results in posteromedial olecranon osteophytes, fractured osteophytes that may become loose bodies, and chondromalacia [14–16].

5.2 Ulnar Collateral Ligament Injury

Acute UCL injuries usually present with a discrete episode of pain following a pitch or throw, often associated with a popping sensation followed by inability to throw after the injury. Chronic injuries often present in the settings of overuse (e.g., year-round athletes, high pitch count, etc.). These athletes complain of gradual onset of medial-sided elbow pain, usually in the late-cocking and acceleration phases. They may note decreased velocity or loss of accuracy and are usually not able to throw at more than 60 to 80 % of their preinjury velocity [17].

In acute UCL injury, the medial elbow and proximal forearm may become swollen and ecchymotic in the first few days following injury. Palpation will reveal point tenderness 2 cm distal to the medial epicondyle, which lies over the UCL. Active and passive range of motion should then be assessed and compared to the contralateral extremity. Professional baseball players and tennis players may have a baseline flexion contracture and valgus alignment of their dominant elbow [8, 9]. Additionally, examination of the shoulder and scapula is important, as proximal dyskinesis can alter throwing mechanics throughout the entire kinetic chain [17].

Examination of the functional integrity of the UCL is perhaps the most essential part of the physical examination. The classic test is abduction stress testing (see Fig. 5.1). Detecting laxity may be difficult, especially in inexperienced examiners, as shoulder rotation may complicate the assessment; therefore, additional tests have been developed including the modified milking maneuver (Fig. 5.2) and O'Driscoll's moving valgus stress test (Figs. 5.3, 5.4, and 5.5).

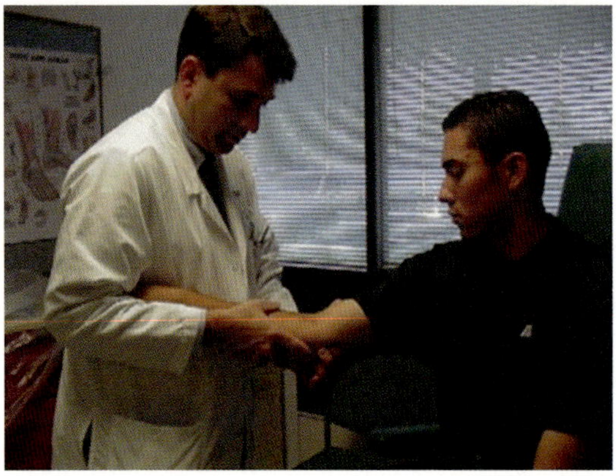

Fig. 5.1 Abduction stress testing of the UCL. This is performed with stabilization of the humerus and applying a valgus-directed force to the elbow. The elbow flexed to 20–30°, and a valgus stress applied to the elbow with the patient's handheld between the examiner's arm and body. A positive test is when there is increased laxity and may be associated with pain and/or lack of firm endpoint [5, 18] (Courtesy of Marc Safran, MD, Redwood City, CA)

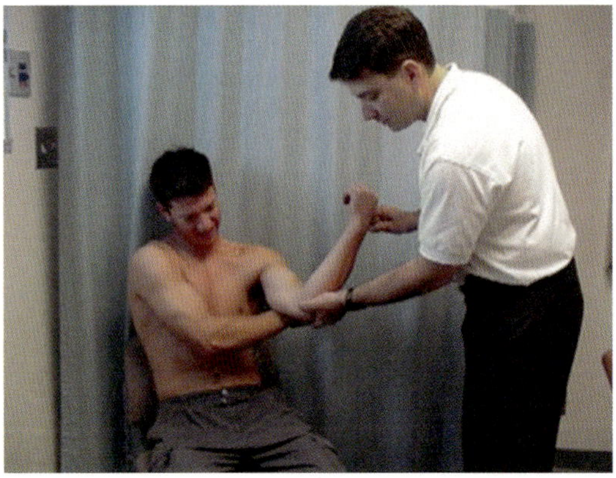

Fig. 5.2 The modified milking maneuver. The patient's arm is adducted and externally rotated. One hand of the examiner stabilizes the patient's elbow while also palpating the medial joint line. The patient's elbow is then flexed to 70° and a valgus stress applied by pulling on the patient's thumb with the contralateral hand. The examiner can then assess joint line gapping and quality of the end point and compare to the contralateral elbow (Courtesy of Marc Safran, MD, Redwood City, CA)

Concomitant injuries (such as medial epicondylosis, flexor-pronator mass avulsion, and cubital tunnel syndrome) should always be evaluated and are addressed later in this chapter.

Plain radiographs should initially be obtained and should include anteroposterior (AP) and lat-

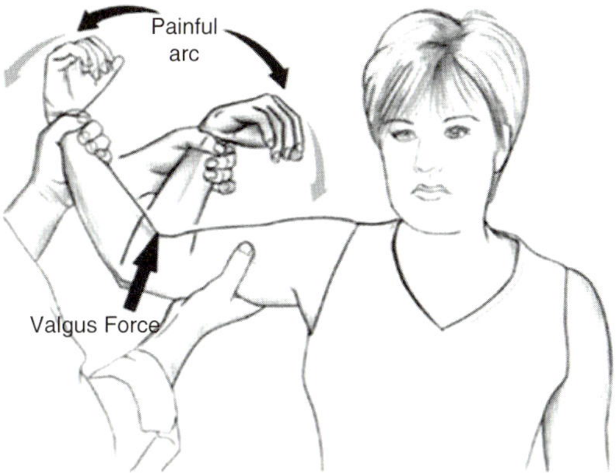

Fig. 5.3 The moving valgus stress test. O'Driscoll described the moving valgus stress test [19], which places the patient's shoulder in 90° of abduction and external rotation. A constant, valgus force is applied to the elbow in full flexion, and then the elbow is extended. A positive test is when the patient complains of maximum elbow pain between 70 and 120 degrees of elbow flexion (Courtesy of Marc Safran, MD, Redwood City, CA)

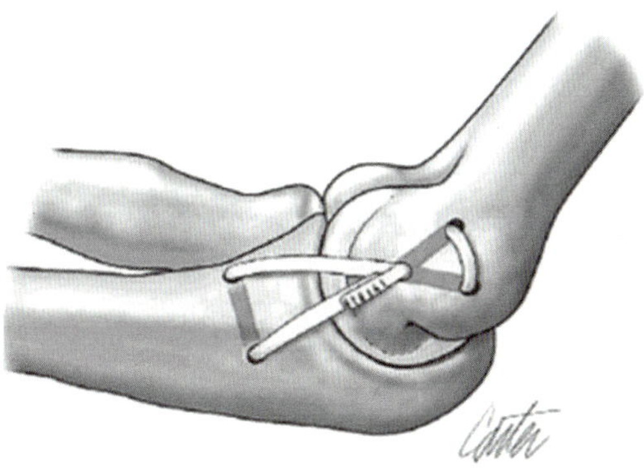

Fig. 5.4 The original figure-of-eight UCL reconstruction technique as developed by Jobe et al. describes transection and subsequent reflection of the flexor-pronator mass of the medial epicondyle and a figure-of-eight graft weave through drill holes in the humerus and ulna, followed by a submuscular ulnar nerve transposition (From Shah et al. [54]; with permission)

eral views. In acute injury, an avulsion fragment may be visible, and in chronic injury, loose bodies, osteophytes of the radiocapitellar and/or ulnohumeral joints, or ossification of the UCL may occur. Stress radiographs of the elbow can also be obtained to assess for widening of the medial joint line. They can be obtained either through manual stress or through commercial devices that apply a uniform force.

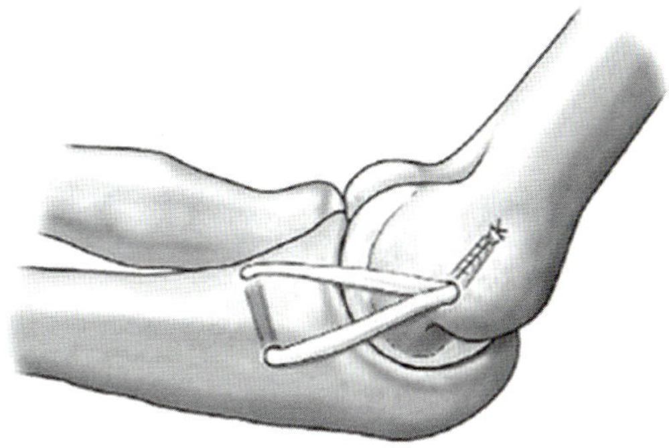

Fig. 5.5 The docking UCL reconstruction technique as developed by Altchek. The two ends of the tendon graft are docked into a single blind-ended humeral tunnel, and the sutures are tied over a humeral bone bridge (From Shah et al. [55]; with permission)

Magnetic resonance imaging (MRI) and MR arthrogram of the elbow have emerged as the most sensitive and specific imaging modality for identifying complete and partial UCL tears. MRI is 57–79 % sensitive and 100 % specific for UCL tears [18, 20]. MR arthrogram is 97 % sensitive for UCL tears and is the senior author's study of choice for suspected UCL tears following completion of plain radiographs [21].

5.2.1 Treatment Options and Results

The initial treatment of UCL injuries includes rest, icing, activity modification, nonsteroidal anti-inflammatory medications, bracing, and physical therapy. Physical therapy should focus on reducing elbow pain and inflammation while also addressing any deficits identified along the throwing kinetic chain, which permits the best chance for successful elbow rehabilitation [22]. After inflammation is reduced and range of motion normalized, strengthening of the wrist and elbow muscles is initiated, followed by a throwing program for gradual return to throwing.

UCL reconstruction is currently the best surgical choice for both acute and chronic UCL ruptures. Indications for reconstruction include (1) acute ruptures in high-level throwers, (2) significant chronic instability, (3) insufficient UCL tissue remaining after UCL debridement for calcifications, and (4) recurrent pain and subtle valgus instability with throwing after supervised rehabilitation [23]. Reconstruction is performed using a free tendon (either autograft or allograft) and tensioning it between the medial humeral epicondyle and the sublime tubercle. Multiple techniques have been described starting with Frank Jobe in 1974 and its subsequent modifications [18, 21, 24–26].

5.2.2 Pearls and Pitfalls of Treatment

The probability of return to sports at the same preinjury level following UCL rupture treated nonoperatively is low (42 % in one study) for overhead athletes. Therefore, for a high-level competitive thrower, surgical reconstruction is usually advocated, as the time to failed nonoperative treatment may be up to 6 months, followed by 12–18 months of postoperative rehabilitation, resulting in up to 2 years time away from sports. Watson et al. in 2014 performed a systematic review comparing the Jobe, modified Jobe, docking, and modified docking techniques of UCL reconstruction [27]. In 1,368 patients, overall results demonstrated a return to play rate of 78.9 %.

5.3 Valgus Extension Overload Syndrome

Athletes with valgus extension overload primarily complain of posterior or posteromedial elbow pain. This is sometimes associated with clicking, grating, or locking if loose bodies are present. The pain is often accentuated during the late acceleration and follow-through phases of throwing, in which the elbow is near full extension [15]. Loose bodies may create temporary locking with a mechanical block to motion, which produces a synovitis that may result in an effusion. On physical examination, palpation may reveal tenderness along the posterior border of the olecranon, and forced extension or applying valgus force against an extended elbow may reproduce the patient's symptoms.

Plain radiographs, including AP and lateral views of the elbow, are helpful for identifying loose bodies, osteophytes, or enlargement of the olecranon. A flexion-axial radiograph can be obtained that may demonstrate posteromedial olecranon osteophytes [14]. A computed tomographic (CT) scan or CT arthrogram may be better at demonstrating both osteophytes and loose bodies present within the elbow.

5.3.1 Treatment Options and Results

Nonoperative treatment should be considered for the early phase of treatment, especially in the absence of loose bodies. The emphasis should initially focus on reducing pain and inflammation. The second phase of treatment should then focus on improving the functional strength of the elbow followed by a progressive throwing program.

Operative treatment is indicated when conservative treatment fails or for those patients who have loose bodies or persistent symptoms which may be caused by chronic valgus instability [16]. Elbow arthroscopy has replaced arthrotomy as the preferred treatment for removing loose bodies and impinging osteophytes. It has low complication rates while allowing earlier and more aggressive rehabilitation and return to sport [28–30].

5.3.2 Pearls and Pitfalls of Treatment

In the setting of UCL insufficiency, a high reoperation rate of up to 41 % has been found when isolated loose body removal or osteophyte resection has been performed [28]. This is felt to be due to either removal of the osteophyte (1) increases the stresses to the UCL or (2) reveals attenuated/damaged UCL. Therefore, we suggest that careful consideration be given to UCL evaluation for the potential UCL reconstruction in combination with debridement in high-level overhead athletes. Additionally, in the light of unclear evidence regarding how much posteromedial olecranon can be safely resected, we advocate that debridement be limited to removal of the impinging osteophyte, leaving the normal olecranon intact.

5.4 Medial Epicondylosis and Flexor-Pronator Tears

Medial epicondylosis, or golfer's elbow, is a tendinosis primarily involving the origin of the pronator teres (PT) and flexor carpi radialis (FCR) muscles and, occasionally, the tendon of flexor carpi ulnaris (FCU) [31]. Patients will often present with medial-sided elbow pain and can be accentuated during the early acceleration phase of throwing [32]. There may be a history of acute trauma which may result in an avulsion of the flexor-pronator mass; however, the most common presentation is of an insidious onset [33].

Physical examination may include swelling of the flexor-pronator mass, as well as tenderness over the distal, anterior, and lateral aspect of the medial epicondyle. These patients may have pain with resisted wrist flexion and forearm pronation, in addition to grip weakness relative to the contralateral extremity [34]. It is important to examine for ulnar nerve symptoms, as nearly 60 % of athletes with medial epicondylosis also have ulnar neuropathy [35, 36]. Plain radiographs are usually normal in this condition. MRI remains the best imaging modality for radiographic diagnosis and remains the standard of care [33].

5.4.1 Treatment Options and Results

Nonsurgical management is the mainstay of treatment and emphasizes rest, activity modification, icing, and oral anti-inflammatories. Local corticosteroid injections, extracorporeal shock wave therapy, and dry needling have all been utilized to varying success [33, 37–41]. Once the acute inflammatory symptoms have subsided, the athlete should be placed in a rehabilitation program that emphasizes flexor-pronator mass stretching and strengthening. It should be noted that most patients (85–90 %) improve with nonsurgical management [35–37, 42].

If symptoms persist past 4–6 months of appropriate, conservative management, then surgical options can be considered. Surgery involves release of the flexor-pronator origin, excision of the friable granulation tissue, stimulation of bleeding from the medial epicondylar bone, and repair/reconstruction of the medial musculature [43, 44].

5.4.2 Pearls and Pitfalls of Treatment

The exception to initial nonsurgical management is in elite athletes with a demonstrated full-thickness tear of the flexor-pronator mass seen on MRI [38]. During surgical intervention for medial epicondylosis, the UCL must be identified and protected. It lies just deep and is adherent to the flexor-pronator muscle group and serves as a partial origin for one of the muscles. In patients with medial epicondylosis and associated ulnar neuropathy, surgical management has not been shown to be as effective as those without neuropathy [45].

5.5 Cubital Tunnel Syndrome

The ulnar nerve is most commonly injured around the elbow, likely due to its superficial location in the subcutaneous tissue, as well as the relatively tight path it follows when it courses around the medial aspect of the elbow. In throwers, the physical examination for cubital tunnel syndrome does not have the classic presentation – they will usually only be symptomatic while throwing.

Radiographs of the elbow may identify potential bony sources of ulnar nerve compression, and MRI may evaluate for soft tissue masses that may cause nerve compression [46]. Electrodiagnostic testing including electromyography (EMG) may be helpful in identifying cases of advanced neuropathy; however, negative testing does not exclude the diagnosis of ulnar neuropathy [10].

5.5.1 Treatment Options and Results

For mild to moderate cases of ulnar nerve compression, nonoperative treatment should be the initial management. This includes rest, activity modification, and nonsteroidal inflammatory medication [13].

Failure of conservative treatment necessitates surgical intervention. Multiple surgical options exist, including in situ decompression, medial epicondylectomy, and anterior transposition (subcutaneous, submuscular, or intramuscular).

A meta-analysis of four randomized, controlled trials comparing in situ decompression to anterior transposition involving 335 patients found no difference in motor nerve conduction studies or clinical outcome scores between the two groups [47–51]. The authors concluded that in situ decompression of the ulnar nerve is a reasonable alternative to anterior transposition. However, in throwing athletes, the senior author prefers subcutaneous transposition to reduce the risk of ulnar nerve subluxation and, for contact athletes, a submuscular transposition to reduce the risk for injury due to direct contact.

5.5.2 Pearls and Pitfalls of Treatment

During the initial physical examination, close attention should be paid to differentiating ulnar nerve subluxation from snapping triceps syndrome. Failure to identify the latter prior to performing cubital tunnel release may lead to failed surgery [52]. Ulnar neuritis often occurs concomitantly with, or is a result of, valgus elbow instability; thus, it is important to recognize and treat the associated pathology. Finally, intraoperative care and time should be taken to ensure that all potential sites of ulnar nerve compression are adequately released. Persistent ulnar nerve symptoms postoperative are most commonly due to incomplete decompression [53].

5.6 Summary

In summary, medial elbow pain is a common in throwing athletes, and often times, the cause is multifactorial as the symptoms commonly overlap. It is important for the clinician to obtain a detailed history and physical examination to identify the cause of pain and determine appropriate treatment. Often times, nonoperative treatment is successful in managing these patients.

References

1. Safran MR, McGarry MH, Shin S, Han S, Lee TQ. Effects of elbow flexion and forearm rotation on valgus laxity of the elbow. J Bone Joint Surg Am. 2005;87(9):2065–74. doi:10.2106/JBJS.D.02045.
2. Fleisig GS, Andrews JR, Dillman CJ, Escamilla RF. Kinetics of baseball pitching with implications about injury mechanisms. Am J Sports Med. 1995;23(2): 233–9.
3. Davidson PA, Pink M, Perry J, Jobe FW. Functional anatomy of the flexor pronator muscle group in relation to the medial collateral ligament of the elbow. Am J Sports Med. 1995;23(2):245–50.
4. Park MC, Ahmad CS. Dynamic contributions of the flexor-pronator mass to elbow valgus stability. J Bone Joint Surg Am. 2004;86-A(10):2268–74.
5. Norwood LA, Shook JA, Andrews JR. Acute medial elbow ruptures. Am J Sports Med. 1981;9(1):16–9. doi:10.1177/036354658100900103.
6. Osbahr DC, Swaminathan SS, Allen AA, Dines JS, Coleman SH, Altchek DW. Combined flexor-pronator mass and ulnar collateral ligament injuries in the elbows of older baseball players. Am J Sports Med. 2010;38(4):733–9. doi:10.1177/0363546509351558.
7. Pechan J, Juliš I. The pressure measurement in the ulnar nerve. A contribution to the pathophysiology of the cubital tunnel syndrome. J Biomech. 1975;8(1):75–9. doi:10.1016/0021-9290(75)90045-7.
8. King JW, Brelsford HJ, Tullos HS. 17 analysis of the pitching Arm of the professional baseball pitcher. Clin Orthop Relat Res. 1969;67:116.
9. Barnes DA, Tullos HS. An analysis of 100 symptomatic baseball players. Am J Sports Med. 1978;6(2):62–7.
10. Del Pizzo W, Jobe FW, Norwood L. Ulnar nerve entrapment syndrome in baseball players. Am J Sports Med. 1977;5(5):182–5.
11. Glousman RE. Ulnar nerve problems in the athlete's elbow. Clin Sports Med. 1990;9(2):365–77.
12. Sattari S, Emad MR. Changes in ulnar nerve conduction velocity across the elbow in different angles of elbow flexion. Electromyogr Clin Neurophysiol. 2007;47(7-8):373–6.

13. Elhassan B, Steinmann SP. Entrapment neuropathy of the ulnar nerve. J Am Acad Orthop Surg. 2007;15(11):672–81.
14. Wilson FD, Andrews JR, Blackburn TA, Mccluskey G. Valgus extension overload in the pitching elbow. Am J Sports Med. 1983;11(2):83–8.
15. Miller C, Savoie F. Valgus extension injuries of the elbow in the throwing athlete. J Am Acad Orthop Surg. 1994;2(5):261–9.
16. Chen FS, Rokito AS, Jobe FW. Medial elbow problems in the overhead-throwing athlete. J Am Acad Orthop Surg. 2001;9(2):99–113.
17. Hariri S, Safran MR. Ulnar collateral ligament injury in the overhead athlete. Clin Sports Med. 2010;29(4):619–44. doi:10.1016/j.csm.2010.06.007.
18. Thompson WH, Jobe FW, Yocum LA, Pink MM. Ulnar collateral ligament reconstruction in athletes: muscle-splitting approach without transposition of the ulnar nerve. J Shoulder Elbow Surg. 2001;10(2):152–7. doi:10.1067/mse.2001.112881.
19. O'Driscoll SWM, Lawton RL, Smith AM. The "moving valgus stress test" for medial collateral ligament tears of the elbow. Am J Sports Med. 2005;33(2):231–9. doi:10.1177/0363546504267804.
20. Timmerman LA, Schwartz ML, Andrews JR. Preoperative evaluation of the ulnar collateral ligament by magnetic resonance imaging and computed tomography arthrography. Evaluation in 25 baseball players with surgical confirmation. Am J Sports Med. 1994;22(1):26–31; discussion 32.
21. Azar FM, Andrews JR, Wilk KE, Groh D. Operative treatment of ulnar collateral ligament injuries of the elbow in athletes. Am J Sports Med. 2000;28(1):16–23. doi:10.1002/jor.1100050309.
22. Freehill MT, Safran MR. Diagnosis and management of ulnar collateral ligament injuries in throwers. Curr Sports Med Rep. 2011;10(5):271–8. doi:10.1249/JSR.0b013e31822d4000.
23. Safran M, Ahmad CS, ElAttrache NS. Ulnar collateral ligament of the elbow. Arthroscopy. 2005;21(11):1381–95. doi:10.1016/j.arthro.2005.07.001.
24. Jobe FW, Stark H, Lombardo SJ. Reconstruction of the ulnar collateral ligament in athletes. J Bone Joint Surg Am. 1986;68(8):1158–63.
25. Rohrbough JT, Altchek DW, Hyman J, Williams III RJ, Botts JD. Medial collateral ligament reconstruction of the elbow using the docking technique. Am J Sports Med. 2002;30(4):541–8. doi:10.1016/S1058-2746(96)80065-6.
26. Koh JL, Schafer MF, Keuter G, Hsu JE. Ulnar collateral ligament reconstruction in elite throwing athletes. Arthrosc J Arthrosc Relat Surg. 2006;22(11):1187–91. doi:10.1016/j.arthro.2006.07.024.
27. Watson JN, McQueen P, Hutchinson MR. A systematic review of ulnar collateral ligament reconstruction techniques. Am J Sports Med. 2014;42(10):2510–6. doi:10.1177/0363546513509051.
28. Ellenbecker TS, Mattalino AJ, Elam EA, Caplinger RA. Medial elbow joint laxity in professional baseball pitchers. A bilateral comparison using stress radiography. Am J Sports Med. 1998;26(3):420–4.
29. O'Driscoll SW, Morrey BF. Arthroscopy of the elbow. Diagnostic and therapeutic benefits and hazards. J Bone Joint Surg Am. 1992;74(1):84–94.
30. Reddy AS, Kvitne RS, Yocum LA, Elattrache NS, Glousman RE, Jobe FW. Arthroscopy of the elbow: a long-term clinical review. Arthroscopy. 2000;16(6):588–94. doi:10.1053/jars.2000.8953.
31. Leach RE, Miller JK. Lateral and medial epicondylitis of the elbow. Clin Sports Med. 1987;6(2):259–72.
32. Cain EL, Dugas JR, Wolf RS, Andrews JR. Elbow injuries in throwing athletes: a current concepts review. Am J Sports Med. 2003;31(4):621–35.
33. Amin NH, Kumar NS, Schickendantz MS. Medial epicondylitis: evaluation and management. J Am Acad Orthop Surg. 2015;23(6):348–55. doi:10.5435/JAAOS-D-14-00145.
34. Pienimäki T, Siira P, Vanharanta H. Widespread pain in chronic epicondylitis. Eur J Pain. 2011;15(9):921–7. doi:10.1016/j.ejpain.2011.04.002.
35. Nirschl RP. Prevention and treatment of elbow and shoulder injuries in the tennis player. Clin Sports Med. 1988;7(2):289–308.
36. Gabel GT, Morrey BF. Operative treatment of medical epicondylitis. Influence of concomitant ulnar neuropathy at the elbow. J Bone Joint Surg Am. 1995;77(7):1065–9.
37. Stahl S, Kaufman T. The efficacy of an injection of steroids for medial epicondylitis. A prospective study of sixty elbows. J Bone Joint Surg Am. 1997;79(11):1648–52.
38. Ciccotti MG, Ramani MN. Medial epicondylitis. Tech Hand Up Extrem Surg. 2003;7(4):190.
39. Lee SS, Kang S, Park NK, Lee CW. Effectiveness of initial extracorporeal shock wave therapy on the newly diagnosed lateral or medial epicondylitis. ANN Rehabil Med. 2012;36(5):681–87.
40. Krischek O, Hopf C, Nafe B, Rompe JD. Shock-wave therapy for tennis and golfer's elbow – 1 year follow-up. Arch Orthop Trauma Surg. 1999;119(1–2):62–6. doi:10.1007/s004020050356.
41. Suresh SPS, Ali KE, Jones H, Connell DA. Medial epicondylitis: is ultrasound guided autologous blood injection an effective treatment? Br J Sports Med. 2006;40(11):935–9. doi:10.1136/bjsm.2006.029983.
42. Vangsness CT, Jobe FW. Surgical treatment of medial epicondylitis. Results in 35 elbows. J Bone Joint Surg Br. 1991;73(3):409–11.
43. Ollivierre CO, Nirschl RP, Pettrone FA. Resection and repair for medial tennis elbow. A prospective analysis. Am J Sports Med. 1995;23(2):214–21.
44. Safran MR. Elbow tendinopathy – surgical repair of the epicondylitides. In: Craig EV, ed. Clinical orthopaedics. Philadelphia: Lippincott Williams & Wilkins; 1999. p. 274–84.
45. Kurvers H, Verhaar J. The results of operative treatment of medial epicondylitis. JBJS Case Connect. 1995;77(9):1374–9.

46. Dellon AL. Patient evaluation and management considerations in nerve compression. Hand Clin. 1992;8(2):229–39.
47. Zlowodzki M, Chan S, Bhandari M, Kalliainen L, Schubert W. Anterior transposition compared with simple decompression for treatment of cubital tunnel syndrome. A meta-analysis of randomized, controlled trials. J Bone Joint Surg Am. 2007;89(12):2591–8. doi:10.2106/JBJS.G.00183.
48. Bartels RHMA, Verhagen WIM, van der Wilt GJ, Meulstee J, van Rossum LGM, Grotenhuis JA. Prospective randomized controlled study comparing simple decompression versus anterior subcutaneous transposition for idiopathic neuropathy of the ulnar nerve at the elbow: part 1. Neurosurgery. 2005;56(3):522–30. doi:10.1227/01.NEU.0000154131.01167.03.
49. Gervasio O, Gambardella G, Zaccone C, Branca D. Simple decompression versus anterior submuscular transposition of the ulnar nerve in severe cubital tunnel syndrome: a prospective randomized study. Neurosurgery. 2005;56(1):108. doi:10.1227/01.NEU.0000145854.38234.81.
50. Nabhan A, Ahlhelm F, Kelm J, Reith W, Schwerdtfeger K, Steudel WI. Simple decompression or subcutaneous anterior transposition of the ulnar nerve for cubital tunnel syndrome. J Hand Surg Br. 2005;30(5):521–4. doi:10.1016/j.jhsb.2005.05.011.
51. Biggs M, Curtis JA. Randomized, prospective study comparing ulnar neurolysis in situ with submuscular transposition. Neurosurgery. 2006;58(2):296–304. doi:10.1227/01.NEU.0000194847.04143.A1.
52. Spinner RJ, O'Driscoll SW, Jupiter JB, Goldner RD. Unrecognized dislocation of the medial portion of the triceps: another cause of failed ulnar nerve transposition. J Neurosurg. 2000;92(1):52–57. doi:10.3171/jns.2000.92.1.0052. http://dx.doi.org/10.3171/jns.2000.92.1.0052.
53. Rogers MR, Bergreld TG, Aulicino PL. The failed ulnar nerve transposition: etiology and treatment. Clin Orthop Relat Res. 1991;269:193.
54. Shah RP, Lindsey DP, Sungar GW, et al. An analysis of four ulnar collateral ligament reconstruction procedures with cyclic valgus loading. J Shoulder Elbow Surg. 2009;18:59.
55. Shah RP, Lindsey DP, Sungar GW, et al. An analysis of four ulnar collateral ligament reconstruction procedures with cyclic valgus loading. J Shoulder Elbow Surg. 2009;18(1):60.

New Aspects in UCL Stabilization

6

L.A. Pederzini, F. Di Palma, and F. Nicoletta

6.1 Introduction

The elbow is one of the most congruous and stable joints of the body.

The normal range of motion of the elbow is approximately 0° of extension and 140° of flexion. A functional range of motion for activities of the daily living has been described to be of 30–130°, and the functional arc of throwing ranges from 20° to 130°. The normal supination and pronation are both of approximately 80° [1].

Although it is not a weight-bearing joint, it can be subjected to high loads when practicing racket or throwing sports or in gymnastics. As a consequence of these continued sport activities, elbow stability, due to static and dynamic constraints, can be compromised.

The elbow is the second most commonly dislocated major joint [2], and 15–35 % of elbow dislocations can have residual instability [3, 4]. Elbow dislocations represent 11–28 % of all elbow injuries, with an annual incidence of six to eight cases per 100,000 people [5].

The elbow is a very congruous joint with two ligamentous complexes: UCL and LCL. They are involved in the pathoanatomy of throwing athletes or in elbow dislocations and instability.

The symptoms of the instability in athletes can occur following a single traumatic event or may be due to repetitive stress leading to chronic laxity such as in a throwing athlete.

6.2 Anatomy

The elbow joint is one of the most useful joint of the body. Its stability is due to different structures that can be divided in primary and secondary stabilizers [6].

The primary stabilizers are represented by the ulnohumeral joint, the ulnar collateral ligament complex (UCL), and the lateral collateral ligament (LCL).

The secondary stabilizers are represented by radial head, capsule, and anterior and posterior muscles that travel across the elbow and enable flexion and extension mobility.

6.2.1 Ulnar Collateral Ligament Complex Anatomy [7]

The UCL complex consists of three ligaments forming a triangular shape: the anterior oblique (AOL), posterior oblique (POL), and transverse ligaments. The proximal origin of the AOL and POL is from the anteroinferior surface of the medial epicondyle [8] (Fig. 6.1).

L.A. Pederzini (✉) • F. Di Palma • F. Nicoletta
Orthopaedic and Arthroscopic Department, New Sassuolo Hospital, via F. Ruini, 2, 41049 Sassuolo, Modena, Italy
e-mail: gigiped@hotmail.com; felice.dipalma@libero.it; fabionicoletta@yahoo.com

L.A. Pederzini et al. (eds.), *Elbow and Sport*, DOI 10.1007/978-3-662-48742-6_6

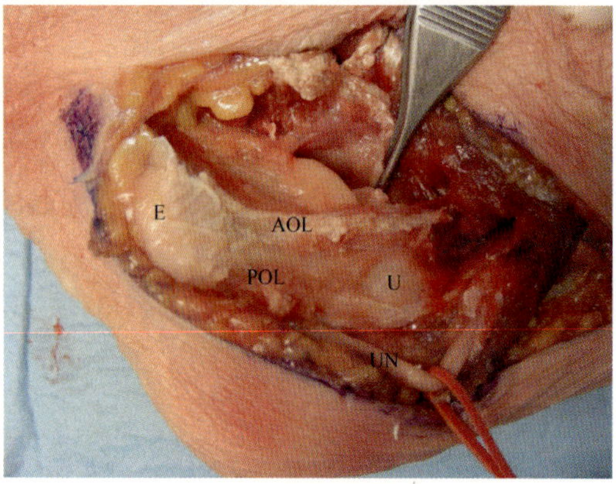

Fig. 6.1 Medial collateral ligament and ulnar nerve. *E* medial epicondyle, *AOL* anterior oblique ligament, *POL* posterior oblique ligament, *U* ulna, *Un* ulnar nerve

The AOL is the strongest component of the UCL [9] and is the primary valgus stabilizer among the different components of the medial ligament complex [9–11].

The AOL is 4–5 mm wide [12] and is histologically divided into two parts, one within the medial capsule and one on the superficial surface of the capsule that also serves as a partial origin of the flexor carpi superficialis [13].

The origin of the AOL is inferior to the axis rotation [14] and inserts 18 mm distal to the coronoid tip, along the medial aspect of the coronoid process, near the sublime tubercle [10, 12].

The AOL is functionally composed of anterior band (AB) and posterior band (PB) that provide a reciprocal function in resisting valgus stress through the range of flexion-extension motion [6, 9]. Recent studies have refuted the concept of an isometric fiber between the AB and PB [15, 16].

The POL is a fan-shaped thickening of the capsule that originates from the medial epicondyle, forms the floor of the cubital canal, and inserts along the midportion of the medial margin of the semilunar notch [15].

It is 5–6 mm wide at its midportion, is thinner than the AOL, and exists within the layers of the medial elbow capsule [13]. The transverse ligament (Cooper's ligament) connects the inferior medial coronoid process with the medial tip of the olecranon [6, 15]. It is generally believed to have little or no contribution to valgus stability [6, 14, 15].

The magnitude and degree of force transmitted across the elbow joint vary based on specific factors which include loading configuration and angular orientation of the joint (degree of elbow flexion) [6, 15].

The athlete is most often exposed to severe, chronic repetitive valgus stresses. Although bony articulation contributes significantly to resisting these stresses with the elbow near full extension (flexed less than 20°) or flexion (greater than 120°) [6, 10, 17, 18], the major restraint to valgus stress between these two ranges is the UCL complex. The anterior half (AB) of the AOL functions as a checkrein from full extension to 85° of flexion, while the PB is taut with elbow flexion beyond 55°. As previously noted, the AB is the most important stabilizer of the UCL complex for valgus throwing forces. The POL functions with the elbow flexed beyond 90° [17–20].

When the UCL is completely sectioned, elbow laxity is greatest at 70° of flexion [10, 21, 22].

6.2.2 Valgus Instability

Patients with medial instability usually report medial elbow pain, decreased strength during overhead activity. Sometimes there may be symptoms of ulnar neuropathy from either acute or chronic UCL injury caused by edema/hemorrhage of the medial elbow or excessive traction on the nerve.

The UCL stability can be assessed with specific physical exam tests.

Patients with isolated UCL injury often have point tenderness 2 cm distal to the medial epicondyle, slightly posterior to the common flexor origin.

The "milking maneuver" involves having the patient apply a valgus torque to the elbow by pulling down on the thumb of the injured extremity with the contralateral limb providing stability [23]. With the modified milking maneuver, the examiner provides stability to the patient's elbow and pulls the thumb to create a valgus stress on the UCL [24]. In cases of UCL insufficiency, these tests result in pain and widening at the medial joint line.

O'Driscoll and coworkers described the moving valgus stress test, in which the valgus torque is maintained constantly to the fully flexed elbow and then quickly extends the elbow [25]. This test is positive if medial elbow pain is elicited and has a 100 % sensitivity and 75 % specificity [25]. The abduction valgus stress test is performed by stabilizing the patient's abducted and externally rotated arm with the examiners axilla and applying a valgus force to the elbow at 30° of flexion. Testing with the forearm in neutral rotation has been shown to elicit the greatest valgus instability [26]. A positive test results in medial elbow pain and widening along the medial joint line. Even so, valgus laxity can be subtle on physical exam, and the range of preoperative detection is between 26 % and 82 % of patients [27, 28]. Furthermore, Timmerman and colleagues found valgus stress testing to be only 66 % sensitive and 60 % specific for detecting abnormality of the anterior bundle of the UCL [29].

6.3 Treatment of UCL Lesions

Initial treatment consists of rest, anti-inflammatory medications, icing, and bracing.

Literature report 42–50 % success rate in returning to previous sport activities after different conservative treatment protocols [30, 31].

These modest results lead to consider surgical treatment, particularly in high-level athletes as treatment of choice.

Surgical treatment for UCL tears has evolved over the time. Early surgical management of UCL insufficiency consisted of transferring the anterior oblique ligament anteriorly and superiorly when the UCL was present but attenuated [20], but this technique was abandoned because the remaining attenuated ligament is believed to be weaker as the result of the repeated microtrauma and because its transferred position is not functionally isometric and could lead to a flexion contracture. This is not acceptable in the high-level athlete.

Primary ligament repair for acute injuries had been supported [32, 33].

Most ligamentous avulsions have traditionally been treated by reattaching the ligament to bone through drill holes, while midsubstance ruptures were repaired primarily [34].

UCL repair is considered only in case of avulsion injuries in younger athletes performing surgery soon after injury and having MRI showing complete avulsion from the bone [35].

In adults, also in acute events, it is frequent to find an intrasubstance damage of the UCL and the reconstruction must be considered.

Conway et al. [32] reported the relative prevalence of injury UCL for locations in 70 athletes with acute UCL injuries: 87 % of the lesions were midsubstance, 10 % were avulsions of the ulna, and only 3 % were avulsions from the humerus [32].

The ability to return to sports at the same level as before injury was reported by Conway et al. to be better with UCL reconstruction with the use of a free graft compared with primary repair [32].

Azar et al. [27] also found better results with UCL reconstruction (81 % able to return to play at the same or higher level) compared with primary UCL repair (63 % return to play at the same or higher level).

Autografts or allografts can be used to perform UCL reconstruction. The graft that can usually be used are:

- Palmaris longus – the absence of the palmaris longus occurs approximately 6–25 % in the general population [36].
- Gracilis.
- Plantaris.
- Extensor toe.
- Achilles.

Dr. Frank Jobe was the first in 1986 to report on a reconstruction technique of MCL [37]. It is often called "Tommy John" surgery after that Los Angeles Dodgers pitcher was the first athlete to undergo this procedure in 1974. Dr. Frank Jobe used bony tunnels in the humerus and ulna to secure a free graft. Exposure of the ligament was achieved through transection of the common flexor- pronator muscle group, from the medial epicondyle, combined with a submuscular ulnar nerve transposition. The ligament was reconstructed by the use of a tendon graft woven through three drill holes in the medial epicondyle and two drill holes in the ulna, in the form of a figure eight, and sutured to itself.

Conway et al. [32] reported that 68 % of patients returned to the previous level of sports participation with this reconstruction technique. There was a high incidence (21 %) of ulnar nerve symptoms after this procedure, requiring a revision procedure of the ulnar nerve in 58 % of these patients.

To minimize trauma to the flexor-pronator muscle group and reduce the incidence of ulnar nerve symptoms, Smith et al. [38] in 1996 described a more limited approach, which involved splitting the flexor-pronator muscle group instead of dividing it completely from the medial epicondyle. Muscle splitting approach is created by incising the raphe of the flexor carpi ulnaris and then is applied valgus stress. Converging 3.2-mm drill holes are made in the ulna anterior and posterior to the sublime tubercle with a minimum 5-mm bridge. A 4.5-mm drill hole is made at the site of the anatomic origin of the anterior bundle of MCL on medial epicondyle that does not penetrate the posterior cortex. A 3.2-mm drill hole is placed just anterior to the epicondylar attachment of the medial intermuscular septum and directed to communicate with the 4.5-mm drill hole in the epicondyle. A second 3.2-mm drill hole is made in the anterosuperior surface of the epicondyle approximately 1 cm from the previous 3.2-mm hole.

The ipsilateral palmaris longus is harvested through a series of small transverse incisions beginning at the distal flexor crease of the wrist. The graft is passed through the proximal ulnar bone tunnel and through medial epicondyle in a figure-eight configuration. With the elbow placed with varus stress, 60° of elbow flexion, and the forearm in supination, tension is applied to the graft. The ulnar side of the graft is sutured to the remnants of the ulnar collateral ligament adjacent to the sublime tubercle. The proximal limb of the graft is sutured to the medial intermuscular septum outside the drill hole. Simple sutures are placed in the crossing limbs of the graft which further tension graft and enhances fixation.

With this modified technique, it was unnecessary to mobilize and transpose the ulnar nerve routinely.

Good results with this modified Jobe technique, in which a muscle-splitting approach is used for exposure, have been reported; Azar et al. [27] reported that 79 % of patients had returned to previous levels of sporting competition, and Thompson et al. [28] reported a rate of 82 %.

Another alternative to transecting the flexor-pronator mass that has been used with good success was elevating the flexor-pronator tendon without detaching or splitting it [39].

In 2001, Altchek et al. [40] and Rohrbough et al. [41] in 2002 described a new reconstruction technique called "docking technique."

The docking technique is a modification of the Jobe technique that simplifies graft passage, tensioning, and fixation. The exposure is obtained by muscle-splitting approach.

This reconstruction is based on a single medial epicondylar drill hole and two drill holes in the ulna similar to the Jobe technique. Humeral tunnel position is located in the anterior half of the medial epicondyle at the anatomic insertion of the native MCL similar to the Jobe technique depth of 15 mm using a 4-mm bur or drill. Two exit tunnels separated by 5 mm to 1 cm.

Graft is passed through the ulnar tunnel from anterior to posterior. Posterior limb of the graft is passed into the humeral tunnel. Final length of the anterior limb of the graft is determined by placing it adjacent to the humeral tunnel and visually estimating the length of the graft that would allow the graft to be tensioned within the humeral tunnel.

A No. 1 braided nonabsorbable suture is placed in a Krackow fashion. Excess graft is excised and graft limb is passed into the humeral tunnel with sutures exiting the small tunnels. Graft tensioning is performed by placing the elbow through a full range of motion with varus stress placed on the elbow. Sutures are tied over the bony bridge on the humeral epicondyle with the elbow in 60° of flexion, supination, and varus stress applied.

Medial epicondylar fixation is based on sutures tied over a bone bridge.

It has been suggested that the docking technique allows for better tensioning of the ligament graft. Rohrbough et al. [41] have reported that

92 % of their patients were able to return to pre-injury levels of competition.

Afterwards, other MCL reconstruction techniques have been evaluated in the laboratory that reconstruct the central isometric fibers of the native ligament. Single drill holes located in the isometric and anatomic location of the anterior bundle of the MCL on the medial epicondyle and ulna have been proposed (single-strand technique), which would reduce the risk of injury to the ulnar nerve and simplify the procedure [42].

A single-strand technique minimizes the risk of injury to the ulnar nerve from a second more posterior drill hole and reduces trauma to the flexor-pronator muscles by allowing a more limited exposure.

Ahmad et al. described the use of an interference screw for fixation of a single-stranded tendon graft in blind osseous tunnels at the origin and insertion of the native ulnar collateral ligament [42]. Armstrong et al. determined the contribution of the central portion of the anterior bundle of the MCL to elbow stability and evaluated the effectiveness of a single-strand MCL reconstruction in restoring elbow stability [16].

Various fixation methods have been proposed and used: interference screws for ulna and humerus fixation; interference screw for ulna fixation and docking technique for humerus fixation (Dane TJ/hybrid), endobutton for ulnar fixation, and docking for humerus fixation.

In 2005, Armstrong et al. [43] reported a biomechanical comparison of the strength of four reconstruction techniques to that of the native ulnar collateral ligament in valgus stress. No difference in strength was found between the docking and single-strand medial collateral reconstruction with the use of an EndoButton for ulnar fixation. Both of these reconstruction methods were stronger than the interference screw or figure-eight technique. The optimal fixation method for a single-strand MCL reconstruction may require improved interference screws or a modified EndoButton procedure [43].

In 2006, a modified docking technique for MCL reconstruction involving a double anterior bundle and a single posterior bundle was described and evaluated [44].

Large et al. in 2007 compared a traditional Jobe bone tunnel ulnar collateral ligament reconstruction to an interference screw reconstruction [45]. The failure strength and initial and overall stiffness of a traditional Jobe bone tunnel UCL reconstruction are superior to those of an interference screw reconstruction (ISR), and only traditional Jobe bone tunnel reconstruction reproduces the initial and overall stiffness of an intact UCL.

Many UCL reconstruction techniques have been described, and a paucity of biomechanical data supports their use. This study found the Jobe bone tunnel technique to be biomechanically superior to the ISR technique.

McAdams et al. compared the docking procedure and the bioabsorbable interference screw procedure [46]. In this study, bioabsorbable interference screw fixation resulted in less valgus angle widening in response to early cyclic valgus load as compared with the docking technique.

The hybrid technique or Dane TJ procedure allows reconstruction and independent tensioning of the anterior and posterior bands of the anterior oblique ligament of the MCL that are not accomplished with the other described techniques. This technique is a hybrid of the interference screw technique distally (in the ulna) and docking procedure proximally (in the humeral epicondyle) [47, 48].

In 2008, Seiber et al. [49] performed a biomechanical evaluation of a new reconstruction technique of the ulnar collateral ligament with modified bone tunnel placement and interference screw fixation.

In 2009, an alternative hybrid technique was proposed by Bennett et al. using small bone tunnels in the medial epicondyle and a single, bioabsorbable screw in the ulna for anatomic reconstruction of both bundles of the MCL that can be tensioned before fixation [50].

There has also been a report published on the biomechanical results of MCL reconstruction with suture anchors to provide graft fixation onto bone as compared with tunnels [51]. The use of allograft for MCL reconstruction and the use of synthetic ligament is now only an area of interest as well [7].

Taking into account the different methods proposed over the years by various authors, some details of technique that are essential for anatomic reconstruction are evident:

1. Minimize trauma to the flexor-pronator muscle group without transection from the medial epicondyle.
2. Reduce the incidence of ulnar nerve symptoms.
3. Use transbone fixation methods (tunnels).
4. Avoid interference of such tunnels or stitches suture with the course of ulnar nerve.
5. Possibility of anatomical reconstruction of both bands of AOL.
6. Tensioning independently at different degrees of flexion of the two bands.
7. Easy measurement of the length of the bands.
8. Intraoperative change of the bands tension.
9. Proximal and distal anatomical intraosseous fixation.

More recently we presented a new double bundles technique [52] using usually gracilis from omolateral knee, that in our opinion simplifies graft passage, tensioning, and fixation.

The exposure is obtained by muscle-splitting approach.

The graft is prepared with a Krackow suture at the two ends of the tendon by use of No. 2 TiCron suture.

A 7-mm drill hole is made at the sublime tubercle directed toward the lateral and posterior cortex of the ulna, away from the proximal radioulnar joint. The far cortex is not disturbed.

The graft is folded over onto itself and introduced into the drill hole so that at least 1 cm of the graft fill the drill hole (Fig. 6.2). A 6–7-mm bioabsorbable interference screw is positioned in the drill hole to stabilize the graft (Fig. 6.3).

One drill hole (7 mm) is positioned on the medial epicondyle at the most isometric point for the anterior bundle of the MCL at the anterior-inferior surface of the medial epicondyle.

This drill hole did not broach the far cortex and is oriented anterior-superior so as to void ulnar nerve damages.

Two 4.5-mm drill holes are placed superiorly and independently convergent to the 7-mm graft hole away from ulnar nerve. The two ends of the tendon first pass together into the 7-mm graft hole, and then each single bundle is retrieved through the 4.5-mm drill hole (Fig. 6.4a, b) and is sutured over itself at different degrees of flexion: anterior bundle at 30° and posterior bundle at 70° (Fig. 6.5).

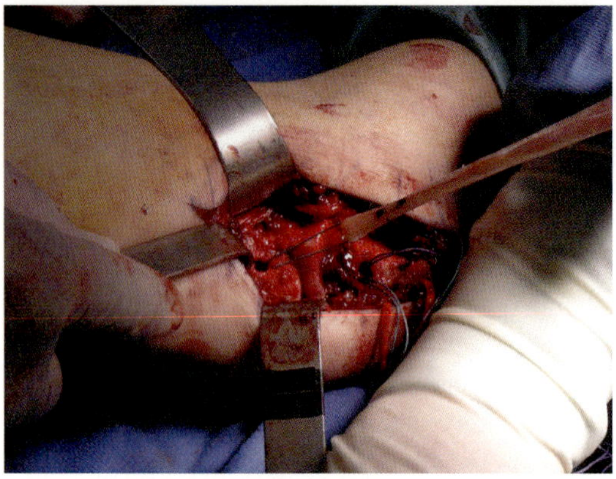

Fig. 6.2 The graft is folded over onto itself and introduced into the drill hole so that at least 1 cm of the graft fill the drill hole

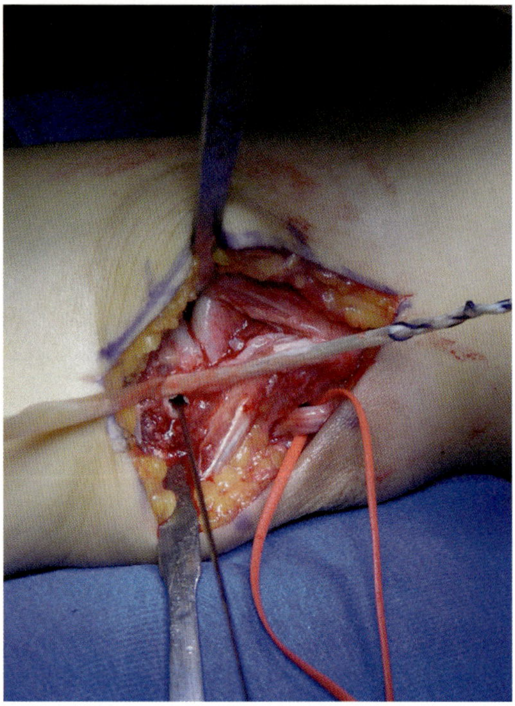

Fig. 6.3 A 6–7-mm bioabsorbable interference screw is positioned in the drill hole to stabilize the graft

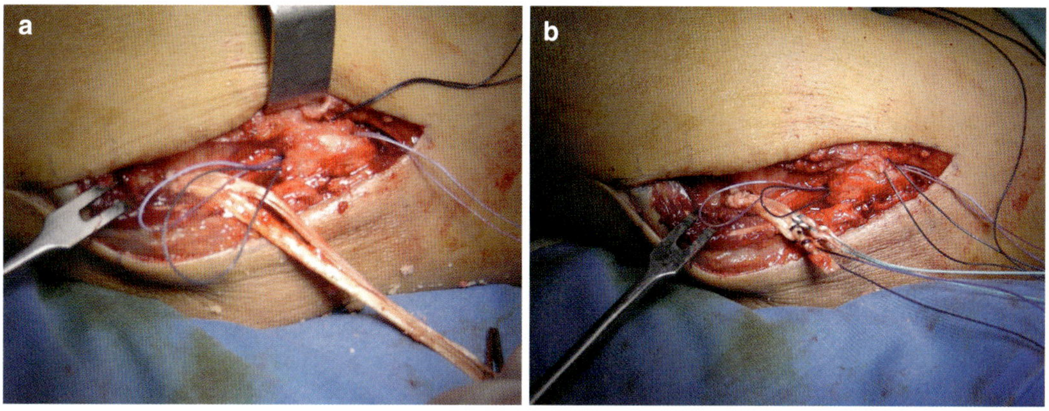

Fig. 6.4 (**a**, **b**) The two ends of the tendon first pass together into the 7-mm graft hole and then each single bundle is retrieved through the 4–5-mm drill hole

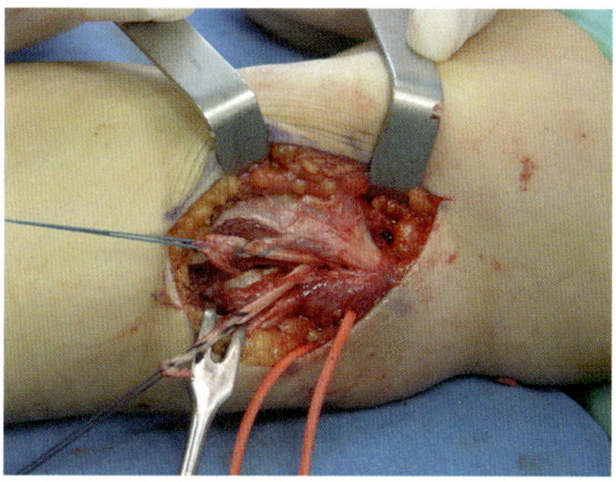

Fig. 6.5 The two ends of the tendon are sutured over itself at different degrees of flexion: anterior bundle at 30° and posterior bundle at 70°

This technique allows to reconstruct a new ligament tensed in all arc of motion and thick enough to reproduced the original UCL.

Postoperatively, the elbow is positioned in brace for 6 weeks and rehabilitative protocols start in 2 weeks.

Sport activity progression is initiated at 3–4 months and return to sport is allowed at 6–8 months post-op.

Reported outcomes of UCL surgery are generally favorable, and in our study, 85 % of 90 athletes were able to return to a previous or higher level of competition. The most common complications are (often temporary) ulnar nerve dysfunction, medial epicondyle fracture, stiffness, and nonspecific elbow pain.

References

1. Morrey BF, Askew LJ, Chao EY. A biomechanical study of normal functional elbow motion. J Bone Joint Surg Am. 1981;63(6):872–7.
2. Safran MR, Baillargeon D. Soft-tissue stabilizers of the elbow. J Shoulder Elbow Surg. 2005;14(1 Suppl S): 179S–85.
3. Mehlhoff TL, Noble PC, Bennett JB, Tullos HS. Simple dislocation of the elbow in the adult. Results after closed treatment. J Bone Joint Surg Am. 1988; 70(2):244–9.
4. Murthi AM, Keener JD, Armstrong AD, Getz CL. The recurrent unstable elbow: diagnosis and treatment. Instr Course Lect. 2011;60:215–26.
5. Hildebrand KA, Patterson SD, King GJ. Acute elbow dislocations simple and complex. Orthop Clin North Am. 1999;30:63–79.
6. Morrey BF, An KN. Articular and ligamentous contributions to the stability of the elbow joint. Am J Sports Med. 1983;11(5):315–9.
7. Safran M M.D., et al. Current concepts ulnar collateral ligament of the elbow. Arthrosc: J Arthrosc Relat Surg. 2005;21(11):1381–95.
8. O'Driscoll SW, Jaloszynski R, Morrey BF, An KN. Origin of the medial ulnar collateral ligament. J Hand Surg [Am]. 1992;17:164–8.
9. Regan WD, Korinek SL, Morrey BF, An K-N. Biomechanical study of ligaments around the elbow joint. Clin Orthop Relat Res. 1991;271:170–9.
10. Callaway GH, Field LD, Deng XH, et al. Biomechanical evaluation of the medial collateral ligament of the elbow. J Bone Joint Surg Am. 1997; 79:1223–31.
11. Morrey BF, Tanaka S, An KN. Valgus stability of the elbow. A definition of primary and secondary constraints. Clin Orthop. 1991;265:187–95.
12. Neill-Cage DJ, Abrams RA, Callahan JJ, et al. Soft tissue attachments of the ulnar coronoid process: an

anatomic study with radiographic correlation. Clin Orthop. 1995;320:154–8.
13. Timmerman LA, Andrews JR. Histology and arthroscopic anatomy of the ulnar collateral ligament of the elbow. Am J Sports Med. 1994;22:667–73.
14. Morrey BF. Anatomy of the elbow joint. In: Morrey BF, editor. The elbow and its disorders. 3rd ed. Philadelphia: WB Saunders; 2000. p. 13–42.
15. Morrey BF, An KN. Functional anatomy of the ligaments of the elbow. Clin Orthop. 1985;201:84–90.
16. Armstrong AD, Ferreira LM, Dunning CE, Johnson JA, King GJW. The medial collateral ligament of the elbow is not isometric. Poster exhibit at the 49th annual meeting of the Orthopaedic Research Society, New Orleans; 2003.
17. An K-N, Morrey BF. Biomechanics of the elbow. In: Morrey BF, editor. The elbow and its disorders. Philadelphia: WB Saunders; 1985. p. 43–61.
18. Fuss FK. The ulnar collateral ligament of the human elbow joint. Anatomy, function and biomechanics. J Anat. 1991;175:203–12.
19. Tullos HS, Schwab GH, Bennett JB, Woods GW. Factors influencing elbow stability. Instr Course Lect. 1982;8:185–99.
20. Schwab GH, Bennett JB, Woods GW, Tullos HS. The biomechanics of elbow stability: the role of the medial collateral ligament. Clin Orthop. 1980;146:42–52.
21. Floris S, Olsen BS, Dalstra M, Sojbjerg JO, Sneppen O. The medial collateral ligament of the elbow joint: anatomy and kinematics. J Shoulder Elbow Surg. 1998;7:345–51.
22. Sojbjerg JO, Oveson J, Nielsen S. Experimental elbow stability after transection of the medial collateral ligament. Clin Orthop. 1987;218:186–90.
23. Safran MR. Ulnar collateral ligament injury in the overhead athlete: diagnosis and treatment. Clin Sports Med. 2004;23:643–63.
24. Safran MR, Caldwell GL, Fu FH. Chronic instability of the elbow. In: Peimer CA, editor. Surgery of the hand and upper extremity. New York: McGraw-Hill; 1996. p. 467–90.
25. O'Driscoll SWM, Lawton RL, Smith AM. the moving valgus stress test for medial collateral ligament tears of the elbow. Am J Sports Med. 2005;33:231–9.
26. Safran MR, Mcgarry MH, Shin S, et al. Effects of elbow flexion and forearm rotation on valgus laxity of the elbow. J Bone Joint Surg Am. 2005;87:2065–74.
27. Azar FM, Andrews JR, Wilk KE, et al. Operative treatment of ulnar collateral ligament injuries of the elbow in athletes. Am J Sports Med. 2000;28:16–23.
28. Thompson W. Ulnar collateral ligament reconstruction in athletes: muscle-splitting approach without transposition of the ulnar nerve. J Shoulder Elbow Surg. 2001;10:152–7.
29. Timmerman LA, Schwartz ML, Andrews JR. Preoperative evaluation of the ulnar collateral ligament by magnetic resonance imaging and computed tomography arthrography. Evaluation in 25 baseball players with surgical confirmation. Am J Sports Med. 1994;32:26–31.
30. Barnes DA, Tullos HS. An analysis of 100 symptomatic baseball players. Am J Sports Med. 1978;6:62–7.
31. Rettig AC, Sherrill C, Snead DS, Mendler JC, Mieling P. Nonoperative treatment of ulnar collateral ligament injuries in throwing athletes. Am J Sports Med. 2001;29:15–7.
32. Conway JE, Jobe FW, Glousman RE, Pink M. Medial instability of the elbow in throwing athletes: treatment by repair or reconstruction of the ulnar collateral ligament. J Bone Joint Surg Am. 1992;74:67–83.
33. Bennett JB, Tullos HS. Ligamentous and articular injuries in the athlete. In: Morrey BF, editor. The elbow and its disorders. Philadelphia: WB Saunders; 1985. p. 502–22.
34. Norwood LA, Shook JA, Andrews JR. Acute medial elbow ruptures. Am J Sports Med. 1981;9:16–9.
35. Freehill MT, Safran MR. Diagnosis and management of ulnar collateral ligament injuries in throwers. Curr Sports Med Rep. 2011;10(5):271–8.
36. Vanderhooft E. The frequency of and relationship between the palmaris longus and plantaris tendons. Am J Orthop. 1996;25(1):38–41.
37. Jobe FW, Stark H, Lombardo SJ. Reconstruction of the ulnar collateral ligament in athletes. J Bone Joint Surg Am. 1986;68:1158–63.
38. Smith GR, Altchek DW, Pagnani MJ, Keeley JR. A muscle-splitting approach to the ulnar collateral ligament of the elbow. Neuroanatomy and operative technique. Am J Sports Med. 1996;24:575–80.
39. Andrews JR, Timmerman LA. Outcome of elbow surgery in professional baseball players. Am J Sports Med. 1995;23:407–13.
40. Altchek DW, Andrew JR. Medial collateral ligament injuries. In: Altchek DW, Andrew JR, editors. The athlete's elbow. Philadelphia: Lippincott Williams and Wilkins; 2001. p. 153–73.
41. Rohrbough JT, Altchek DW, Hyman J, Williams III RJ, Butts JD. Medial collateral ligament reconstruction of the elbow using the docking technique. Am J Sports Med. 2002;30:541–8.
42. Ahmad CS, Lee TQ, Elattrache NS. Biomechanical evaluation of a new elbow ulnar collateral ligament reconstruction using interference screw fixation. Am J Sports Med. 2003;31:332–7.
43. Armstrong AD, Dunning CE, Ferreira LM, Faber KJ, Johnson JA, King GJ. A biomechanical comparison of four reconstruction techniques for the medial collateral ligament–deficient. Elbow J Shoulder Elbow Surg. 2005;14:207–15.
44. Koh JL, Schafer MF, Keuter G, Hsu JE. Ulnar collateral ligament reconstruction in elite throwing athletes. Arthrosc: J Arthrosc Relat Surg. 2006;22(11):1187–91.
45. Large TM, Coley ER, Peindl RD, Fleischli JE. A biomechanical comparison of 2 ulnar collateral ligament reconstruction techniques. Arthroscopy. 2007;23:141–50.

46. McAdams TR, Lee AT, Centeno J, Giori NJ, Lindsey DP. Two ulnar collateral ligament reconstruction methods: the docking technique versus bioabsorbable interference screw fixation–a biomechanical evaluation with cyclic loading. J Shoulder Elbow Surg. 2007;16:224–8.
47. Conway J. The Dane TJ procedure for elbow medial ulnar collateral ligament insufficiency. Tech Should Elbow Surg. 2006;7:36–43.
48. Ahmad CS, ElAttrache NS. Elbow valgus instability in the throwing athlete. J Am Acad Orthop Surg. 2006;14:693–700.
49. Seiber KS, Savoie FH, McGarry MH, Gupta R, Lee TQ. Biomechanical evaluation of a new reconstruction technique of the ulnar collateral ligament in the elbow with modified bone tunnel placement and interference screw fixation. Clin Biomech. 2010;25:37.
50. Bennett JM, Mehlhoff TL. Reconstruction of the medial collateral ligament of the elbow. J Hand Surg. 2009;34A:1729–33.
51. Hechtman KS, Tjin-A-Tsoi EW, Zvijac JE, Uribe JW, Latta LL. Biomechanics of a less invasive procedure for reconstruction of the ulnar collateral ligament of the elbow. Am J Sports Med. 1998;26:620–4.
52. Pederzini L, Prandini M, Tosi M, Nicoletta F. The acute lesions of the medial collateral ligament of the elbow S14 GIOT Agosto. GIOT. 2012;38(Suppl 2):14–18.

Evaluation of UCL by Ultrasound

7

Giovanni Merolla, Giuseppe Porcellini,
Gianluca Bullitta, and Giuseppe Giannicola

7.1 Introduction

Ulnar collateral ligament (UCL) has a complex anatomy and is the most important stabilizing structure to valgus and internal rotatory forces across the elbow joint [1, 2]. It is anatomically divided in three components: the anterior medial collateral ligament (AMCL), the posterior medial collateral ligament (PMCL), and the transverse ligament [3]. The AMCL consists of an anterior bundle and a posterior bundle; the anterior bundle primarily stabilizes the elbow from 30 to 120° of flexion, while the posterior bundle has the same function at the terminal phase of the elbow flexion [4]. The UCL can be injured after repeated valgus force applied to the elbow, as it happens in overhead sports or working activities or as a result of direct or indirect acute trauma [4]. Such trauma may be associated with bone injuries including fractures of the radial head, olecranon, and medial epicondyle [5]. Ultrasound (US) is an excellent imaging modality for evaluation of elbow joint, the integrity of the surrounding soft tissues, and the assessment of the UCL after trauma or after surgical reconstruction.

7.2 Ultrasound Technique and Normal Elbow Anatomy

US examination of the elbow can be performed on the patient supine or seated and the elbow placed on an examination table [6, 7]. We use a high-frequency linear transducer of 7.5–14 MHz. Tendons and ligaments demonstrate characteristic hyperechoic fibrillar echotexture when imaged perpendicular to the ultrasound beam; iso- to hypoechoic echogenicity of ligaments and tendons may be diagnosed as abnormalities [6]. Assessment of the contralateral elbow is useful as comparison, and dynamic imaging helps to evaluate the integrity of the collateral ligaments, subluxation of the ulnar nerve or triceps tendon, and intra-articular bodies. US examination begins with the assessment of anterior elbow where the key structures to be evaluated include the anterior joint recess, distal brachialis muscle, distal biceps brachii muscle and tendon, and the median nerve. The elbow is extended and the forearm is supinated and the examination should include both transverse and longitudinal planes extending at

G. Merolla (✉) • G. Porcellini
Unit of Shoulder and Elbow Surgery, D. Cervesi Hospital, Cattolica – AUSL della Romagna Ambito Territoriale di Rimini, Cattolica, Italy
e-mail: giovannimerolla@hotmail.com; giovanni.merolla@auslrn.net

G. Bullitta MD • G. Giannicola MD, PhD
Orthopedics and Traumatology, "Sapienza" University of Rome, Rome, Italy
e-mail: giannicola.giuseppe@gmail.com; gbullitta@alice.it

L.A. Pederzini et al. (eds.), *Elbow and Sport*, DOI 10.1007/978-3-662-48742-6_7

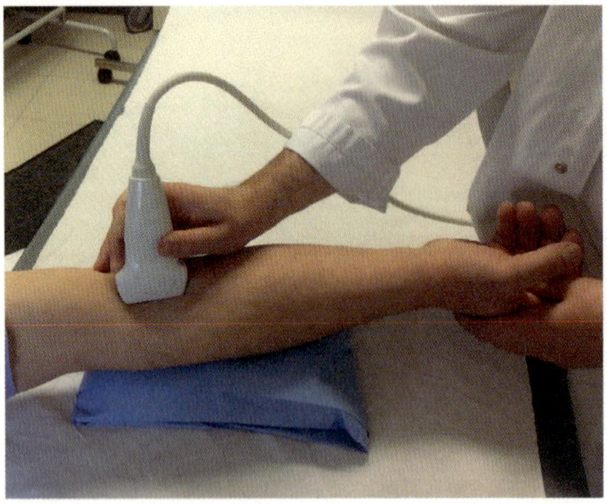

Fig. 7.1 Anterior elbow examination. The patient is seated with the elbow extended and the forearm supinated. The probe is placed on the longitudinal plane (long axis). A slight bending of the patient's body toward the examined side makes full supination and assessment of the anterior compartment easier. Full elbow extension can be facilitated by placing a pillow under the joint

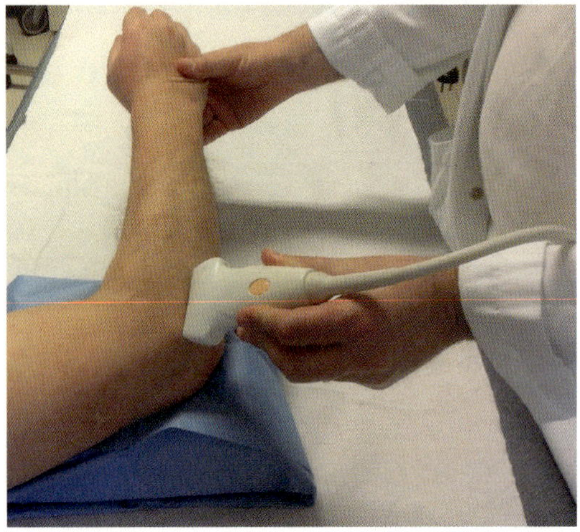

Fig. 7.2 The lateral aspect of the elbow is examined with the elbow in extension or in slight flexion. The probe is on the long axis to evaluate the common extensor tendon origin

least 5 cm proximal and 5 cm distal to the joint (Fig. 7.1) [7]. The lateral elbow structures to be evaluated include the common extensor tendon, lateral collateral ligamentous complex, radiocapitellar joint, annular ligament, capitellum, and radial nerve, including the posterior interosseus nerve, which is its deep motor branch. The lateral elbow is evaluated by placing the elbow in flexion with the forearm pronated (Fig. 7.2). Structures of interest in the medial compartment include the common flexor tendon and the UCL, the ulnar nerve, the medial part of the triceps tendon, and the anterior band of the UCL. The medial elbow is evaluated with the patient's forearm placed in supination and extension or slight flexion (Fig. 7.3a) [7]. The transducer is placed in the long axis (coronal plane), over the medial epicondyle; this allows to show the hyperechoic bony contours of the medial epicondyle and ulnotrochlear articulation (Fig. 7.3a). An additional evaluation will include transverse US to identify common flexor-pronator mass (pronator teres and common flexor tendon, flexor carpi radialis, palmaris longus, flexor carpi ulnaris, and flexor digitorum superficialis) that originates from the medial epicondyle and anterior band of the UCL [8]. The origin of the common flexor-pronator mass has a hyperechoic fibrillar pattern comparable to that of the common extensor tendon [9]. Anterior band of UCL appears on US as hyperechoic, thin, compact fibrillar band just deep to the common flexor tendon; it originates from the anteroinferior aspect of the medial epicondyle to insert on the sublime tubercle of the coronoid process of the ulna (Fig. 7.3b) [8, 10]. Less commonly, the proximal attachment of the anterior band has a cordlike or broad-based appearance [11]. Dynamic US by application of valgus stress on the elbow allow to evaluate for ligamentous laxity, and comparison with the uninjured side is mandatory [12]. As with all ligaments, the anterior band of the UCL is susceptible to anisotropy.

7.3 US Assessment of UCL Injuries

Injuries of UCL are often injured concomitantly with the overlying common flexor-pronator mass [12]. Partial UCL tears appear as focal hypoechoic heterogeneity and ligamentous thickening [8, 11, 12]. Disruption of the UCL with widening of the ulnotrochlear joint indicates a full-thickness tear [8, 11, 12]. Dynamic valgus stress assessment allows differentiation between complete and

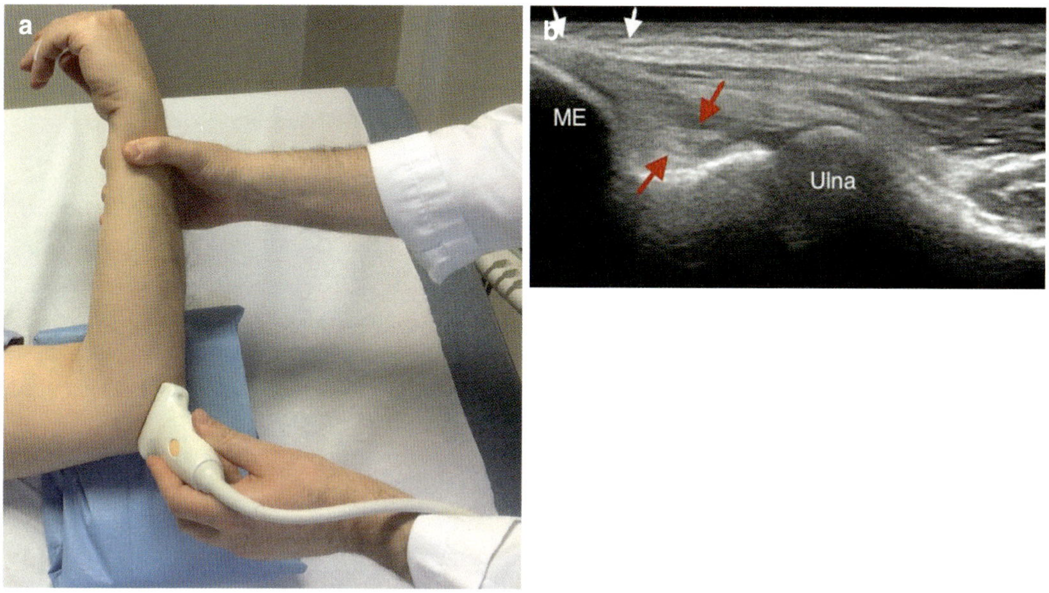

Fig. 7.3 (**a**, **b**) Examination of the medial elbow. (**a**) The forearm is supinated and the elbow extended or slightly flexed, resting on a table with a pillow under the joint. (**b**) The cranial edge of the probe is placed over the medial epicondyle in the coronal plane to reveal the common flexor tendon in its long axis and the anterior bundle of the medial collateral ligament deep to this tendon. *ME* medial epicondyle, *white arrows* common flexor tendon origin; *red arrows* anterior bundle of the medial

incomplete UCL by asymmetrical widening of the ulnohumeral joint [11, 12]. Assessment of the contralateral UCL provides useful information on the normal morphology of UCL and the inherent stability of the ulnohumeral joint. This is in line with the findings during arthroscopic evaluation of widening of the ulnohumeral joint in case of a tear of the deep layer of the UCL while visually remaining intact externally [13]. US can be useful in the assessment of ulnar nerve entrapment (cubital tunnel syndrome) by demonstrating a hypoechoic thickened ulnar nerve with a cross-sectional area greater than 7.5 mm^2 at the level of the medial epicondyle. A thickened, hypoechoic ulnar nerve with loss of its fascicular appearance may be seen in ulnar nerve subluxation as a result of irritation from friction during translocation. Dynamic imaging during active elbow flexion will demonstrate medial and anterior dislocation of the ulnar nerve over the medial epicondyle. Typically, the ulnar nerve will relocate within the cubital tunnel during elbow extension. Correlation with symptoms and the appearance of the contralateral nerve is important, as ulnar nerve subluxation is seen in up to 20 % of asymptomatic patients. In some patients, especially overhead athletes, the subluxation of the ulnar nerve is accompanied with a subluxation of the medial part of the triceps tendon.

The ulnar nerve, in general, subluxates over the medial epicondyle between 70° and 90° of flexion, and the triceps subluxates between 110 and 120° of flexion.

7.4 US Evaluation of Reconstructed UCL

The surgical procedure require the identification of the isometric origin of the anterior band of the MCL on the anteroinferior aspect of the medial epicondyle be identified, preserving the origin of flexor-pronator tendons. After exposure of the sublime tubercle on the medial aspect of the proximal ulna, humeral and ulnar tunnels are prepared for the passage of the tendon graft, which is then fixed using a figure-of-eight configuration or a docking technique (see Chap. 7). US is performed

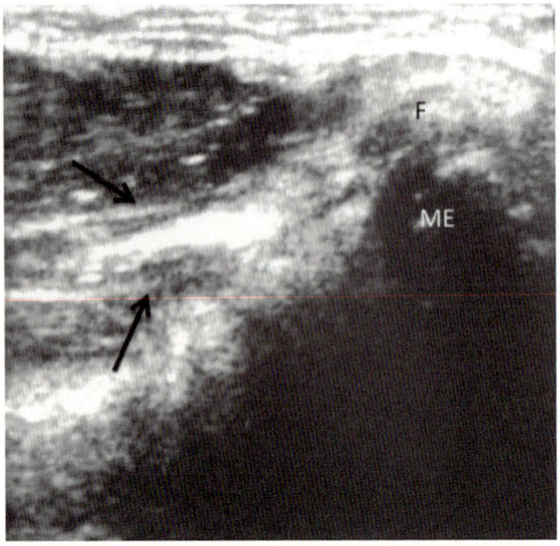

Fig. 7.4 Ultrasound assessment of the right reconstructed UCL. The graft appears as a hyperechoic cordlike structure (*black arrows*) that lay deep to the common flexor tendon surrounded by scar tissues. *ME* medial epicondyle, *F* common flexor tendon

with the transducer placed in the long axis, with its cranial aspect over the medial epicondyle so that the hyperechoic bony contours of the medial epicondyle and ulnotrochlear articulation are seen [8]. Compared to the original anterior fibrillar band of the UCL, the graft appears as a more hyperechoic compact "cordlike" band that lay just deep to the common flexor tendon (Fig. 7.4). The US allows to follow the course of the graft from the isometric origin on the anteroinferior aspect of the medial epicondyle to the ulnar insertion close to the sublime tubercle [14]. Dynamic US is also performed to evaluate the tensile properties and the resistance of the graft with application of valgus stress on the elbow. Merolla et al. [14] in a recent research article reported good to excellent results with graft reconstruction techniques in subjects with chronic UCL insufficiency, showing similar clinical and radiographic results of allograft vs. autograft; the same authors highlights the efficacy of musculoskeletal US to evaluate the reconstructed UCL.

Conclusions

US is an effective diagnostic tool in terms of cost-effectiveness, accessibility, and patient comfort and can be used as an alternative for patients who have contraindications to magnetic resonance imaging (MRI). The high image resolution is facilitated by the superficial location of the elbow. US is effective and reliable in the assessment of postoperative elbow after UCL reconstruction as shown in recent research articles.

Although it is operator dependent and requires a learning curve, it remains an excellent imaging tool, and the advantages are such that it continues to be increasingly used as an alternative or adjunct to MR imaging.

References

1. Regan WD, Korinek SL, Morrey BF, An KN. Biomechanical study of ligaments around the elbow joint. Clin Orthop Relat Res. 1991;271:170–9.
2. Hotchkiss RN, Weiland AJ. Valgus stability of the elbow. J Orthop Res: Off Publ Orthop Res Soc. 1987;5:372–7. doi:10.1002/jor.1100050309.
3. Fuss FK. The ulnar collateral ligament of the human elbow joint. Anatomy, function and biomechanics. J Anat. 1991;175:203–12.
4. Morrey BF, An KN. Articular and ligamentous contributions to the stability of the elbow joint. Am J Sports Med. 1983;11:315–9.
5. Forthman C, Henket M, Ring DC. Elbow dislocation with intra-articular fracture: the results of operative treatment without repair of the medial collateral ligament. J Hand Surg. 2007;32:1200–9. doi:10.1016/j.jhsa.2007.06.019.
6. Beggs I. Ultrasound of the shoulder and elbow. Orthop Clin North Am. 2006;37:277–85. doi:10.1016/j.ocl.2006.03.004. v.
7. Beggs I, et al. Musculoskeletal ultrasound technical guidelines. II. Elbow. European Society of Musculoskeletal Radiology. 2006. http://www.essr.org/html/img/pool/elbow.pdf. Accessed 26 Feb 2015.
8. Konin GP, Nazarian LN, Walz DM. US of the elbow: indications, technique, normal anatomy, and pathologic conditions. Radiographics. 33:E125–47. doi:10.1148/rg.334125059.
9. Ciccotti MC, Schwartz MA, Ciccotti MG. Diagnosis and treatment of medial epicondylitis of the elbow. Clin Sports Med. 2004;23:693–705. doi:10.1016/j.csm.2004.04.011. xi.
10. Ward SI, Teefey SA, Paletta GA, et al. Sonography of the medial collateral ligament of the elbow: a study of cadavers and healthy adult male volunteers. AJR Am J Roentgenol. 2003;180:389–94. doi:10.2214/ajr.180.2.1800389.
11. Jacobson JA, Propeck T, Jamadar DA, et al. US of the anterior bundle of the ulnar collateral ligament: findings in five cadaver elbows with MR arthrographic

and anatomic comparison – initial observations. Radiology. 2003;227:561–6. doi:10.1148/radiol.2272020462.
12. Nazarian LN, McShane JM, Ciccotti MG, et al. Dynamic US of the anterior band of the ulnar collateral ligament of the elbow in asymptomatic major league baseball pitchers. Radiology. 2003;227:149–54. doi:10.1148/radiol.2271020288.
13. Timmerman LA, Andrews JR. Arthroscopic treatment of posttraumatic elbow pain and stiffness. Am J Sports Med. 1994;22:230–5.
14. Merolla G, Del Sordo S, Paladini P, Porcellini G. Elbow ulnar collateral ligament reconstruction: clinical, radiographic, and ultrasound outcomes at a mean 3-year follow-up. Musculoskelet Surg. 2014. doi:10.1007/s12306-014-0325-0.

Olecranon Elbow Pain in Sportsmen

8

Roberto Rotini, Michele Cavaciocchi, Krishna Kumar, and Enrico Guerra

8.1 Which Sports and Why

Various sports can create an elbow functional overload with olecranon pain; throwing sports (i.e., baseball, softball, javelin, handball, water polo, football), "racket" sports (i.e., tennis, golf, cricket, etc.), and superior limb-bearing sports (i.e., gymnastics, dive) can cause functional overload of the olecranon and consequent pain [1–9]. Gymnasts and wrestlers show high risk for olecranon stress fractures, related to high weight-bearing across the elbow and sudden extension forces associated with triceps-demanding maneuvers [5].

8.2 Introduction

In modern sports, the elbow sustains a critical load. Children and teenager can run the risk of significant lesions, thinking that 55 % of US high school students take part in sports, like baseball and softball (third and fourth most practiced) [10]. This risk level drove US Baseball Little League to define guidelines for pitchers, to avoid excess of stress to these young athletes.

Based on these considerations, an epidemiological increase of elbow overuse is evident and covers a wide part of the general population.

Pain resolution and sport restart in few times are the goals of treatment.

Roughly, in athletes, elbow lesions can find their origin in a high-energy trauma (sprains, dislocations, fracture-dislocations) or in a low-energy trauma or microtrauma. A high-energy trauma shows a very typical presentation, it is difficult to miss its diagnosis, and it requires an early and careful treatment to minimize the sequelae. Microtrauma and overuse lesions have an insidious onset and the clinician must pay a great attention to avoid underestimating them.

8.2.1 Notes of Elbow Biomechanic

In the daily activities, the elbow sustains a load which is three times of body weight, with a peak at 90° of flexion. The joint is inherently in valgus, so the forces are not well distributed on the articular structures, which must support a continuous valgus stress along the entire range of movement.

Several cadaveric studies described some particular elbow features: intrinsic valgism is controlled, in maximum extension and maximum flexion, by the osseous ulnohumeral congruence [11]. Histological and biomechanical studies underline the different tensions of the two bundles (anterior and posterior) of the medial/ulnar collateral complex (UCL) during the elbow

R. Rotini (✉) • M. Cavaciocchi • K. Kumar
E. Guerra
Shoulder and Elbow Unit, Rizzoli Institute, Bologna, Italy
e-mail: roberto.rotini@ior.it

L.A. Pederzini et al. (eds.), *Elbow and Sport*, DOI 10.1007/978-3-662-48742-6_8

motion in flexion and extension [12]: the anterior bundle provides valgus stability throughout the entire range of motion and consists of anterior and posterior bands that originate from the inferior aspect of the medial epicondyle and insert at the sublime tubercle on the medial aspect of the coronoid process [13–16]. The anterior band of the UCL is the primary restraint to valgus rotation at 30, 60, and 90° of flexion and was a co-primary restraint at 120° of flexion. The posterior band of the anterior UCL is a co-primary restraint at 120° of flexion and a secondary restraint at 30 and 90° of flexion [12, 17]. The oblique bundle (transverse ligament) lies at the distal-medial aspect of the joint capsule and does not cross the elbow joint. The posterior bundle is thinner and weaker than the anterior bundle and provides secondary elbow stability over 90° of flexion [13, 14, 17]. In cadaveric models, the incision of the anterior bundle of the UCL creates medial elbow instability, most of all at 70° of flexion [18], so if UCL is not sufficient, the radiohumeral joint becomes a primary valgus stabilizer of the elbow [11]; the olecranon resection improves the stress over UCL [19].

In athletes, a repetitive valgus stress is well defined for pitchers and creates a high tension of the medial compartment, a compression of the lateral compartment, and a posteromedial compression between olecranon and fossa; proceeding on this vicious circle, the UCL looses its tension, increasing the stress on the joint, leading to osteochondral lesions, and determining pain, swelling, and stiffness.

8.2.2 Causes of Olecranon Pain in the Athlete

1. Valgus extension overload syndrome (or posteromedial elbow impingement)
2. Olecranon stress fractures
3. Persistence of the olecranon physis
4. "Boxer's elbow"
5. "Handball goalie's elbow"
6. Triceps tendon lesions/tendonitis
7. Triceps snapping
8. Olecranon bursitis

8.2.2.1 Valgus Extension Overload Syndrome (VEOS)

Firstly described by Wilson et al. in 1983 [20], VEOS is a condition that results from impingement of the posteromedial tip of the olecranon process on the medial wall of the olecranon fossa. Incidence data show that VEOS can affect the 65 % of the overhead athletes [21, 22].

The throwing mechanism bring the elbow, in the acceleration phase, to 3,000 deg/s of angular speed and to 64 N/m of torque force, passing from 110 flexion degrees to 20 extension degrees [23, 24]; in addition, during the throwing, the valgus torque concentrates to the medial elbow a shear force of approximately 300 N [23, 25, 26].

Concomitantly, compressive forces at the lateral radiocapitellar joint reach 500 N. The rapid elbow extension that occurs with throwing is one of the fastest recorded human motions [27].

This functional overload determines a tensile stress on the medial elbow, a shear force on the posterior elbow, and a compression force on the lateral elbow. A repetitive performance of this action creates lesions on the various elbow districts, with symptoms beginning on the medial side (UCL disease, medial instability) and extending to the posterior (impingement of olecranon fossa) and to the lateral compartment (cartilage and bone lesions, OCD) [28–30].

As explained by Dugas [27], in the overhead or throwing athlete, increase of medial elbow laxity may predispose the athlete to micromotion of the olecranon tip within the fossa as the elbow is forcibly extended.

King and colleagues [31] suggested that with excessive valgus force, ligamentous laxity on the medial aspect of the elbow accentuates the impingement of the posteromedial olecranon within the olecranon fossa. This posteromedial impingement leads to osteophyte formation on the posteromedial tip of the olecranon as an attempt to create more stability. The impingement and the symptoms worsen with continued throwing or overhead delivery.

Aguinaldo and Chambers [32] reported in 2009 several mechanical factors in the throwing motion that predispose the elbow to high valgus load. These factors include late trunk rotation, reduced shoulder external rotation, and increased elbow flexion. Sidearm pitchers were found to be more susceptible than overhead pitchers. In many throwers and overhead athletes, there never appears a clinical problem with VEOS because they discontinue throwing in high volumes as the result of increasing age and decreasing opportunity to play competitive overhead sports. In higher-level athletes, and in people who continue to enjoy overhead sports into adulthood, the appearance of symptomatic VEOS is increased. Recurrent UCL injuries, such as strains or minimal tears, can lead to increased laxity and pressure in the posteromedial side of the elbow.

8.2.2.2 Olecranon Stress Fractures

Stress fractures are partial or complete fractures of a bone resulting from its inability to resist a stress applied in a repeated manner [33]. The first olecranon stress fracture description belongs to Waris in 1946 that described the lesion of a javelin thrower [34]. Charlton [35] underlines that this kind of lesions affects patients with a closed physis; similarly, Rettig [36] emphasized how stress fractures represent a different clinical picture from the olecranon physis persistence, basing on the differences in physiopathology of mature and immature skeleton.

As explained by Nakaji [37] and by Lu [38], the olecranon stress fractures are an uncommon source of elbow pain in athletes, mostly occurring in throwing athletes including baseball players, gymnasts, javelin players, wrestlers, and lifters.

Lu [38] underlines that the stress fractures and tip fractures of the olecranon are not the same entity although they are both seen in throwing athletes.

The location of the stress fracture can be the olecranon tip or the mid-articular portion; usually, these fractures show a nondisplaced pattern. The possible cause of olecranon stress fracture may be the result of intrinsic forces from the muscle contraction during the terminal phase of throwing and impingement of the olecranon against the medial wall of the olecranon fossa.

Analyzing the causes of the olecranon stress fractures, Paci et al. [39] sustain that the cause of the tip lesions is impingement into the fossa; transverse lesions are caused by a combine between extension forces and triceps pull (typical of weight lifters); oblique fractures are due to a VEOS mechanism, with both valgus and extension forces (typical of throwers, as confirmed by Ahmad [40] and Kancherla [21]). Some authors show different opinions on the olecranon stress fracture pathogenesis: Nakaji [37] affirms that these lesions originate from violent triceps tractions, without association with VEOS mechanism. Ahmad [40] confirms the hypothesis postulated by King [31] that the pathomechanics of olecranon stress fractures are also similar to injuries due to a valgus extension overload. Stress injury across the olecranon is caused by repetitive abutment of the olecranon into the olecranon fossa, traction from triceps activity during the deceleration phase of throwing, and impaction of the medial olecranon onto the medial wall of the olecranon fossa from valgus forces. Both repetitive microtrauma caused by olecranon impingement or excessive triceps tensile stress have also been implicated as etiologies [41]. Schickendantz [42] supposes that the origin of the olecranon stress fractures can be found in the failure of the olecranon trabecular bone during cyclic loads, most of all without signs of medial instability. Furushima in a recent paper [43] made a literature review and purposed a new classification of olecranon stress fracture, based on the origin and the direction of the fracture plane; this classification is based on five different kind of fracture: physeal, classic, transitional, sclerotic, and distal; the patient age at the beginning of the symptoms influence the characteristic pattern of fracture.

8.2.2.3 Persistence of the Olecranon Physis

The olecranon physis has two ossification centers, one posterior, responsible for the longitudinal axis of the ulna, and one anterior at the olecranon tip, that contributes to the joint surface. These two centers fuse and create a single physis that persists until age 16 in boys and age 14 in girls. A persistent olecranon physis, although similar to an olecranon stress fracture, is a result of repetitive elbow stress leading to sclerotic changes during physeal closing [21].

A posterior elbow pain in childhood can direct the diagnosis to apophysitis, but in late childhood, it can refer to a persistence of the olecranon physis.

Charlton affirms that this pathology can derive from repetitive isolated stress forces of the triceps insertion on the olecranon, as the ones that can occur in gymnasts and divers [35]; rare is its origin from VEOS mechanism.

8.2.2.4 "Boxer's Elbow"

This is a rare condition that finds its pathogenetic mechanism in repetitive high-force hyperextensions of the elbow, causing posterior or posterolateral osteophyte with impingement into the olecranon fossa and posterior and/or posterolateral pain. The boxers are prone to hyperextension with missed punches. Boxer's elbow is not associated with instability, unlike handball goalie's elbow, that has been associated with medial instability [44].

8.2.2.5 "Handball Goalie's Elbow"

The serial studies done by Tyrdal [45] and the study done by Popovic and Lemaire [46] suggested that the mechanism underlying the problem of handball goalkeepers' elbow is increased load in hyperextension. However, in a study based on the video analysis to evaluate the loads on handball goalkeepers in the moment of the save, Akgun [47] suggests that handball goalkeepers are subject to valgus loads more than hyperextension loads on their elbows. During the impact between the ball and the hand, a valgus load on the elbow is well depicted. Similarities between symptoms of baseball pitchers, valgus extension overload syndrome, and the handball goalkeepers elbow complaints confirm the theory that the pathogenesis in these sports motion is the same [48].

8.2.2.6 Triceps Tendon Lesions/Tendonitis

A pattern of posterior elbow pain in the athlete can find its origin in the triceps tendon pathology. Triceps tendon rupture is rare: as reported by Morrey [49], on 856 upper extremity tendon injuries treated at Mayo Clinic, 8 injuries were reported on triceps tendon. In this population, the possible kind of triceps lesions are partial and complete ruptures, that are linked with local steroid injection, use of steroid drugs with anabolic aims, and metabolic diseases. The injury can derive from a direct hit, from an eccentric load on a contracted tendon, or, rarely, from a fall on the outstretched hand.

8.2.2.7 Triceps Snapping

Triceps snapping is a well-defined disorder of the elbow, typical of the second decade of life. The main symptom is a lateral or medial snapping of the triceps, caused often by sport activities that involve upper limbs. Causes can be represented by triceps hypertrophy, triceps anomalous slipping propensity, epicondyle hypoplasia, or post-traumatic bone malalignment. The most common feature is a subluxation of the medial head of the triceps over medial epicondyle [49]. The medial snapping can be the cause of ulnar nerve irritation or compression.

8.2.2.8 Olecranon Bursitis

Olecranon bursitis can be a rare cause of posterior elbow pain in sportsmen, because it typically affects middle-aged men and it is often correlated with comorbidities, that are uncommon in athletes, like rheumatoid arthritis, gout or pseudogout, systemic lupus erythematosus, pigmented villonodular synovitis, diseases causing impaired immunity, or with several other systemic causes. Nevertheless, repetitive low-level elbow trauma represents the main pathogenesis of the olecranon bursitis. At the origin of this disease can be found upper limb weight-bearing sports (wrestlers, gymnasts). Olecranon bursitis can appear as aseptic or septic: in the last case, the most common cause of infection is *Staphylococcus aureus*, but several other different organisms (Gram-positive, Gram- negative, atypical bacteria, and fungi) have been reported [50].

8.3 Physical Examination

A thorough evaluation starts with knowing the patients, their sport, and their level of competition. Complaints may include pain, decreased motion, mechanical symptoms (clicking, locking, popping, etc.), instability, and paresthesias as well as throwing-specific symptoms. Changes in accuracy, velocity, endurance, and strength aid in diagnosis and will be used as markers to measure improvement. Any changes in a training or throwing regimen should be noted, including pitch counts, innings, games pitched, and rest between pitching for baseball players.

Physical examination starts with inspection of the posture, arm position, muscle mass, skin, and asymmetries compared with contralateral extremity. Tenderness on palpation of olecranon, medial and lateral epicondyles, radial head, and soft spot may indicate acute fracture, stress fracture, or tendonitis. Lateral olecranon tenderness on palpation may indicate a stress fracture, proximal medial tenderness, and impingement. Tenderness over the tendons can indicate microtrauma or inflammation. Palpation of the ulnar nerve along its course should not elicit any pain, but a positive Tinel sign can be found as indication of ulnar nerve pathology. In skeletally immature athletes, tenderness may indicate injury to the apophysis or physis.

8.3.1 Valgus Extension Overload Syndrome

The typical presentation symptoms are a posteromedial pain, most of all in deceleration phase with maximum extension, a limitation in complete elbow extension, and a joint crackling. The athlete usually refers a long history of elbow pain, during or immediately after the sport, resolved with drugs or rest in the same way, pain is never complained during the normal daily activities. The medical evaluation is usually required when the athlete's performance is bluntly insufficient (i.e., the loss of 30 % of speed in baseball pitching); rarely, a medical evaluation is required for the loss of the last 10–20° of extension, generally because this loss is necessary in few sports (shot put).

The most important question to ask a thrower is in which phase of throwing the symptons occur. If the athlete experiences pain medially at the onset of arm acceleration, there should be concern about the UCL. If the athlete experiences posterior pain at ball release when the elbow nears terminal extension, VEOS is more likely to be the cause. Posteromedial pain with resisted arm extension may be more likely with distal triceps tendonitis rather than VEOS [27]. The range of movement can be normal or just slightly limited [42].

A complete evaluation must be carried out, because, the elbow overload could derive from a defect in foot-hand kinetic chain [51].

It is important to perform the clinical test for medial instability (valgus stress test, milking test, Mayo valgus movement test, valgus extension overload test). These tests are not easy in execution, usually create pain and apprehension, and cannot give information to the clinician, also on the basis of the constitutional and asymptomatic laxity of many thrower, that are not easy to understand. Suzuki suggested the milking maneuver at 90° of flexion, where the olecranon does not engage the olecranon fossa, to differentiate valgus extension overload syndrome from medial collateral ligament injury [7].

It is common for a thrower to have some loss of elbow extension in the dominant throwing elbow, and this finding should not appear during the examination. When an injury is suspected to the UCL, a VEOS. The presence or absence of posteromedial pain in forced extension should be noted in the physical examination of each thrower.

Imaging is useful in the evaluation of VEOS: standard and oblique X-ray can help to assess the presence of osteophytes; X-ray under stress and arthrography has low practical utility. The 2D and 3D CT scan can underline the osteophytes or loose bodies. The MRI, most of all with contrast inside the joint, can help in the diagnosis of UCL lesions and is, nowadays, the gold standard in the study of an athlete with posterior elbow pain.

Cohen underlines MRI as an important diagnostic aid in confirming the proper diagnosis of elbow injury in the throwing athlete. His study identifies distinct bony and articular changes to the posterior trochlea and olecranon along with posteromedial synovitis in athletes with VEOS. Other associated findings may include loose bodies, as well as chronic changes to the UCL or to the flexor/pronator tendon origins. MRI identifies a reproducible pattern of pathology in throwing athletes with this disorder and these MRI findings correlate highly with arthroscopic evaluation [52].

The same author affirms that throwing athletes with MRI changes to the olecranon but pain in the early acceleration phase of throwing are more likely to have UCL insufficiency, whereas throwing athletes with similar MRI changes but pain during full extension and the follow-through phase of throwing are more likely to have posteromedial impingement.

As Dugas noted, VEOS is a syndrome, not a radiographic condition. The absence of osteophytes or loose bodies does not eliminate VEOS as a cause of the athletes' symptoms, because the condition of posteromedial impingement predates the formation of osteophytes [27].

8.3.2 Olecranon Stress Fractures

The presentation of this disease is a progressive pain impairment in a period of some weeks during the pitching [37]. Usually, the pain is absent at rest. Pain and tenderness can be located at both posterolateral and posteromedial region [53].

The ROM can be limited in maximum extension and the maneuvers of extension against resistance determine pain [21].

Schickendantz suggests the utility of olecranon percussion in differential diagnosis of posterior elbow pain: in his study, all cases with stress olecranon fractures were positive with this maneuver [42]; it has been proved by Anderson [54] that tibial percussion inducing local vibration can unmask the symptoms of a stress fracture, mainly if incomplete.

Rare findings of associated proximal radial stress fracture are described [42], while UCL lesions have not been described in association with olecranon stress fractures.

X-ray imaging (usually performed both in the affected elbow and in healthy one) is adequate to study these lesions.

8.3.3 Persistence of the Olecranon Physis

Adolescents typically present with posterior elbow pain at terminal elbow extension in the follow-through phase of throwing with a strength loss. Sometimes, a loss of the complete elbow ROM and a mild medial instability can be found [21, 35]; the mean period of symptoms is 26 months (4–60 months) [35].

Plain radiographs of bilateral elbows may show a sclerotic physis, widened as high as 5 mm on the affected side. A T2-weighted MRI may show physeal edema. In a recent study looking at the utility of radiographic criteria for guiding nonoperative versus operative treatment, sclerotic change was found to be a highly predictive variable for requiring operative intervention [55].

8.3.4 "Boxer's Elbow"

In boxers, the onset of the complaints was acute after a missed punch. The complaints in the acute phase were pain dorsally and swelling of the elbow directly after the trauma. Recurrence of symptoms occurred after similar trauma of the elbow and led to chronic complaints in these patients. In the chronic phase, all patients had posterior elbow pain, stiffness, and loss of extension. They were unable to continue training or to compete. The imaging usually underlines the typical posterolateral osteophytes, useful for the differential diagnosis with VEOS.

8.3.5 "Handball Goalie's Elbow"

The diagnosis of "handball goalie's elbow" covers a wide pattern of symptoms: pain, weakness, reduced range of motion, apprehension, numbness, swelling, clicking, locking, and instability [56]. As for VEOS, the imaging aids the diagnosis (X-ray, CT, MRI).

8.3.6 Triceps Tendon Lesions/ Tendonitis

The history of the trauma is fundamental in the diagnosis of triceps tendon lesions: in most cases, the lesion is preceded by a period of tendon pain. The assessment of these patients must be accurate: range of motion is usually reduced and the palpation of the triceps tendon insertion can show a defect; in the opinion of Bach [57], these signs are pathognomonic of triceps tendon disruption. Active elbow extension can be present, but extension against gravity is not allowed in the complete ruptures. It is important to execute a provocative maneuver such as the "modified" T. Campbell Thompson test [58] (Image 8.1).

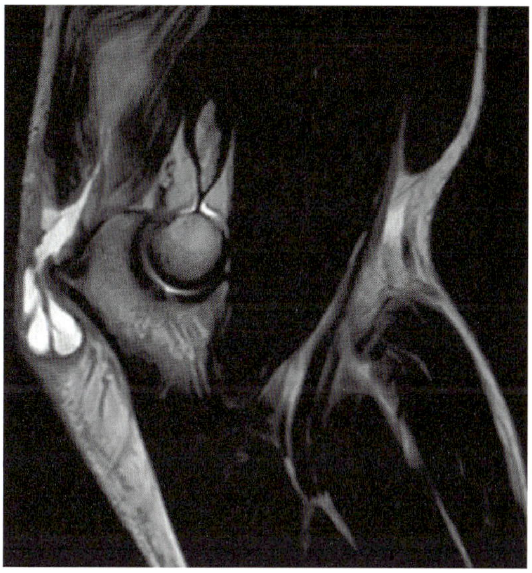

Image 8.1 MRI sagittal T2 view of a complete triceps tendon lesion

8.3.7 Triceps Snapping

The clinical study of the triceps snapping is usually performed with the patient's elbow on the examiner's open hand, with the thumb over the medial epicondyle; a passive movement from extension into flexion can reveal a single or double snap with anterior direction; if a double snap is found, the ulnar nerve determine the first one, followed by the medial head of the biceps [59]. The imaging study of triceps snapping can benefit of ultrasounds, most of all with a direct dynamic evaluation [60] of the ulnar nerve and/or of the medial head of the triceps; the MRI finds its utility, if the study is performed with the elbow in flexion [61] (Image 8.2).

8.3.8 Olecranon Bursitis

The diagnosis is clinical, based on a conspicuous swelling on the posterior elbow, caused by the effusion that develops because of bursal inflammation. Dealing with pain, in septic bursitis, all the elbow movements are painful, while in aseptic bursitis, pain is low or absent. The features of

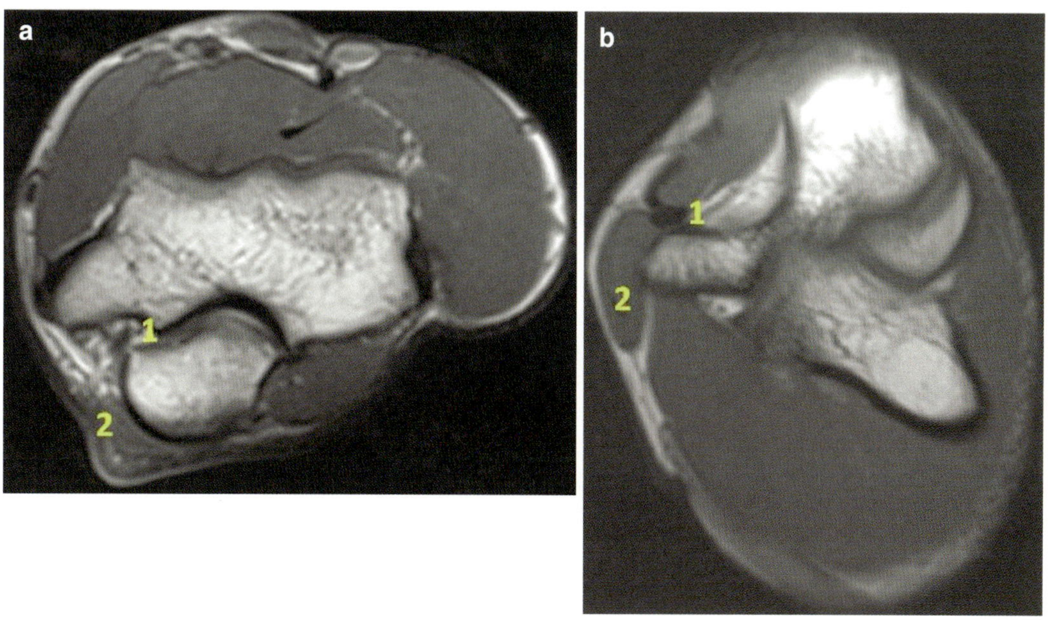

Image 8.2 MRI coronal T1 view of a case of triceps snapping: (**a**) in full extension, the snapping is not demonstrable; (**b**) in 120° of flexion, the MRI demonstrates a triceps snapping and dislocating ulnar nerve

aseptic and septic olecranon bursitis, if compared, do not show significant differences.

The skin temperature over the bursitis is higher in septic cases and normal in aseptic. Ultrasound scanning can be used for differential diagnosis in elbow swelling (synovial proliferations, calcifications, loose bodies, rheumatoid nodules, gouty tophi) and to evaluate the general quality of the fluid. Standard X-ray of the affected elbow is useful to exclude bony lesions and to study the joint. Rare is the use of MRI [50].

8.4 Treatments

8.4.1 Valgus Extension Overload Syndrome

The first treatment is conservative: rest from sport, NSAIDs, ice, and rehabilitation therapies, at least for the first 4 weeks. From the fifth week, a program of strengthening of active elbow stabilizers, the full elbow movement recovery, and a plyometric rehabilitation can be started. The restart of the sport-specific gesture with a specific and progressive program can be planned between the 16th and the 24th week from the beginning of rest.

Kancherla suggests rest and pitching limitation for 2–6 weeks, followed by a sport-specific rehabilitation (dynamic stabilization, reinforcement of flexor/pronator mass, in particular with eccentric exercises) and an interval throwing program; if this program is not effective in pain resolution, this author suggests to evaluate for surgical treatment [21].

An imaging evidence of posteromedial spurs should drive the choice toward surgical removal. Arthroscopy is very useful in this disorder, because it gives the possibility to assess the anterior compartment, looking for chondral lesions, loose bodies, and instability signs (by direct view of UCL anterior bundle or by the indirect sign of the medial joint side opening of 1 mm at 70° of flexion) [62].

Cohen underlined that arthroscopic debridement, olecranon spur excision, and loose body removal allow return to throwing sports and reliable subjective and objective results in carefully selected patients [52].

The posterior compartment study gives the possibility to treat olecranon spurs and analyze olecranon fossa. In literature, it has been proved that an olecranon resection lower than 8 mm. is not dangerous for an iatrogenic loss of ulnohumeral constraint and a consequential strain increasing on UCL, but we consider prudent to remove just the spurs and the posterior scar. After an arthroscopic arthrolysis, the rehabilitation program can be started after 2 weeks with the aim of coming back to the field between 3 and 6 months.

8.4.2 Olecranon Stress Fracture

Both conservative and surgical modalities have been purposed for the treatment of olecranon stress fractures. Several authors refer good results with conservative treatment based on rest, splint, and progressive return to sport [2, 42, 53]. Surgical treatment, however, is considered by some authors the better option for these patients, primarily with the aim of a quick competitive sport return [7] and secondly because the incidence of nonunion and delayed union is higher after conservative treatment and requires secondary intervention [7, 63, 64].

Lu suggests that minimally or nondisplaced transverse fractures respond successfully to conservative measures, including activity restriction or immobilization with splint/cast [38]. For those with displacement greater than 2 mm, surgical treatment leads to good results and lower nonunion rates. Lu also agree with Suzuki's statements [7] suggesting an early surgical approach for oblique olecranon stress fractures. Symptomatic tip fragments should be excised [2, 65].

Orava proposed the use of tension band for transverse fractures and screw in compression for the oblique ones [6]. Furthermore, arthroscopically assisted procedures can allow for additional diagnosis of associated lesions (loose bodies, osteophytes, ligament injury, and chondral damage). The postoperative treatment for olecranon stress fractures is based on splint with 90° of flexion for 7–10 days, followed by a 4-week rehabilitation with passive and then active flexion and extension and active pronation and supination, full active movement allowed at the sixth week, strengthening exercises during the eighth week, and interval throwing program in the 12th week.

8.4.3 Persistence of the Olecranon Physis

As for the previously described disorders, the initial management consists of rest, cessation of throwing, nonsteroidal anti-inflammatory drugs (NSAIDs) and ice, that can be successful in most patients. Surgical treatment may be beneficial after failing conservative management for 3 or 4 months, preferring low-profile systems, as tension-band wire construct and a single lag screw have been described as successful fixation options [35, 66]. Arthroscopy is not routinely used but can be useful in the cases of associated chondral lesions, that need a treatment.

After the surgery, a removable splint is usually used for 3 weeks, with passive and active movement from the second week; interval throwing program is allowed after 8 weeks and return to competition usually needs 4 months.

8.4.4 "Boxer's Elbow"

The treatment of boxer's elbow is based, firstly, on nonsurgical treatment (rest, ice, compression, elevation), physical therapy, NSAIDs, and eventually corticosteroid injections of the posterior side of the elbow. If this approach fails, surgical treatment can be considered. Elbow arthroscopy with debridement of the olecranon is usually the first choice, because it allows scar tissue and loose bodies removal, resection of posterolateral osteophytes, and partial resection of the olecranon tip. An arthroscopic stress test, to evaluate the medial opening, should always be performed [44].

8.4.5 "Handball Goalie's Elbow"

Basing on similar pathogenesis and clinical onset, handball goalie's elbow is treated in the same manner as VEOS.

8.4.6 Triceps Tendon Lesions/Tendonitis

Historically, partial tears of the triceps have been treated conservatively [57, 67, 68]. In his work on professional American football players, Mair [69] evaluated 11 complete ruptures and 10 partial ruptures; the author underlines that the extent of the tear may help to decide whether early surgery is necessary: MRI lesions of 90–100 % of the triceps tendon should be treated with early surgical repair. Partial tears (involving 75 % of the tendon on MRI or less) show the capacity to heal in some instances.

According to Morrey, partial tears can be treated nonoperatively for 6–8 weeks: if the symptoms does not disappear after this period, the patient should be surgically treated; for complete ruptures, immediate surgery is the treatment of choice. If the lesion is treated acutely, a direct suture of the tendon to the olecranon with nonabsorbable sutures is indicated. If a delayed reconstruction must be performed, Morrey suggest the anconeus slide, in the cases with minor defects and if this muscle is intact, or the Achilles tendon allograft for major lesions [49].

8.4.7 Triceps Snapping

Triceps snapping in athletes, when the symptoms are not tolerated and negatively affect the performance, can be surgically treated: a release of the medial head of the triceps is followed by a reattachment in a more lateral position, so to avoid its snapping over medial epicondyle. In some cases, a simple removal of the medial head of the triceps can be performed without compromising the triceps strength. Ulnar nerve decompression is usually performed, its anterior transposition is evaluated basing on the symptoms and on the specific findings on the surgical field (Image 8.3).

8.4.8 Olecranon Bursitis

Conservative management is indicated, as the first step, in non-painful cases: the patient should

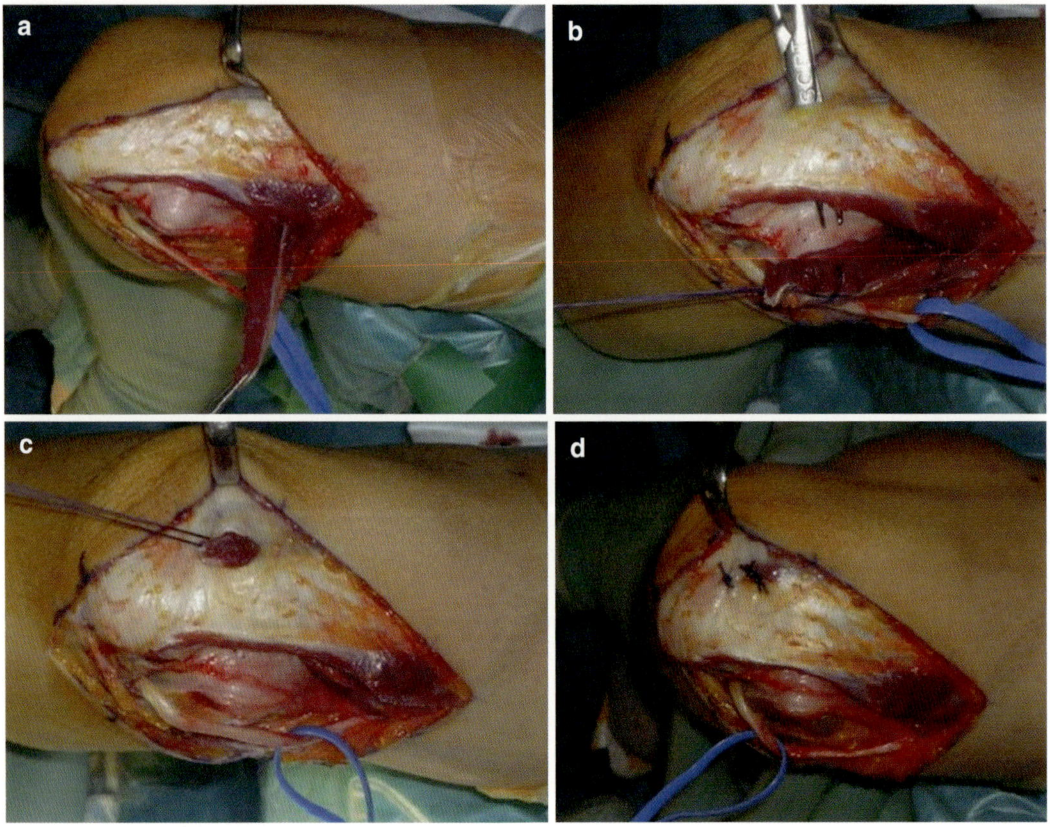

Image 8.3 Surgical images of the triceps snapping case, reported in the MRI of Fig. 2: (**a**) portion of the medial head of the triceps detached; (**b**) preparation for transposition; (**c**) portion of the medial head of the triceps transposed in a more lateral position; (**d**) suture of the portion of the medial head of the triceps into the new position with clinical disappearance of snapping

be advised to avoid repetitive movements and the elbow should be protected with a bandage or, in cases of major swelling, with a brace. Comorbidities have to be treated with specific therapies.

In painful conditions or in the cases where the suspect of infection is high, a liquid aspiration from bursitis should be performed in aseptic conditions, for microbiological study, white cell counts, and glucose level quantification; a concomitant blood sample is desirable, because it is useful to compare the amount of white cells and glucose in the two samples: a fluid glucose level of less than 50 % of the serum level is suggestive for infection. Steroid injection into the bursa must be carefully evaluated, because of the high complication rate (infections, skin atrophy, chronic pain), that with aspiration alone are absent. After the aspiration, a compressive bandage is needed. We prefer to use a splint with 90° of flexion for 5–7 days, with the aim to aid soft tissue healing, avoiding the movement.

Aseptic olecranon bursitis that cannot find a solution with these treatments and septic bursitis need surgical excision; in the septic cases, specific antibiotic therapy must be extended as necessary [50].

8.5 Pearls of the Treatment/Prevention

Based on biomechanical and epidemiological considerations, the posterior elbow pain can be determined from a set of traumatic factors, that can create several lesions over the whole elbow.

Once defined the surgical indication in the athlete with olecranon posterior pain, Paci suggests that the surgeon keeps a prudential attitude, treating the whole pattern of elbow lesions (loose bodies removal, spurs resections, UCL reconstruction), considering that these lesions find a common pathogenesis, with the aim to recreate a correct biomechanics, that is the base for a maximum sport-oriented recovery [39].

The key to success with VEOS and "handball goalie's elbow" is the early recognition of the condition and the careful conservative management of the symptoms with appropriate periods of rest. If those conservative measures fail, arthroscopic surgical management is typically successful in returning the athlete to competitive sports at every level. Modification to throwing biomechanics may not necessarily improve clinical outcomes because the stresses from repetitive throwing may be the driving force to injury.

Olecranon stress fractures must be correctly diagnosed, classified, and treated, keeping in mind that a conservative treatment can be successful but that in high-level athletes, an aggressive approach can accelerate the return to sport and prevent delayed union and nonunion.

Persistence of the olecranon physis is treated without surgery in the majority of cases; if surgery is required, after the failure of conservative treatment, a synthesis with low-profile systems should be preferred; some authors suggest the use of bone graft to improve healing.

The boxer's elbow is rare and can find its solution with conservative treatment, but often, arthroscopy of the posterior elbow is useful to obtain a quick sport return.

The approach for the posterior elbow pain in patients with skeletal immaturity must keep in highest importance the prevention [70] that needs a multidisciplinary approach (pediatrics, sports medicine, orthopedics, physiotherapy, etc.), aiming to preserve joint integrity and function and conciliating a healthy and harmonious growth with the sport. The prevention is the keystone of the athlete's treatment, most of all for the younger ones, as well established with Baseball Little League for pitchers.

The surgery must be the last step of an articulated treatment and should be performed in the ideal physical and mental conditions (end of season, high motivation in return, etc.); the medical team must take care of every athlete "like a professional athlete," well defining from the beginning all the steps of the treatment.

8.6 Results after Treatment (Evidence Based)

8.6.1 Valgus Extension Overload Syndrome

Reddy [71] refers a return to competitive sport after arthroscopy treatment of VEOS for 85 % of the athletes treated.

In case of medial instability, the arthroscopic treatment should be followed by a UCL reconstruction that can warrant a return to competitive sport in a percentage of cases from 81 to 95 in literature [72–74]. After a UCL reconstruction, the mean time to come back in competitive sport is at least 12 months. Dugas refers that the recurrence of the symptoms or clinical findings of VEOS are rare and have not been reported in any of the large series of elbow procedures in athletes. In his clinical experience, recurrence of posteromedial impingement is secondary to an underappreciation of the underlying medial ligamentous laxity and other predisposing pathology [27].

8.6.2 Olecranon Stress Fracture

Several authors refer good results with conservative treatment: Nuber suggests a treatment based on rest, splint, and progressive return to sport with good results [2]; Schickendantz refers that seven professional athletes with olecranon stress fractures came back to competitive sport with a personalized conservative treatment [42]. Patel expresses good results with rest, pitching avoidance, and limitation to complete extension for 4 weeks with splints; after this period, he allows full ROM and resistance, limiting the valgus stresses for 6 weeks; from the sixth week, sport-specific exercises are begun and from the eighth week, the interval throwing program can start [53].

Suzuki [7] and Nakaji [37], based on the good results obtained in their cases, suggest an early ORIF for olecranon stress fractures in the athletes. Paci performed an ORIF with a compression screw in 18 high-level athletes (in addition, two patients underwent a medial compartment reconstruction), that had poor results after conservative treatment, with a mean FU of 6.2 years. All cases showed the fracture healing and 94 % of patients return to the same or higher level of competition in a mean of 28 weeks. Despite the percentage of sport return and the good functional results, this study shows a high rate of concomitant surgical procedures and additional procedures: 6 of the 18 patients underwent hardware removal (two because of infection), two needed a second time reconstruction of the medial compartment because of persistent instability, and two patients needed olecranon spurs or loose bodies removal for unresolved pain. In the case series described by Paci, the return to competitive sport has been reached in a mean of 29 weeks (8–45) [39].

8.6.3 Persistence of the Olecranon Physis

As underlined by Charlton, the conservative treatment is successful in most patients [35]. However, resolution of symptoms can take as long as 4 months [75].

Dealing with surgery, the highest rates of successful union have been shown in patients undergoing bone grafting [35, 75], with the aim of filling the bone gap that this patients usually present. Charlton and Chandler found that operative stabilization with internal fixation and autogenous iliac crest bone grafting can resolve symptoms and allow a skeletally mature overhead athlete to return to previous throwing performance, maintained to a 32 months FU. Fixation alone, however, may lead to a 66 % failure rate [35].

8.6.4 "Boxer's Elbow"

In [Valkering] case series, the arthroscopic treatment of five professional boxers with partial resection of the olecranon tip and removal of scar tissue and loose bodies brought to an improvement in ROM and a return to their preexisting level of boxing activity [44].

8.6.5 Triceps Tendon Lesions/Tendonitis

Mair [69] recommends early surgical repair of complete or near complete tears of the triceps tendon; in his case series, all of the 11 players with complete tears underwent early surgery with a direct tendon to bone repair, with a full range of motion at the final follow-up (3 years). Ten of these 11 athletes returned to the same sport level. Nine athletes with partial tears of the triceps had conservative treatment: the healing was obtained in six cases and a delayed surgery was necessary for the other three.

8.6.6 Triceps Snapping

At our knowledge, no definitive results of the treatment of this disorder have been published in long FU case series.

8.7 Pitfalls of the Treatment

In VEOS, it is important to note that significant posteromedial olecranon resection can lead to increased elbow valgus, as suggested by Kamineni and Ahmad [19, 40], increasing strain on the UCL. Goals of surgical treatment are osteophyte removal with preservation of normal bone. If a valgus stress test is positive, suggesting UCL insufficiency, reconstruction can be performed at the same time.

In the treatment of olecranon stress fractures with metal wires, it is important to avoid a secondary hardware pullout: to prevent this complication, we are used to reach the anterior ulnar cortex with the wires, under intensifier; moreover, to minimize pin migration, we adopt pins built with a proximal eyelet for the cerclage, so to secure the pins by the cerclage itself.

In the triceps tendon reconstruction is important to exploit a bone fragment if it is present, we can perform a bone synthesis, that can help the surgeon in the tendon repair; if no olecranon fragment is seen, the triceps tendon should be well basted with high-strength wires, that should be divergent, with the aim of recreating a wide "footprint" of the triceps on the olecranon.

Approaching a triceps snapping, the ulnar nerve must be carefully studied: if, as usual, also the ulnar nerve snaps with triceps, during the surgery, it should be transposed.

Great attention is necessary with olecranon bursitis: a liquid aspiration should be performed only when necessary, in the cases of suspect infection and in conditions of absolute asepsis. Steroid injection into the bursa must be carefully evaluated, because of the high complication rates (infections, skin atrophy, chronic pain) that with aspiration alone are absent.

References

1. Waris W. Elbow injuries in javelin throwers. Acta Chir Scand. 1946;93:563–75.
2. Nuber GW, Diment MT. Olecranon stress fractures in throwers. A report of two cases and a review of the literature. Clin Orthop. 1992;278:58–61.
3. Rao PS, Rao SK, Navadgi BC. Olecranon stress fracture in a weight lifter: a case report. Br J Sports Med. 2001;35:72–3.
4. Wilkerson RD, Johns JC. Nonunion of an olecranon stress fracture in an adolescent gymnast. A case report. Am J Sports Med. 1990;18:432–4.
5. Maffulli N, Chan D, Aldridge MJ. Overuse injuries of the olecranon in young gymnasts. J Bone Joint Surg Br. 1992;74:305–8.
6. Orava S, Hulkko A. Delayed unions and nonunions of stress fractures in athletes. Am J Sports Med. 1988; 16:378–82.
7. Suzuki K, Minami A, Suenaga N, Kondoh M. Oblique stress fracture of the olecranon in baseball pitchers. J Shoulder Elbow Surg. 1997;6:491–4.
8. Barnes DA, Tullos HS. An analysis of 100 symptomatic baseball players. Am J Sports Med. 1978;6:62–7.
9. Miller JE. Javelin thrower's elbow. J Bone Joint Surg. 1960;42B:788–92.
10. National Federation of State High School Associations. National Federation of State High School Associations 2012–2013 High school athletics participation survey. 2013.
11. An K-N, Morrey BF. Biomechanics of the elbow. In: Morrey BF, editor. The elbow and its disorders. Philadelphia: WB Saunders; 1985. p. 43–61.
12. Regan WD, Korinek SL, Morrey BF, An K-N. Biomechanical study of ligaments around the elbow joint. Clin Orthop. 1991;271:170–9.
13. Schwab GH, Bennett JB, Woods GW, et al. Biomechanics of elbow instability: the role of the medial collateral ligament. Clin Orthop Relat Res. 1980;146:42–52.
14. Morrey BF. Applied anatomy and biomechanics of the elbow joint. Instr Course Lect. 1986;35:59–68.
15. Jobe FW, Kvitne RS. Elbow instability in the athlete. Instr Course Lect. 1991;40:17–23.
16. Sojbjerg JO, Ovesen J, Nielsen S. Experimental elbow instability after transection of the medial collateral ligament. Clin Orthop Relat Res. 1987;218:186–90.
17. Callaway GH, Field LD, Deng XH, et al. Biomechanical evaluation of the medial collateral ligament of the elbow. J Bone Joint Surg Am. 1997;79(8):1223–31.
18. Floris S, Olsen BS, Dalstra M, Sojbjerg JO, Sneppen O. The medial collateral ligament of the elbow joint: anatomy and kinematics. J Shoulder Elbow Surg. 1998;7:345–51.
19. Kamineni S, Hirahara H, Pomianowski S, et al. Partial posteromedial olecranon resection: a kinematic study. J Bone Joint Surg Am. 2004;85:1005–11.
20. Wilson FD, Andrews JR, Blackburn TA, McCluskey G. Valgus extension overload in the pitching elbow. Am J Sports Med. 1983;11:83–8.
21. Kancherla VK, Caggiano NM, Matullo KS. Elbow injuries in the throwing athlete. Orthop Clin North Am. 2014;45(4):571–85. doi:10.1016/j.ocl.2014.06.012. Review.
22. Andrews JR, Timmerman LA. Outcome of elbow surgery in professional baseball players. Am J Sports Med. 1995;23:407–13.
23. Fleisig GS, Andrews JR, Dillman CJ, Escamilla RF. Kinetics of baseball pitching with implications about injury mechanisms. Am J Sports Med. 1995;23:233–9.
24. Werner SL, Fleisig GS, Dillman CJ. Biomechanics of the elbow during baseball pitching. J Orthop Sports Phys Ther. 1993;17:274–8.
25. Davidson PA, Pink M, Perry J, et al. Functional anatomy of the flexor pronator muscle group in relation to the medial collateral ligament of the elbow. Am J Sports Med. 1995;23(2):245–50.
26. Glousman RE, Barron J, Jobe FW, et al. An electromyographic analysis of the elbow in normal and injured pitchers with medial collateral ligament insufficiency. Am J Sports Med. 1992;20(3):311–7.
27. Dugas JR. Valgus extension overload: diagnosis and treatment. Clin Sports Med. 2010;29(4):645–54. doi:10.1016/j.csm.2010.07.001. Review.
28. Ahmad CS, Park MC, ElAttrache NS. Elbow medial ulnar collateral ligament insufficiency alters posteromedial olecranon contact. Am J Sports Med. 2004; 32:1607–12.

29. Auer M, Jansson K, Josefsson PO, Linden B. Osteochondritis dissecans of the elbow. Clin Orthop. 1992;284:156–60.
30. Takahara M, Shundo M, Kondo M, Suzuki K, Nambu T, Ogino T. Early detection of osteochondritis dissecans of the capitellum in young baseball players. Report of three cases. J Bone Joint Surg Am. 1998; 80:892–7.
31. King JW, Brelsford HJ, Tullos HS. Analysis of the pitching arm of the professional baseball pitcher. Clin Orthop. 1969;67:116–23.
32. Aguinaldo AL, Chambers H. Correlation of throwing mechanics with elbow valgus load in adult baseball pitchers. Am J Sports Med. 2009;37:2043–8.
33. Brukner P. Stress fractures of the upper limb. Sports Med. 1998;26(6):415–24. Review.
34. Waris W. Elbow injuries of javelin-throwers. Acta Chir Scand. 1946;93:563–75.
35. Charlton WP, Chandler RW. Persistence of the olecranon physis in baseball players: results following operative management. J Shoulder Elbow Surg. 2003; 12(1):59–62.
36. Rettig AC, Wurth TR, Mieling P. Nonunion of olecranon stress fractures in adolescent baseball pitchers: a case series of 5 athletes. Am J Sports Med. 2006;34(4): 653–6.
37. Nakaji N, Fujioka H, Tanaka J, Sugimoto K, Yoshiya S, Fujita K, Kurosaka M. Stress fracture of the olecranon in an adult baseball player. Knee Surg Sports Traumatol Arthrosc. 2006;14(4):390–3. Epub 2005 Apr 26.
38. Lu CC, Chen SK, Wang CW, Chou PH. Chondromalacia of trochlear notch after healing of olecranon stress fracture: a case report. Arch Orthop Trauma Surg. 2006;126(4):271–4. Epub 2005 Oct 20.
39. Paci JM, Dugas JR, Guy JA, Cain Jr EL, Fleisig GS, Hurst C, Wilk KE, Andrews JR. Cannulated screw fixation of refractory olecranon stress fractures with and without associated injuries allows a return to baseball. Am J Sports Med. 2013;41(2):306–12. doi:10.1177/0363546512469089. Epub 2012 Dec 6.
40. Ahmad CS, ElAttrache NS. Valgus extension overload syndrome and stress injury of the olecranon. Clin Sports Med. 2004;23(4):665–76. x. Review.
41. Cain Jr EL, Dugas JR, Wolf RS, et al. Elbow injuries in throwing athletes: a current concepts review. Am J Sports Med. 2003;31(4):621–35.
42. Schickendantz MS, Ho CP, Koh J. Stress injury of the proximal ulna in professional baseball players. Am J Sports Med. 2002;30(5):737–41.
43. Furushima K, Itoh Y, Iwabu S, Yamamoto Y, Koga R, Shimizu M. Classification of olecranon stress fractures in baseball players. Am J Sports Med. 2014;42(6):1343–51 [Epub ahead of print].
44. Valkering KP, van der Hoeven H, Pijnenburg BC. Posterolateral elbow impingement in professional boxers. Am J Sports Med. 2008;36(2):328–32. Epub 2007 Nov 6.
45. Tyrdal S, Olsen BS. Hyperextension of the elbow joint: pathoanatomy and kinematics of ligament injuries. J Shoulder Elbow Surg. 1998;7(3):272–83.
46. Popovic N, Lemaire R. Hyperextension trauma to the elbow: radiological and ultrasonographic evaluation in handball goalkeepers. Br J Sports Med. 2002;36(6):452–6.
47. Akgun U, Karahan M, Tiryaki C, Erol B, Engebretsen L. Direction of the load on the elbow of the ball blocking handball goalie. Knee Surg Sports Traumatol Arthrosc. 2008;16(5):522–30.
48. Sabick MB, Torry MR, Lawton RL, Hawkins RJ. Valgus torque in youth baseball pitchers: a biomechanical study. J Shoulder Elbow Surg. 2004;13(3): 349–55.
49. Morrey BF. Rupture of the triceps tendon. In: Morrey BF, editor. The elbow and its disorders. 4th ed. Philadelphia: Saunders Elsevier; 2009. p. 359–88. ISBN 978-1-4160-2902-1.
50. Elliott J. Olecranon bursitis. In: Stanley D, Trail IA, editors. Operative elbow surgery. Edinburgh: Churchill Livingstone Elsevier; 2012. p. 547–54.
51. Kibler WB, Sciascia A. Kinetic chain contributions to elbow function and dysfunction in sports. Clin Sports Med. 2004;23:545–52.
52. Cohen SB, Valko C, Zoga A, Dodson CC, Ciccotti MG. Posteromedial elbow impingement: magnetic resonance imaging findings in overhead throwing athletes and results of arthroscopic treatment. Arthroscopy. 2011;27(10):1364–70. doi:10.1016/j.arthro.2011.06.012. Epub 2011 Aug 27.
53. Patel RM, Lynch TS, Amin NH, Calabrese G, Gryzlo SM, Schickendantz MS. The thrower's elbow. Orthop Clin North Am. 2014;45(3):355–76. doi:10.1016/j.ocl.2014.03.007.
54. Andrews JR, Clancy WG, Whiteside JA. On-field evaluation and treatment of common athletic injuries. St Louis: Mosby; 1997. p. 202.
55. Matsuura T, Kashiwaguchi S, Iwase T, et al. The value of using radiographic criteria for the treatment of persistent symptomatic olecranon physis in adolescent throwing athletes. Am J Sports Med. 2010;38(1): 141–5.
56. Tyrdal S, Bahr R. High prevalence of elbow problems among goalkeepers in European team handball 'handball goalie's elbow'. Scand J Med Sci Sports. 1996; 6:297–302.
57. Bach Jr BR, Warren RF, Wickiewicz TL. Triceps rupture, a case report and literature review. Am J Sports Med. 1987;15:285–9.
58. Viegas SF. Avulsion of the triceps tendon. Orthop Rev. 1990;19:533–6.
59. Benson EC, Athwal GS, King GJW. Clinical assessment of the elbow. In: Stanley D, Trail IA, editors. Operative elbow surgery. Edinburgh: Churchill Livingstone Elsevier; 2012. p. 45–65.
60. Spinner RJ, Goldner RD, Lee RA. Diagnosis of snapping triceps with US. Radiology. 2002;224(3):933–4. author reply 934. No abstract available.
61. Spinner RJ, Goldner RD. Snapping of the medial head of the triceps and recurrent dislocation of the ulnar nerve. Anatomical and dynamic factors. J Bone Joint Surg Am. 1998;80(2):239–47.

62. Field L, Savoie F. The arthroscopic evaluation and management of elbow trauma and instability. Oper Tech Sports Med. 1998;6(1).
63. Wilkerson RD, Johns JC. Nonunion of an olecranon stress fracture in an adolescent gymnast. A case report. Am J Sport Med. 1990;18:432–4.
64. Banas MP, Lewis RA. Nonunion of an olecranon epiphyseal plate stress fracture in an adolescent. Orthopedics. 1995;18:1111–2.
65. Hulkko A, Orava S, Nikula P. Stress fractures of the olecranon in javelin throwers. Int J Sport Med. 1986;7:210–3.
66. Lowery Jr WD, Kurzweil PR, Forman SK, et al. Persistence of the olecranon physis: a cause of "little league elbow". J Shoulder Elbow Surg. 1995;4(2):143–7.
67. Anderson RL. Traumatic rupture of the triceps tendon. J Trauma. 1979;19:134.
68. Levy M, Goldberg I, Meir I. Fracture of the head of the radius with a tear or avulsion of the triceps tendon. J Bone Joint Surg. 1982;64B:70–2.
69. Mair SD, Isbell WM, Gill TJ, Schlegel TF, Hawkins RJ. Triceps tendon ruptures in professional football players. Am J Sports Med. 2004;32(2):431–4.
70. Olsen SJ, Fleisig GS, Dun S, Andrews JR. Risk factors for shoulder and elbow injuries in adolescent baseball pitchers. Am J Sports Med. 2006; 34:905.
71. Reddy AS, Kvitne RS, Yocum LA, et al. Arthroscopy of the elbow: a long-term clinical review. Arthroscopy. 2000;16(6):588–94.
72. Azar FM, Andrews JR, Wilk KE, Groh D. Operative treatment of ulnar collateral ligament injuries of the elbow in athletes. Am J Sports Med. 2000;28: 16–23.
73. Thompson WH, Jobe FW, Yocum LA, Pink MM. Ulnar collateral ligament reconstruction in athletes: muscle splitting approach without transposition of the ulnar nerve. J Shoulder Elbow Surg. 2001; 10:152–7.
74. Wong AS, Baratz ME. Sports injuries of the elbow. In: Stanley D, Trail IA, editors. Operative elbow surgery. Edinburgh: Churchill Livingstone Elsevier; 2012. p. 493–509.
75. Skak SV. Fracture of the olecranon through a persistent physis in an adult. A case report. J Bone Joint Surg Am. 1993;75(2):272–5.

9 Lateral-Sided Elbow Pain

Paolo Arrigoni, Riccardo D'Ambrosi,
and Pietro Randelli

9.1 Introduction

Lateral epicondylitis is a common source of pain on the lateral side of the elbow. This tendinopathy has an incidence of 1.3 % in the population between 30 and 64 years, with a peak between 45 and 54 [1]. It typically affects the dominant upper extremity and is associated with a repetitive and forceful activity [2]. Lateral epicondylitis is believed to be a degenerative process, which originates from repetitive microtraumas. Typically, samples from the affected tissue show angiofibroblastic hyperplasia at the origin of the extensor tendons [3]. Activities requiring repeated contraction of the wrist extensors are implicated, with the extensor carpi radialis brevis (ECRB) tendon most commonly involved. Studies comparing cadaveric and surgical specimens indicate that lateral epicondylitis evolves through several stages, beginning with degenerative angiogenesis up to fibrosis and calcification [3–5]. Although the lateral epicondylitis is commonly known as tennis elbow, this term is not entirely correct. This tendinopathy is frequently work related and occurs in patients not playing tennis [6]; however, it has been estimated that 10–50 % of people who regularly play tennis do develop the condition at some time during their careers [7]. Epicondylitis is more common in male than female tennis players, unlike what happens in the general population (Table 9.1). Lateral epicondylitis is more frequent than medial-sided elbow pain, with ratios reportedly ranging from 4:1 to 7:1 [8]. Dominant elbow is commonly involved. Acute onsets of symptoms occur more often in young athletes; chronic recalcitrant symptoms typically occur in older patients.

P. Arrigoni, MD (✉) • R. D'Ambrosi, MD
P. Randelli, MD
U.O. Ortopedia e Traumatologia II,
IRCCS Policlinico San Donato,
San Donato Milanese, Milan, Italy
e-mail: arrigoni.p@gmail.com

9.2 Anatomy

In order to better understand the etiology of this tendinopathy, it is essential to analyze the anatomic relationships of the lateral compartment of the elbow. Cohen and Romeo [9] showed the relationships that exist between the extensor carpi radialis longus (ECL) and ECRB. The

Table 9.1 Risk factors for lateral epicondylitis

Risk factors
Overuse in sport
Smoking
Obesity
Oral steroid use
Age 45–54 years
Other tendinopathies
Repetitive movement
Diabetes
White race

L.A. Pederzini et al. (eds.), *Elbow and Sport*, DOI 10.1007/978-3-662-48742-6_9

ECRL origin is entirely muscular along the lateral supracondylar ridge of the humerus. The shape of the muscle is triangular, with the apex positioned proximally. Instead, the origin of the ECRB is entirely tendinous. Although the origin of the ECRB is mixed with that of the extensor digitorum communis, the authors showed [9] how dissecting from distal to proximal and following their under surface the two tendons can be isolated behind the humerus. The origin of the ECRB is located just below the distal-most tip of the lateral supracondylar ridge. The footprint of the tendon has a diamond shape of about 13×7 mm (Fig. 9.1). At the radiocapitellar joint, the tendon lies at the level of the front portion of the capsule, but it is possible to easily isolate the two structures at this level.

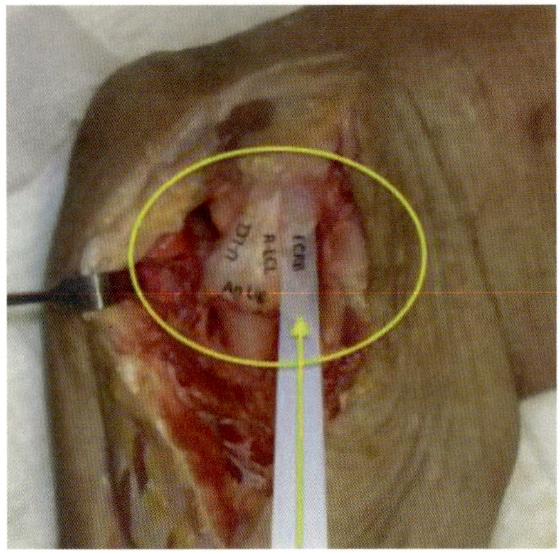

Fig. 9.1 Cadaveric preparation in right elbow: in the *yellow circle* the anatomy of LCL complex; the *yellow arrow* shows ECRB and close relation with R-LCL (An Lig. = Annular ligament)

9.3 Pathomechanics

Biomechanical analysis has shown that eccentric contractions of the extensor carpi radialis brevis (ECRB) muscle during backhand tennis swings are the cause of repetitive microtraumas that result in microtears in the origin of the tendon [10]. Other authors have suggested different causes like direct trauma in the lateral region of the elbow or relative hypovascularity of the region, fluoroquinolone antibiotics, and anatomic predisposition [11–13]. Cyriax was the first to theorize that tears of the common extensor origin were involved in the disease process [14]. Subsequently, other authors showed that the nature of the disease is actually a degenerative tendinopathy. Goldie described the histological presence of granulation tissue found at the origin of the ECRB [15]. Macroscopic tearing in association with the histological findings was described by Coonrad and Hooper [6]. Nirschl called these histological changes "angiofibroblastic hyperplasia [16, 17]." In his study, he noted gray friable tissue characterized by disorganized collagen formation with immature fibroblastic and vascular elements. Subsequently, increased rates of apoptosis and cellular autophagy have been observed in tenocytes, resulting in disruption of extracellular collagen matrix and weakening of the tendon [18]. These changes at the tendon's origin are the pathologic healing response to microtears caused by repetitive eccentric or concentric overloading of the extensor muscle mass [19]. Several studies have suggested that the origin of the extensor digitorum communis (EDC) is also implicated in lateral epicondylitis [20, 21].

9.4 Clinical Presentation

Patients complain of pain that radiates from the lateral epicondyle down to the forearm, often associated with weakness and difficulty in the handgrip.

Nirschl has divided symptoms into seven phases [22, 23]. A history of previous occurrence of tennis elbow also suggests tendinopathy. Imaging techniques such as magnetic resonance or diagnostic ultrasound are useful to identify the calcifications, tears, or ruptures of the ECRB [24, 25]. Physical examination should begin with cervical spine and be followed by the entire upper extremity. The examination proceeds then to the elbow. The elbow is tender over the lateral epicondyle and slightly distal, into the extensor mass.

Table 9.2 Different diagnoses of lateral elbow pain

Pathology	History	Physical examination
Cervical spondylosis	Neck pain Radicular pain to the elbow	Symptoms with spine compression extension
Radial tunnel syndrome	Insidious pain at lateral elbow	Pain 2–4 cm distal to epicondyle
Posterior interosseous nerve compression	Insidious pain at lateral elbow and weakness	Weakness of wrist and finger extensors
Intra-articular bodies	Trauma	Clicking or limitation of range of motion
Chondral lesions	Trauma	Clicking or limitation of range of motion
Tumors	Night pain Prior malignancy	Palpable mass
Avascular necrosis	Alcohol abuse HIV Sickle cell anemia Corticosteroids	Joint effusion, mechanical symptoms
Osteochondritis dissecans	Gymnast Throwers, adolescent	Joint effusion, mechanical symptoms

Thomsen maneuver (resisted wrist extension with the elbow in full extension and forearm in pronation) or maximal wrist flexion can exacerbate pain at the lateral epicondyle. The first maneuver causes painful eccentric contraction at the origin of the ECRB. The second maneuver places the ECRB on maximal stretch, passively tensioning the muscle origin and thus causing pain. In order to exclude the presence of a plica, the elbow must be flexed passively with the forearm pronated and supinated. If a plica is involved, the point of maximal tenderness is usually located more distally and posteriorly, over the radiocapitellar joint, compared to lateral epicondylitis. Other causes of lateral sided elbow pain can be nerve entrapments at one or more sites, such as radial tunnel syndrome or posterior interosseous nerve (PIN) syndrome. Up to 5 % of patients with lateral epicondylitis presents radial nerve entrapment [26].

Pain elicited with resisted supination (when the nerve is trapped in the supinator muscle) or with resisted long-finger extension (when the nerve is trapped at the ECRB) can indicate PIN entrapment. Differential diagnosis between nerve entrapment and lateral epicondylitis can be difficult. The treatment of the two conditions is entirely different. The elbow examination is completed with a standard evaluation of elbow effusion, stability, and range of motion. The examination then moves distally toward the forearm and the hand. Grip strength should be tested to determine whether it decreases compared with the unaffected side or causes significant discomfort. Neurovascular status is a basic component of the examination and should be noted. Differential diagnosis for atraumatic lateral elbow pain may include radicular cervical spine disease, radial nerve compression, intra-articular loose bodies, and chondral lesions. Tumors, avascular necrosis, and osteochondritis dissecans of the capitellum, even if less common, may be considered as well (Table 9.2).

9.5 Surgical Treatment

Conservative treatment is the gold standard. However, between 5 % and 10 % of these patients develop persistent symptoms that may require surgical treatment. Particularly, persistent pain at night can determine the choice of surgical treatment. Surgical treatment with tendon release should be reserved in case of failure of the conservative treatment that should not last less than 6 months.

Surgical treatment can be percutaneous, open, or arthroscopic, with success rates ranging between 65 % and 95 % [27].

9.6 Percutaneous Treatment

A blade, often number 11, is inserted perpendicular to the skin anterior to the lateral epicondyle, then a one-centimeter-long skin incision is performed. A complete release of the common extensor origin is performed moving the tip of the blade anteriorly and inferiorly from the lateral epicondyle. A further displacement is then achieved by the Mill's manipulation, consisting of a forcible, full extension of the elbow with the forearm fully pronated and the wrist and fingers held in flexion. At the end of the procedure, a gap of one centimeter, on average, is easily palpable between the lateral epicondyle and the retracted tendons. This procedure is preferred by many authors because it's less invasive and the surgical results are similar to those of more elaborated procedures [28]. Baumgard and Schwartz [28] reported 91 % excellent (no symptoms under any circumstances), 0 % fair (improvement but still symptomatic), and 9 % unsatisfactory (no improvement) after an average follow-up of 34 months (range: 14–81 months). Another case series of percutaneous release reported similar results [29]. Powell and Burke [30] reviewed 20 patients after a follow-up raging from 5 to 36 months. They showed 85 % excellent or good results. Grundberg and Dobson [31] presented the results of percutaneous release in 32 cases of tennis elbow. With a mean follow-up of 26 months, he had 90.6 % of excellent and good results. More recently, Nazar et al. [32] showed how percutaneous release of the epicondylar muscles has a high rate of success: it is relatively simple to perform, it is done as a day-case procedure, and it doesn't show complications. As a matter of fact, the postoperative outcome was between good and excellent in most patients. Eighty-seven percent of patients had complete pain relief with no complications reported.

All the patients returned to their normal jobs and hobbies such as gardening, horse riding, and playing musical instruments. We personally do not routinely choose this technique because of the theoretical risk of damaging part of the radial component of the lateral collateral ligament, although this is not supported by the available literature.

9.7 Open Treatment

Several open techniques have been described. The original technique (1955 Bosworth) [33] involves the identification and removal of the abnormal tissue that surrounds the common origin of the extensor tendons, the creation of a bone bed that promotes healing, and finally the reconstruction of the overlying aponeurosis. First of all, it is necessary to identify the ERCB tendon: its origin is located below the lateral epicondylar prominence, along a longitudinal ridge, and is directed from the upper part of the capitellum to the level of the radiohumeral joint.

Its tendon runs below the extensor digitorum communis and its aponeurosis, distally to the epicondyle. It can be easily isolated, proceeding from anterior to posterior and starting at the junction between the ECRL and EDC aponeurosis. The undersurface of the ECRB tendon can be elevated from the ECRL muscle in oblique fashion. The aponeurosis of the EDC lies on top of the ECRB and is tightly opposed. The ECRB tendon is debrided and the epicondylar origin denuded or drilled. The open approach leads to greater visualization of the operative field and the pathologic tissue; however, it is associated with a higher incidence of complications and a longer time to return to work [34].

9.8 Arthroscopic Treatment

Arthroscopic release is especially indicated when a concomitant intra-articular pathology is suspected. The advantage of exploring the joint is recently increasing the indications. Patient is placed in lateral decubitus position with the operative arm supported by an arm holder at 100° of flexion/90° of abduction at the level of the shoulder. The elbow is positioned at 90° of flexion, with the forearm hanging free from gravity (Fig. 9.2). Forty milliliter of sterile saline solution is injected

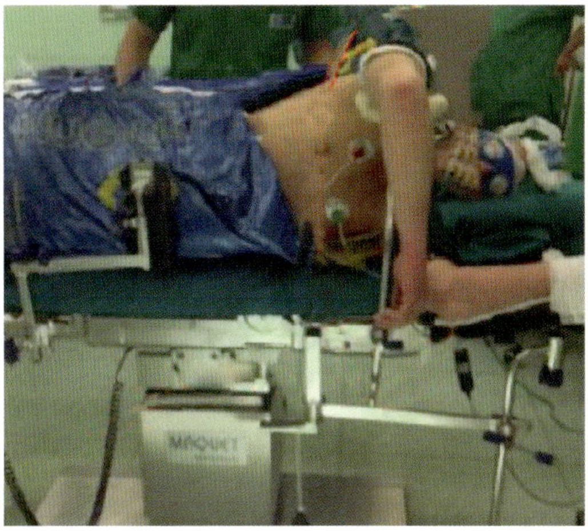

Fig. 9.2 Arthroscopic set-up: patient is placed in a modified lateral decubitus position with the operative arm positioned in 100° of flexion/90° of abduction at the level of the shoulder by any holder. The elbow is positioned in 90° of flexion, with the forearm hanging free to gravity

before placing the portals to distend the elbow joint. A proximal anteromedial portal is created 2–3 cm proximal to the medial humeral epicondyle and 1 cm anterior to the intramuscular septum. Then a 30° arthroscope is inserted into this portal. This allows intra-articular diagnostic evaluation of the anterior compartment. The proximal anterolateral portal is located approximately 3 cm proximal and 1 cm anterior to the lateral epicondyle. A retractor, aimed at the radiocapitellar joint to protect the posterior interosseous nerve, can be inserted through this portal. The instruments are introduced through the anterolateral portal, located 1.5–2 cm proximal and 1 cm anterior to the lateral epicondyle.

9.8.1 Standard Procedure

As decribed by Baker and Jones [27], any lateral synovitis is debrided and the lateral capsule is released. The capsule is usually intact, but occasionally it is possible to identify a disruption of the underlying capsule. A monopolar thermal release of the lateral soft tissues is performed. With this method, the capsule is first incised or released from the humerus. After the capsule is retracted distally, the ECRB tendon is visualized posteriorly and the ECRL can be identified more anteriorly. Once the capsule is adequately resected, the ECRB origin is released from the epicondyle: starting at the top of the capitellum, the release is then carried posteriorly [35]. Typically, the entire ECRB retracts distally away from the humerus. Care is taken not to release the extensor aponeurosis that lies behind the ECRB tendon. This structure can be seen as a striped background of transversely oriented tendon and muscular fibers much less distinct than the ECRB. It is located posterior to the ECRL.

9.8.2 Preferred Technique [36]

A limited anterolateral V-shaped capsulotomy is performed with a hooked electrocautery device, under visualization with a 30° arthroscope. The superior arm of the V is performed parallel to the distal humerus. By tensioning the capsule with pronation, the radial component of the LCL (R-LCL) is better visualized. Care must be taken to perform the capsulotomy with the forearm pronated in order to tension the R-LCL and facilitate its protection. Pronation also offers the advantage of moving the posterior interosseous nerve further medial, away from the surgical area. The inferior limit of the capsulotomy is approximately 0.5–1 cm superior to the radial head. A 70° arthroscope is then inserted through the window created by the capsulotomy. The 70° arthroscope offers a frontal view of the most lateral aspect of the lateral compartment with the capsule/R-LCL defining the articular side and the tendon fibers of the ECRB on the extracapsular side. With the 70° scope in the anteromedial portal, an accurate soft-tissue dissection between the capsule/R-LCL and ECRB is then performed. This allows an accurate definition of the surgical plane between the ECRB and R-LCL.

These two structures must be clearly visualized as distinct and independent in order to proceed with a safer resection. Then a hooked electrocautery device is advanced through the anterolateral portal.

The hooked shape allows the surgeon to "hook" the ECRB tendon and to perform the

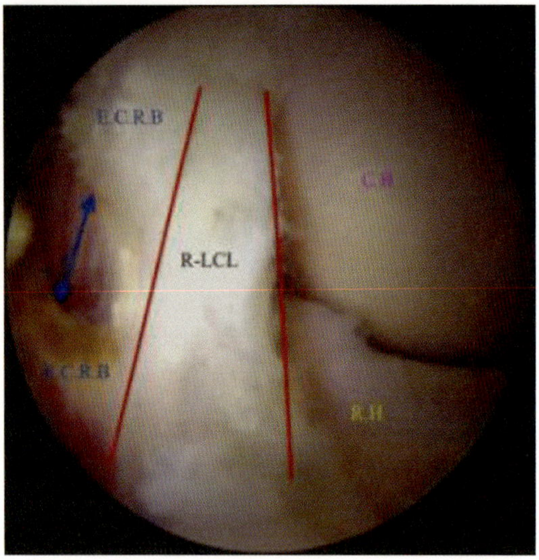

Fig. 9.3 Arthroscopic intraoperative picture after ECRB release of right elbow. The *arrow* shows the gap left after tendon release. The ECRB tendon stump is visible in the upper part of the figure (*CH* capitulum humeri, *RH* radial head)

release from the inner/anterior part to the outer/posterior aspect, approximately 1 cm from the proximal bone insertion (Fig. 9.3), while protecting and preserving the R-LCL. This step is the main difference compared to the standard technique. The posterior common extensors origin is then assessed. This independent structure is more posterior to the ECRB tendon. The common tendon is probed to check its condition. During the first 48 h, active elbow, wrist, and hand range of motion is encouraged. As symptoms regress, stretching exercises are initiated, and after 4–6 weeks from surgery, the patient begins a strengthening program.

9.9 Synovial Fringe

An hypertrophic radiocapitellar plica can cause impingement at the posterolateral side of the elbow. Thickening and fibrosis of the plica, which represent a congenitally originated fold, are related to repetitive microtraumas [37]. The plica can occur in association with capitellar osteochondritis dissecans and often presents with painful clicking, catching, effusions, and snapping with pronated elbow flexion greater than 90° [38, 39]. In most cases, physical examination is negative, although the patient may refer tenderness posterior to the lateral epicondyle and centered over the joint. Plain radiographs and MRI are often negative. Other associated pathological conditions can include chondromalacia of the anterolateral radial head and the capitellum [38]. Conditions that may mimic symptomatic plicae, including lateral epicondylitis, proximal radial head dislocation, and radial tunnel syndrome, must always be considered in differential diagnosis because they often show similar clinical findings [40]. Conservative management with rest, NSAIDs, and gentle motion with the addition of an intra-articular steroid injection can diminish symptoms and reduce inflammation. When such measures have failed, arthroscopy can confirm diagnosis and allow the resection of the plica with good to excellent results [38, 41, 42]. During arthroscopy, after the debridement of the synovitis surrounding the radial neck and the anterior capsule, the lateral plica can be seen as a fibrous band folding over the radial head, which can snap over the radial neck and head during elbow flexion/extension. Postoperative management consists of early range of motion, progressive strengthening followed by an interval throwing program of 8 weeks until symptoms resolution. Synovial plica in the radiocapitellar compartment as a cause of posterolateral elbow impingement has been described for the first time by Clarke. In his study, he reported successful arthroscopic excision in three cases [43]. All three patients had an area of chondromalacia on the margin of the radial head [43]. Commandre et al. [44] described a single case of successful arthroscopic removal of a plica that was causing pain but no mechanical symptoms. Akagi and Nakamura [45] reported a hypertrophic synovial plica causing pain and snapping with elbow flexion after repetitive microtraumas. They performed an open resection of the plica and found cartilage damage of the anterolateral aspect of the radial head. Antuna and O'Driscoll [38] published a case series including 14 patients with painful snapping elbows caused by synovial hypertrophic plicae. Twelve of 14 patients had successful arthroscopic treatment. Thirteen patients suffered erosion of the radial head, while three patients showed some degree of damage also at the capitulum humeri [38]. The high incidence of chondromalacia might be due to long-standing symptoms before surgery (13 months): during this period, the mechanical snapping of the synovial folds may lead to cartilage degeneration [38]. Early diagnosis and prompt surgical treatment of a hypertrophic synovial plica as a cause of snapping elbow are therefore crucial to avoid subsequent mechanical degeneration of the adjacent cartilage. Ruch et al. [46] presented a case series of ten patients with initial symptomatic radiocapitellar plica. All patients underwent successful arthroscopic plica removal after failed conservative treatment. Excellent results were reported, with postoperative free range of motion in all patients [9]. This study also underlines that hypertrophic synovial folds as causes of posterolateral elbow impingement are frequently under- or misdiagnosed. Kim et al. [42] reported on 12 relatively young, throwing athletes and golfers suffering from posterolateral elbow impingement caused by synovial plica. All patients underwent successful arthroscopic debridement of the thickened plica with excellent outcomes, except one patient who developed medial elbow instability and underwent subsequent reconstructive surgery.

References

1. Sims SE, Miller K, Elfar JC, Hammert WC. Non-surgical treatment of lateral epicondylitis: a systematic review of randomized controlled trials. Hand (N Y). 2014;9(4):419–46.
2. Shiri R, Viikari-Juntura E, Varonen H, et al. Prevalence and determinants of lateral and medial epicondylitis: a population study. Am J Epidemiol. 2006;164(11): 1065–74.
3. Taylor SA, Hannafin JA. Evaluation and management of elbow tendinopathy. Sports Health. 2012;4(5): 384–93.
4. Nirschl RP, Pettrone FA. Tennis elbow. The surgical treatment of lateral epicondylitis. J Bone Joint Surg Am. 1979;61(6A):832–9.
5. Regan W, Wold LE, Coonrad R, et al. Microscopic histopathology of chronic refractory lateral epicondylitis. Am J Sports Med. 1992;20(6):746–9.
6. Coonrad RW, Hooper WR. Tennis elbow: its courses, natural history, conservative and surgical management. J Bone Joint Surg Am. 1973;55:1177–82.
7. Nirschl RP. Soft-tissue injuries about the elbow. Clin Sports Med. 1986;5:637–52.
8. Gabel GT, Morrey BF. Tennis elbow. Instr Course Lect. 1998;47:165–72.
9. Cohen MS, Romeo AA. Open and arthroscopic management of lateral epicondylitis in the athlete. Hand Clin. 2009;25(3):331–8.
10. Riek S, Chapman AE, Milner T. A simulation of muscle force and internal kinematics of extensor carpi radialis brevis during backhand tennis stroke: implications for injury. Clin Biomech (Bristol, Avon). 1999;14:477–83.
11. Schneeberger AG, Masquelet AC. Arterial vascularization of the proximal extensor carpi radialis brevis tendon. Clin Orthop Relat Res. 2002;398:239–44.
12. LeHuec JC, Schaeverbeke T, Chauveaux D, et al. Epicondylitis after treatment with fluoroquinolone antibiotics. J Bone Joint Surg Br. 1995;77:293–5.
13. Bunata RE, Brown DS, Capelo R. Anatomic factors related to the causes of tennis elbow. J Bone Joint Surg Am. 2007;89:1955–63.
14. Cyriax JH. The pathology and treatment of tennis elbow. J Bone Joint Surg. 1936;18:921–40.
15. Goldie I. Epicondylitis lateralis humeri (epicondylalgia or tennis elbow). A pathogenetical study. Acta Chir Scand Suppl. 1964;57:Suppl 339:1+.
16. Nirschl RP. Elbow tendinosis/tennis elbow. Clin Sports Med. 1992;11:851–70.
17. Nirschl RP. Muscle and tendon trauma: tennis elbow. In: Morrey BF, editor. The elbow and its disorders. 1st ed. Philadelphia: WB Saunders; 1985. p. 537–52.
18. Chen J, Wang A, Xu J, et al. In chronic lateral epicondylitis, apoptosis and autophagic cell death occur in the extensor carpi radialis brevis tendon. J Shoulder Elbow Surg. 2010;19:355–62.
19. Tuite MJ, Kijowski R. Sports-related injuries of the elbow: an approach to MRI interpretation. Clin Sports Med. 2006;25:387–408, v.
20. Fairbank SM, Corlett RJ. The role of the extensor digitorum communis muscle in lateral epicondylitis. J Hand Surg Br. 2002;27(5):405–9.
21. Greenbaum B, Itamura J, Vangsness CT, et al. Extensor carpi radialis brevis. An anatomical analysis of its origin. J Bone Joint Surg Br. 1999;81:926–9.
22. Van Hofwegen C, Baker 3rd CL, Baker Jr CL. Epicondylitis in the athlete's elbow. Clin Sports Med. 2010;29(4):577–97.
23. Martinez-Silvestrini JA, Newcomer KL, et al. Sensitivity of the patient-rated forearm evaluation questionnaire in lateralepicondylitis. J Hand Ther. 2005;18:400–6.
24. Potter HG, Hannafin JA, et al. Lateral epicondylitis: correlation of MR imaging, surgical and histopathological finding. Radiology. 1995;196:43–6.
25. Steinborn M, Phaler M, Jessel C, et al. Magnetic resonance imaging in lateral epicondylitis of the elbow. Arch Orthop Trauma Surg. 1998;118:121–5.

26. Field LD, Savoie FH. Common elbow injuries in sport. Sports Med. 1998;26:193–205.
27. Baker Jr CL, Jones GL. Arthroscopy of the elbow. Am J Sports Med. 1999;27(2):251–64. Review.
28. Baumgard SH, Schwartz DR. Percutaneous release of the epicondylar muscles for humeral epicondylitis. Am J Sports Med. 1982;10:233–6.
29. Yerger B, Turner T. Percutaneous extensor tenotomy for chronic tennis elbow: an office procedure. Orthopedics. 1985;8:1261–3.
30. Powell SG, Burke AL. Surgical and therapeutic management of tennis elbow: an update. J Hand Ther. 1991;4:64–8.
31. Grundberg AB, Dobson JF. Percutaneous release of the common extensor origin for tennis elbow. Clin Orthop Relat Res. 2000;376:137–40.
32. Nazar M, Lipscombe S, Morapudi S, Tuvo G, Kebrle R, Marlow W, Waseem M. Percutaneous tennis elbow release under local anaesthesia. Open Orthop J. 2012; 6:129–32.
33. Bosworth DM. The role of the orbicular ligament in tennis elbow. J Bone Joint Surg Am. 1955;37-A(3): 527–33.
34. Dunkow PD, Jatti M, Muddu BN. A comparison of open and percutaneous techniques in the surgical treatment of tennis elbow. J Bone Joint Surg Br. 2004; 86-B:701–4.
35. Cohen MS, Romeo AA, Hennigan SP, Gordon M. Lateral epicondylitis: anatomic relationships of the extensor tendon origins and implications for arthroscopic treatment. J Shoulder Elbow Surg. 2008;17(6):954–60.
36. Arrigoni P, Fossati C, Zottarelli L, Brady PC, Cabitza P, Randelli P. 70° frontal visualization of lateral compartment of the elbow allows extensor carpi radialis brevis tendon release with preservation of the radial lateral collateral ligament. Arthroscopy. 2014;30(1): 29–35.
37. Ruch DS, Papadonikolakis A, Campolattaro RM. The posterolateral plica: a cause of refractory lateral elbow pain. J Shoulder Elbow Surg. 2006;15(3):367–70.
38. Antuna SA, O'Driscoll SW. Snapping plicae associated with radiocapitellar chondromalacia. Arthroscopy. 2001;17(5):491–5.
39. Steinert AF, Goebel S, Rucker A, et al. Snapping elbow caused by hypertrophic synovial plica in the radiohumeral joint: a report of three cases and review of literature. Arch Orthop Trauma Surg. 2010;130(3): 347–51.
40. Lowery Jr WD, Kurzweil PR, Forman SK, et al. Persistence of the olecranon physis: a cause of "little league elbow". J Shoulder Elbow Surg. 1995;4(2): 143–7.
41. Ahmad CS, Vitale MA, ElAttrache NS. Elbow arthroscopy: capitellar osteochondritis dissecans and radiocapitellar plica. Instr Course Lect. 2011;60: 181–90.
42. Kim DH, Gambardella RA, Elattrache NS, et al. Arthroscopic treatment of posterolateral elbow impingement from lateral synovial plicae in throwing athletes and golfers. Am J Sports Med. 2006;34(3):438–44.
43. Clarke RP. Symptomatic, lateral synovial fringe (plica) of the elbow joint. Arthroscopy. 1988;2:112–6.
44. Commandre FA, Taillan B, Benezis C, et al. Plica synovialis (synovial fold) of the elbow report on one case. J Sports Med Phys Fitness. 1988;2:209–10.
45. Akagi M, Nakamura T. Snapping elbow caused by the synovial fold in the radiohumeral joint. J Shoulder Elbow Surg. 1998;4:427–9.
46. Ruch DS, Papadonikolakis A, Campolattaro RM. The posterolateral plica: a cause of refractory lateral elbow pain. J Shoulder Elbow Surg. 2006;3:367–70.

PRP in Lateral Elbow Pain

10

Jorge Guadilla, Emilio Lopez-Vidriero, Rosa Lopez-Vidriero, Sabino Padilla, Diego Delgado, Rafael Arriaza, and Mikel Sanchez

10.1 Introduction

The lateral elbow pain has been named differently along the years.

Lateral epicondylitis was first described in the medical literature by Runge in 1873 [1].

The term "tennis elbow" appeared ten years later and remained since its initial description by Major who in 1883 described the "lawn tennis arm" [2].

Nevertheless, it is known that less than 10 % of patients consulting for this condition are actually tennis or racquet sport players [3].

Also called "lateral elbow pain" or "chronic lateral elbow pain," this term is wide enough to include different clinical conditions. In the literature other names as "lateral epicondylalgia," "shooter's elbow," or "archer's elbow" can be found to describe conditions that have in common the lateral elbow pain [4].

J. Guadilla • S. Padilla • D. Delgado • M. Sanchez
Unidad de Cirugia Artroscopica, VItoria, Spain

E. Lopez-Vidriero, MD, PhD (✉)
Chief of Traumatology, Department at Ibermutuamur Sevilla, ISMEC. International Sports Medicine Clinic, Arjona 10. Bajo, Sevilla 41001, Spain
e-mail: director@ismec.es

R. Lopez-Vidriero
ISMEC. International Sports Medicine Clinic, Arjona 10. Bajo, Sevilla 41001, Spain

R. Arriaza
Arriaza Asociados, La Coruña, Spain

The most used term is "lateral epicondylitis" and was previously considered to be a tendinitis, arising as inflammation of the tendon [5–7]. However, the current consensus is that microtrauma from excessive and repetitive use of the forearm extensors initiates a degenerative process with a paucity of inflammatory cells. Therefore, histologically it is said to be more a tendinosis (epicondylosis) than a tendinitis [8–10]. However, there is a last years' trend that establishes that inflammation plays a role in general tendinopathy more than suspected. Thus, degeneration (osis) and inflammation (itis) could both be involved in the origin and progression of tendinopathies triggered by stressful stimuli such as mechanical stress present in the lateral epicondylitis [11, 12].

The condition which is going to be described along this chapter is an enthesopathy of the lateral epicondyle, and the most commonly affected muscle is the extensor carpi radialis brevis (ECRB) [13].

In the remainder of this chapter, the term lateral epicondylitis (LE) is going to be used.

10.2 Incidence and Related Sports

Tendon injuries, both acute and chronic (or tendinopathy), affect the quality of life, increase the costs of health care, and lead to stop sporting activities of a quite high amount of patients and sport professionals.

L.A. Pederzini et al. (eds.), *Elbow and Sport*, DOI 10.1007/978-3-662-48742-6_10

The prevalence of lateral epicondylitis (LE) in the general population has been reported to be between 1 % and 3 % in adults, with no gender differences (es la misma referencia para todo el parrafo, la que aparece al final). This condition is most prevalent in the fifth decade of life, with peak incidence occurring between the ages of 45 and 60 years [14].

However, most publications are available about the incidence of LE. More comprehensive population-based studies are necessary [15].

Occupational risk factors, forceful activities, high force combined with high repetition or awkward posture, and the use of vibratory tools are associated with epicondylitis [16]. Any activity that involves overuse of the wrist extensor or supinator muscles may be the cause of this condition. The most commonly affected muscle is the ECRB [13, 17].

Epicondylitis is more common in the dominant elbow than in the nondominant, which means that exposure to physical load factors is involved in lateral epicondylitis [18, 19].

Despite the fact that less than 10 % of patients with this syndrome are actually tennis players, it is estimated that even more than 50 % of those who play tennis will experience some degree of lateral elbow pain along their lifetimes [20, 21]. In addition, the incidence of lateral epicondylitis is significantly higher in nonexpert than in expert tennis players [22] and those who use a one-handed backhand stroke [23].

The most common cause is overuse or repetitive strain caused by repeated extension or bending back of the wrist against resistance. Therefore, during the practice of tennis in case of a poor forehand or backhand technique, the wrist is bent when striking a backhand and huge forces are transferred through the tendons to the elbow rather than through the entire arm. Also, if the racquet grip is too small, the muscles work harder increasing the forces through the ECRB tendon. Strings that are too tight and playing with wet, heavy balls will transmit more shock and energy to the forearm.

Thus, some authors highlighted that racquet sports may cause the condition due to a combination of (1) incorrect technique, (2) extended duration of play, (3) frequency of play, (4) size of the racquet handle (affecting the lever arm of the force applied through the forearm), and (5) racquet weight [3, 23, 24].

Lateral epicondylitis is common in athletes of all ages and skill levels due to increasing participation in sports involving overhead arm motions. Sports as mentioned tennis, windsurfing, rock climbing, javelin throwing, team handball, and wheelchair modalities have been involved in lateral epicondylitis and other elbow injuries [25].

10.3 Degenerative Tendinopathies

10.3.1 Basic Science on Tendinopathies [26]

The basic components of adult tendon are water, collagen and elastic fibers, and cells (fibroblasts or tenocytes) organized in a tissue of mesenchymal origin. The cell component mainly consists in fibroblasts (tenocytes; 95 %), with synovial and endothelial cells and chondrocytes, making up less than 5 % of the total volume. Tenocytes are responsible for generating and maintaining the extracellular matrix (ECM), with the functionality and viability of the former depending on the quality of the ECM. The extracellular matrix contains 65–80 % of type I collagen and elastin fibers, which together make up 2 % of the dry weight of the tendon (it should be remembered that 50–70 % of a tendon is water). Other elements such as proteoglycans, glycosaminoglycans, various structural proteins such as integrins (which bind to laminin, fibronectin, and tenascin), and a group of enzymes known as matrix metalloproteases (MMPs, mainly collagenases such as MMP1), which play key roles in the maintenance and remodeling of the ECM, are also present.

The tendon presents *three specific characteristics* that are vital for understanding both the fragility and instability of the metabolic balance (remodeling/degradation) and its high mechanical strength.

1. Tendons act as an interface between the muscle and bone; thus they are the tissue transition zones. Mainly the myotendinous junction (MTJ) is subjected to high mechanical stresses. At the same time, the so-called osteotendinous junction (OTJ) also has its own structural and functional properties, which differ from those of the myotendinous junction but are also in a delicate metabolic balance.
2. During rapid growth periods and in early stages of the growth process, both tenoblasts and tenocytes exhibit high aerobic metabolic activity. Once they reach maturity, aerobic metabolism decreases and its anaerobic counterpart predominates.
3. There is a marked asymmetry between the limited number of tenocytes in the tendinous tissue and the large volume of extracellular matrix (ECM). In the adult or mature tendon, this cell/ECM ratio is even lower. Furthermore, this imbalance is amplified by the poor vasculature of the tendinous tissue.

These aspects mean that the tendon, together with the joint cartilage, is one of the structures in the musculoskeletal system that must bear some of the highest mechanical stresses, which are amplified enormously during sporting activity, above all in elite sports, with their endless hours of repetitions and training. It is known that these highly specialized nature tissues pay a price for this specialization in terms of limited ability to repair themselves in the event of rupture, with low metabolic, vascular, nerve resources (Fig. 10.1).

The tendinous degeneration commonly referred to as tendinosis appears to be the end result of the inability of tenocytes (fibroblasts) to maintain the extracellular matrix in physiological conditions, mainly due to disruption of the remodeling/degradation (anabolism/catabolism) balance. This alteration of the extracellular matrix also affects the metabolism and fibroblast activity, thus perpetuating a vicious circle. There have been major immunohistochemical advances and gene expression analysis of pathological tendons showing proinflammatory mediators such as interleukin-1α, interleukin-β, TNF-α, as well as immunocompetent cells that may contribute to tendon inflammation [27]. In addition, extracellular matrix fragments stemmed from the breakdown of tenascin and hyaluronan may act as triggers of tendon resident macrophages, thereby unleashing an inflammatory response [27].

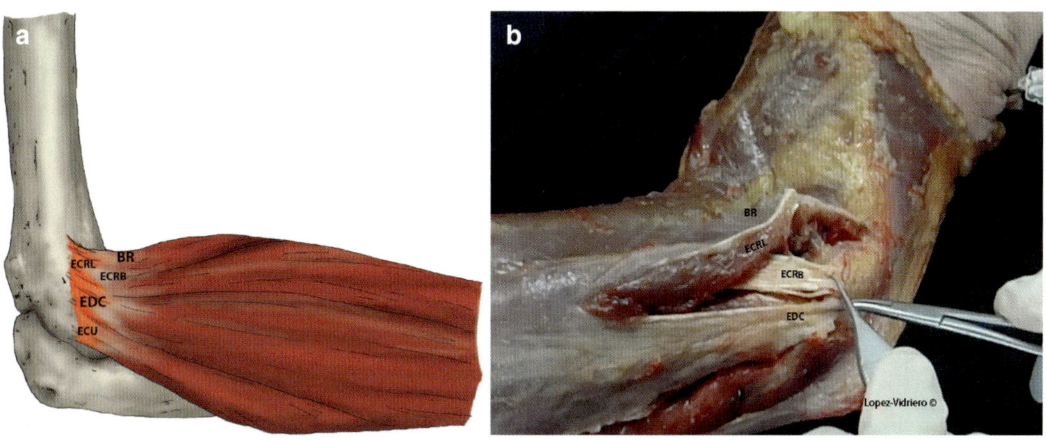

Fig. 10.1 (**a**) Schematic drawing showing the extensor-supinator muscles. BR: Brachiorradialis. ECRL: extensor carpis radialis longus. ECRB: extensor carpis radialis brevis (responsible for most of the pathology). ECD: extensor digitis comunis. ECU: extensor carpis ulnaris. (**b**) Anatomic specimen showing diseccion of the tendons. Notice the deeper location of the ECRB to the ECRL on the surface

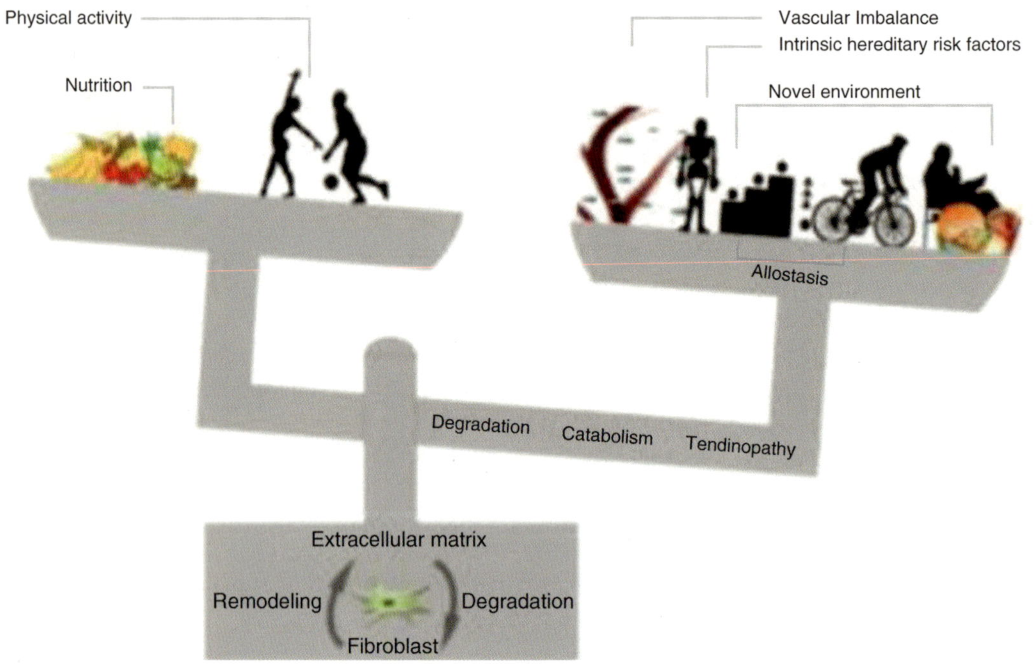

Fig. 10.2 Tendinopathy fisiopathology theory. "With permission of authors of *A new biological Approach to Orthopedic Surgery and Sport Medicine 1st Ed. Teamwork Media*"

These intrinsic and extrinsic factors may determine the workload threshold beyond which the metabolic remodeling ability of tenocytes (fibroblasts) is insufficient to maintain an extracellular matrix. That can adapt to the higher level of mechanical stress resulting from the activity undertaken (allostasis). The most important factors that affect the disruption of the balance are shown in Fig. 10.2.

A number of pathophysiological hypotheses have been proposed to explain the underlying causal mechanism of tendinopathies. Thus, apoptosis, vascular changes, and pain-related inflammation have all been suggested by [28], whereas Alfredson and coworkers [29, 30] have described intratendinous lactate and glutamate alterations, as well as neovascularization phenomena. Thus, suggesting their metabolic/vascular/neural involvement in tendon degeneration, these mechanisms may interact in an overlapping manner (uncompensated vascularization, localized temperature increase, acidosis, new environment, and intrinsic factors).

10.3.2 Pathogenesis of Lateral Epicondylitis

In 1936, Cyriax [12] proposed that microscopic or macroscopic tears of the common extensor origin were involved in the pathogenesis of this condition. Thereafter, other investigators showed that the disease base is actually a degenerative tendinopathy [31–33] (añadir REFERENCIA).

The application of stress to a tendon normally leads to increased cross-linkage and collagen deposition [8]. When the rate of stretching and loads to the tendon exceed the tolerance of the tendon, a micro-tear results. Then the balance is lost, and the adaptation of the tendon to multiple micro-tears leads to tendinosis. Collagen within the tendons gets degraded because it is kept under high stress and it gets degraded in such quantity that the tenocytes are not able to replace it. From a mechanical point of view, these cumulative microtraumas result from repetitive wrist extension and alternating forearm supination and pronation [31, 32]. Histologically four stages are described that result from such repetitive microtrauma [8, 34, 35]:

Stage 1: It starts with an acute inflammatory response, which can sometimes resolve completely.
Stage 2: If the aggression is maintained, a concentration of fibroblasts, vascular hyperplasia, and disorganized collagen, known in conjunction with angiofibroblastic hyperplasia, can be seen histologically.
Stage 3: Continuous accumulation of pathological changes leads to structural failure. In this stage the tendon suffers partial or complete rupture.
Stage 4: To the characteristics described in stage 2 or 3, other changes such as fibrosis are associated, as well as soft matrix calcification within the disorganized loose collagen and hard osseous calcification.

In 1973, Coonrad and Hooper were the first to describe macroscopic tearing in association with the histologic changes within the ECRB [31]. Six years later Nirschl called these histologic findings "angiofibroblastic hyperplasia" [33] as he showed that those findings were characterized by disorganized, immature collagen formation with immature fibroblastic and vascular elements. The term used today is angiofibroblastic tendinosis [36]. Ultrasonographically, tendon thickening or thinning, focal areas of hypoechogenicity, tendon tears, calcification, and even bony irregularity can be demonstrated mostly in the stages 3 and 4 [3, 37].

10.4 Diagnosis

Epicondylitis causes pain and disability, both in general population and in athletes. In addition, it has an economic cost in terms of days off the working activity and training. Thus, proper diagnosis and treatment are of paramount importance. An accurate, detailed, and thorough history and physical examination, combined with appropriate imaging studies in case of need, are essential in understanding the mechanisms and pathophysiology of the injury and making a specific diagnosis [3, 33, 36].

10.4.1 History and Physical Examination

During the history it is advisable to ask the patient for those sporting activities or job circumstances that could cause or exacerbate the symptoms.

Clinically, LE is characterized by tenderness or pain over the lateral humeral epicondyle or, more typically, in the area where the common extensor muscles (specially the ECRB) meet the lateral humeral epicondyle. The patient may refer to a direct trauma to the lateral aspect of the elbow, but often the pain can be gradual and insidious. The pain often radiates down the forearm and unusually is proximal to the elbow. The intensity of the pain can range from intermittent and mild to constant and severe, affecting all daily activities.

The patient usually suffers weakness in grip strength that affects sports practice, working activities, and even activities of daily living as shaking hands, shaving, lifting, or raising a coffee mug.

It is recommended to rule out cervical spine pathology, followed by an examination of the entire upper extremity, with special attention to the shoulder, comparing with the unaffected, contralateral extremity. Palpation of the lateral humeral epicondyle or the origin of the ECRB will reproduce the pain.

A number of tests that could reproduce this pain, helping to the diagnosis, have been described:

- Resisted third finger extension can be painful because of selective recruitment of the ECRB tendon (Maudsley's test)
- Resisted wrist extension with the elbow fully extended and in pronation stresses the whole common extensor origin and can reproduce the pain (Thompson maneuver).
- Asking the patient to lift a chair with the forearm pronated recreates the combination

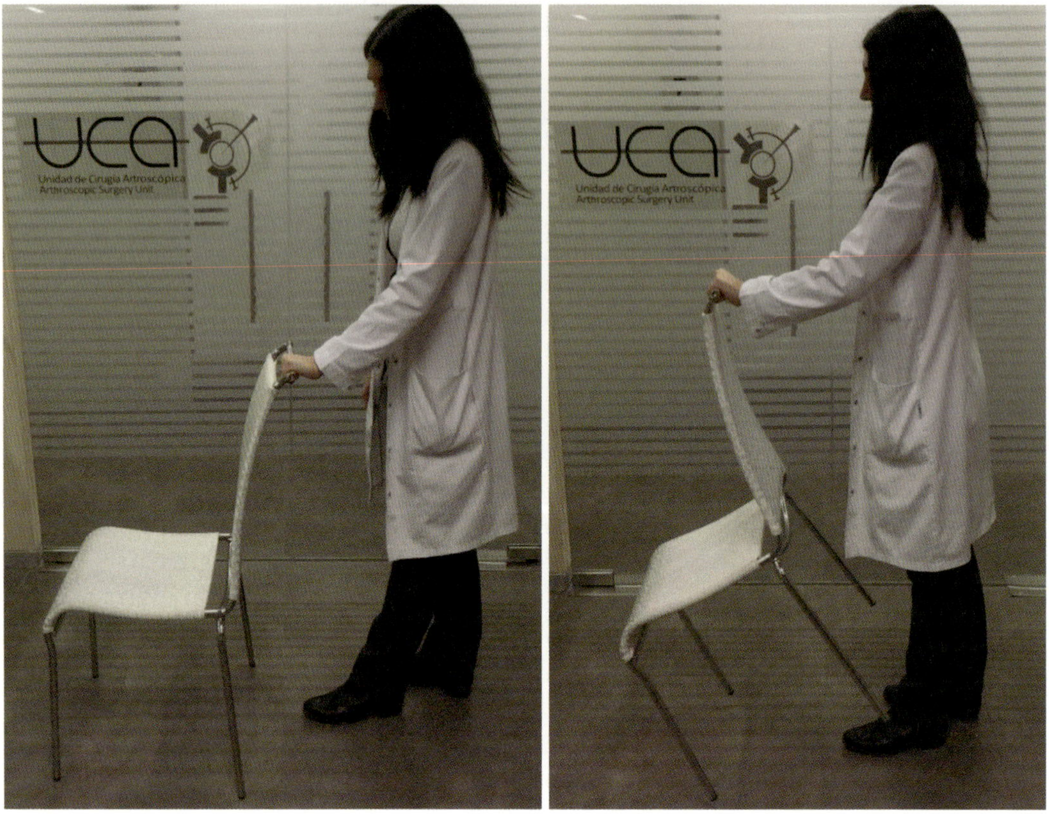

Fig. 10.3 Chair test or Gardner test

described above and also causes lateral elbow pain ("chair test" or Gardner test, Fig. 10.3) [38–40].

- Others like Bowden test, Cozen's test, and Mill's test can be helpful.

Generally, range of motion at the wrist and elbow is not affected. Grip strength may be decreased as a result of pain.

10.4.2 Imaging and Complementary Test

In most cases a diagnosis of lateral epicondylitis can be made clinically. The X-rays can be helpful in demonstrating calcifications in the soft tissue at or near the insertion of the ECRB (found in 25 % of the cases [41]). They are helpful to rule out other potential causes of pain (including loose bodies, osteoarthritis, and osteochondritis dissecans) (Figs. 10.4 and 10.5).

Ultrasound imaging can be useful by identifying structural changes in the affected tendons (thickening or thinning, tendon tears, calcification, bony irregularity, etc.). Doppler ultrasound is able to detect neovascularization.

MRI can help to confirm diagnoses involving the extensor tendon origin. MRI has 90–100 % sensitivity and 83–100 % specificity for detecting epicondylitis [42]. Magnetic resonance imaging may also be useful if concomitant intra-articular pathology or ligamentous injuries are suspected.

Electromyography can be useful in excluding posterior interosseous nerve entrapment (radial tunnel syndrome).

10.4.3 Differential Diagnosis

Accurate diagnosis of lateral epicondylitis may be difficult since there are other conditions with similar symptoms (pain and reduced strength).

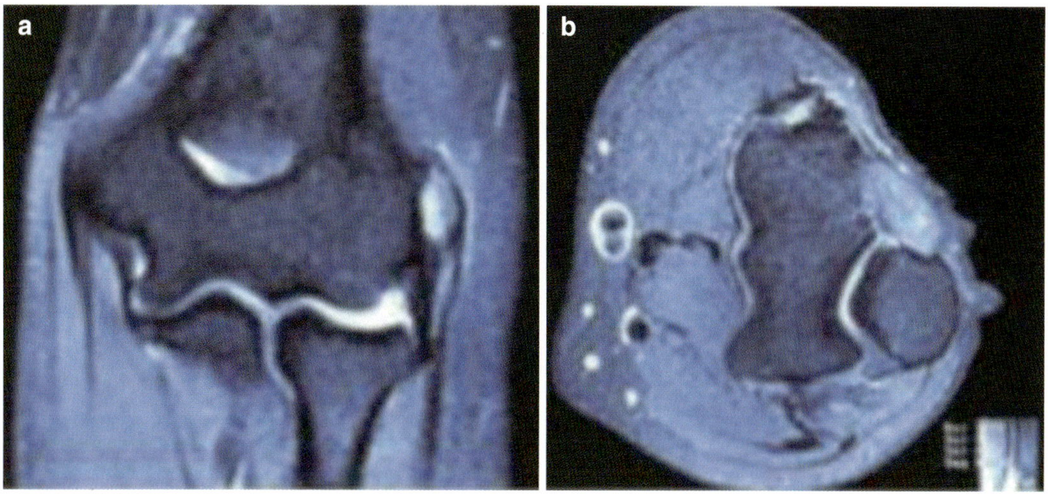

Fig. 10.4 MRI images of a lateral epicondylitis

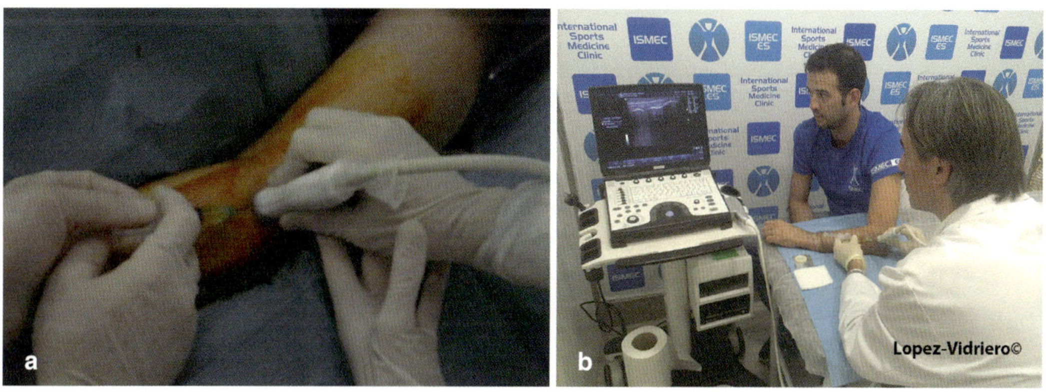

Fig. 10.5 (**a**) Ultrasound guided inyection with 4 hands. The surgeon injects while is helped by the radiologist using the probe. (**b**) Ultrasound guided injection with 2 hands. The surgeon triangulates by himself injecting with one hand while the other holds the probe. The skin is prepared with clorhexidine. Notice that sterile gel is used. The probe is protected with sterile latex sheath. The needle in the screen generates the typical reverberance due to the fact that is made of metal

Differential diagnosis for lateral epicondylitis has to include [3, 24, 33, 36]:

1. Cervical radiculopathy with pain irradiated to elbow and forearm.
2. Elbow overuse due to an ipsilateral shoulder malfunction (compensatory mechanism).
3. Entrapment of the posterior interosseous nerve (PIN), also known as radial tunnel syndrome, which affects 5 % of LE patients, does not cause increased pain with resisted wrist extension (see Sect. 4.1). Pain may be caused by resisted forearm supination as the supinator muscle is one of the areas of compression of this nerve. Electromyography and local injection of anesthetic to the region of the PIN may relieve the pain [43].
4. Joint problems: Ulnar collateral ligament injury, loose bodies, degenerative changes at the radiocapitellar joint, and osteochondritis dissecans. Rajeev and Pooley found 59 % of degenerative changes in 117 elbow arthroscopies performed for LE treatment [44]. It should be taken into account for the treatment of LE either in young or in middle-aged population.

5. Infection or tumors around or within the joint may also mimic LE clinical features and sometimes could appear as a mass.

10.5 Treatment of Lateral Epicondylitis

The aims of treatment for LE should be:

- Pain control
- Preservation of movement-function of the joint and upper limb
- Improvement in grip strength and endurance
- Return to normal function and activity
- Avoidance of further histological and clinical deterioration

Some studies have reported unpredictable healing patterns and have identified factors linked to poor outcomes. In this way, high baseline pain scores, manual work, and involvement of the dominant extremity have directly seen related to worse outcomes [14].

10.5.1 Described Treatment Options

Some authors have shown that the lateral elbow tendinopathy is a self-limited condition, and rest with or even without the use of some analgesic or anti-inflammatory medication in the acute phase of pain could resolve the symptoms.

The average duration of a typical episode is about 6 months to 2 years, but most patients (89 %) recover within 1 year [45].

To date, a standardized, universally accepted program for LE treatment has not been established by the orthopedic surgeon's community [3]. It leads to a wide diversity of treatment ranging from an expectant waiting approach, nonsteroidal anti-inflammatory drugs (NSAIDs), physical therapies, bracing, acupuncture, laser therapy, extracorporeal shock wave therapy, percutaneous radiofrequency thermal lesioning, topical nitrates, injection of glucocorticoid, botulinum toxin, autologous blood injection, and platelet-rich plasma therapies to surgery.

The choice, as reported by some studies depends on experience, expertise, and equipment at any given clinic or center. What is quite clear is that patient education is usually one of the important core elements of any plan or protocol.

The evidence indicates that wait and see policy would be enough for most patients [45, 46]. Injection with glucocorticoids has been used since the 1950s and has been the treatment of choice for most of the physicians. However, nowadays its efficacy and utility are considered controversial, since some studies addressed that long-term outcome of steroid injections is poorer than expected and could even alter the ability to heal and damage the tendon and tissues around. It is reported that 72 % of patients treated with steroid injections experience a recurrence within 12 months, compared with 9 % in those treated with a wait and see strategy [47–49].

Furthermore, as confirmed by the systematic review by Dean et al. [50], the local administration of glucocorticoid has significant negative effects on tendon cells, including reduced cell viability, cell proliferation and collagen synthesis, collagen disorganization, and cell necrosis, leading to a reduction of mechanical properties of the tendon. This should mean that in case of planning an infiltration of glucocorticoids for any tendinopathy and the use of an ultrasound guidance would be of paramount importance to avoid intratendinous injection.

It is well established that surgery is reserved for patients who fail to respond to nonoperative treatments, and multiple variations on open approach as percutaneous and arthroscopic procedures have been described. Studies of Nirschl and Pettrone [33] are considering that a range of 4–11 % of patients ultimately could require surgical treatment for relief of their symptoms.

Until today, the evidence about surgical treatment for LE is lacking, and the Cochrane Library has classified surgical treatment as having insufficient evidence to support or refute its use [51]. Despite exhaustive nonsurgical management and even correct surgical intervention, there is a small percent of patients who continue to feel symptoms, usually in terms of pain. In such cases the possibility of a wrong initial diagnosis or an associated pathology should be considered and ruled out.

10.5.2 Biological Therapies for Tendinopathies: PRP

Despite the fact that there are many options to treat injured tendons, as described previously, it is a reality that none of those are foolproof and it leads to the need of further studies and investigations on pathogenesis of tendon damage to understand and develop new strategies of treatments.

Therefore, mainly in the last decade, minimally invasive interventions with the theoretical ability of boosting the healing response or neutralizing degenerative changes in tendinopathy have received the watchful eye of the community and are being investigated.

Among the emerging technologies, with "biologically friendly" or "regenerative" profile, autologous whole blood and platelet-rich plasma (PRP) have been recently used in several clinical studies for the treatment of LE. PRP is defined as "a sample of autologous blood with concentrations of platelets above baseline values" [52].

The management of musculoskeletal injuries with PRP therapies has been advocated since 2003 [53], when Sánchez et al. published, as far as we know, the first paper on the use of PRP to treat an articular osteochondral avulsion of the knee.

Since then, this promising and innovative technology has stimulated translational research and interest among both the scientific and medical communities and has widened PRP applications to several musculoskeletal problems [54–57].

In the other hand, the term "PRP" is wide enough to generate confusion. Due to the fact that different preparations, with unequal cell population and activation method, with different amount of platelets above peripheral blood baseline, and, even more, with a nonconsensual protocol of application, are being used and investigated under the name of PRP [54, 58–60], therefore, different attempts of classification have been described, and some authors [55, 59, 60] have proposed systems that try to classify PRP systems by activation mechanism, platelet number, and/or cell content. The absence of a validated classification system that identifies crucial differences between PRP formulations makes it difficult to compare studies, and it involves that, despite intensive research and huge number of publications in the last years, there is a gap in the basic knowledge necessary to establish the best PRP product for each clinical condition, as well as the guidelines for clinical applications [57].

There is some evidence to state that PRP formulations (number of platelets, presence of white blood cells (WBCs), balance between platelet secreted and plasma proteins, mechanism of plasma activation) and/or application procedures (i.e., number of doses, volume, activation, and injection procedures) could be linked to clinical effect [57, 61, 62]. In this way there are enough reasons to believe that the use of leukocyte-rich PRP (L-PRP) and leukocyte-depleted PRP (pure or P-PRP) should not be the same (L-PRP is more proinflammatory when injected in rabbits [63], it increases the levels of metalloproteases when assayed in tenocyte cultures [64], and it induced more transient postinjection swelling and pain when injected into the knee for treatment of knee osteoarthritis [65]). There are some trials performed with a combination of local anesthetics and PRP. An in vitro study by Carofino et al. concluded that the addition of either anesthetics or corticosteroids to PRP resulted in statistically significant decreases in tenocyte proliferation and cell viability [66].

Even more, there is no consensus about the frequency and number of PRP injections in chronic injuries. The majority of the studies have been performed with a single PRP application, but in our opinion a degenerative process could not be solved with just one intervention, and therefore, two or even three injections would be more efficient than a single PRP application, but, actually, this issue remains to be clarified [67].

Our group has been using from the beginning of our research a 100 % autologous PRP with a standardized composition and dosage (PRGF-Endoret, BTI, Vitoria-Spain). It contains a moderated platelet concentration (2- to 2.5-fold increase compared with peripheral blood) [57], obtained after a single spinning. One of the most relevant and controversial issues is the presence of WBCs in PRP. The first and most widely used classification would define the system we are using, as pure PRP (P-PRP) because it does not contain WBCs [59] The PRGF-Endoret is classified as type 4-B (minimal WBCs, activated with calcium chloride, and platelet concentration below 5) as proposed by Mishra et al. for sports medicine classification [55]. Finally, PRGF would fit in the P2-x-Bb category (platelet count greater than baseline levels to 750,000 platelets/mL, exogenous activation with calcium chloride, with WBCs, and specifically neutrophils, below or equal to baseline levels) according to the PAW (platelets, activation, and WBCs) classification [60].

10.5.2.1 The Scientific Rationale behind the Use of PRP Use on Tendinopathies and Lateral Epicondylitis

PRP preparations include growth factors, cytokines, and morphogens contained in platelets, as well as fibrinogen and other plasmatic proteins in a biologically balanced aggregate, managed and delivered in a pharmacological manner [68]. This may account for two special features: the resolution of inflammation and avoidance of fibrosis. In addition to containing GFs, PRP provides the damaged tissue with a transient biological fibrin scaffold, which stems from the polymerization of fibrinogen, a pleiotropic blood protein that regulates coagulation, inflammation, and tissue regeneration. PRP tendon infiltrations are aimed at recruiting, activating, and mobilizing satellite cells and resident macrophages which contribute to repair processes by cell signaling soluble factors. Once the activated preparation rich in growth factors is injected, this liquid-to-gel transition 3D injectable scaffold allows a successful filling of the tissue gaps and defects. With a local and gradual activation and a homogeneous distribution through and interaction with the ECM of tissue, it is converted into a matrix-like viscous and malleable structure [69]. This fibrin scaffold formed "in situ" as a provisional extracellular matrix and containing binding sites for cell adhesion as well as proteins such as thrombospondin-1 (TSP-1), alpha-1-antitrypsin fibronectin, acute phase proteins, or proteins related to lipid metabolisms [70] serves as a highway for mechanical energy to transit from the environment to the cell, thereby bridging cell-to-cell tissue transition, promoting multicellular assembly, providing mechanical support and plastic-elastic stiffness which has a drastic impact on fates of different cell types such as fibroblasts [71], and endowing tissues with a suitable mechanical and chemical microenvironment for biological restoration. In addition, fibrin matrix, by heparin-binding domains, may sequester growth factors such as PDGF, FGF, HGF, BBNF, and VEGF [72, 73] and gradually release them later, exerting a synergistic action on tissue repair.

Since this dynamic spongelike fibrin-matrix scaffold is autologous, bio-reabsorbable, biocompatible, and free of leukocytes and red cells, PRP scaffolds might be considered the best tailored among all the tissue engineering materials [74].

There is a great deal of evidence illustrating the anabolic effects of PRPs on tendon cells [75–78]. PRP stimulates the synthesis of several types of collagen and other oligomeric matrix proteins, resulting in a synthesis of extracellular matrix which is conducive to the tendon anabolism and homeostasis. The wide spectrum of cell response in vitro and in vivo in both tendon stem cell differentiation and tendon cell proliferation, together with a substantial expression of VEGF and HGF by tendon cells, thereby generating a balanced angiogenesis, constitutes the rationale for the application of activated liquid and fibrin scaffolds to the injured site of the tendon to prompt the repair events in one area that brings about a great deal of morbidity. The infiltration of activated liquid form of PRP to a tendon damaged area elicits a set of sequential remodeling events that might lead to the tendon healing. Although the TGF-B1 family drives fibrogenesis and potentially might stimulate the formation of scar tissue in the tendon, the fibrotic effect of TGF-B1 present in the PRP would be either modulated, counterbalanced, or even hindered by the presence and local production of VEGF and HGF, a potent antifibrotic and anti-inflammatory agent, as has been shown by our work on cells cultured on fibrin matrices [79].

10.5.2.2 What Does Evidence-Based Literature Say about PRP and Lateral Epicondylitis?

In the last decade and taking into account the promising role of PRP for LE established by Mishra et al. in 2006 [80], different research projects have been developed, comparing PRP to different classically accepted treatments for LE, as corticosteroids, local anesthetics, and autologous blood. To date, all controlled clinical trials in epicondylitis (nine) have been performed with L-PRP [80–88]. So far there are no direct comparisons between L-PRP and pure PRP. There are also two case series papers with 6 and 30 patients and a single injection.

PRP Versus Bupivacaine Injections

Mishra and Pavelko [80] were the first people performing a case-control study with PRP on patients ($n=20$) in which nonsurgical treatment had failed. Fifteen patients were injected with PRP and the other five with bupivacaine, intending these to act as controls. They found a 60 % improvement in VAS in PRP arm at 8 weeks and a 93 % reduction in VAS and function at 24 months of follow-up.

This study opened a way of research on PRP effect for LE, but the real value of it is conditioned by the design itself. In 2014 Mishra et al. [87] published a multicenter randomized and controlled trial (RCT) on 230 patients (116 injected with PRP and 114 with bupivacaine) that had at least 3 months of symptoms and had failed conventional therapy. The injection site was blocked in both cases using 0.5 % bupivacaine with epinephrine, before injecting PRP. At 12 weeks no significant differences between PRP and bupivacaine were found. However, significant VAS improvement and also significant success rates (>25 % reduction in pain score versus baseline) at 24 weeks were encountered in PRP group.

Both studies were performed with a single injection of unactivated L-PRP and without ultrasound guidance.

PRP Versus Corticosteroid Injections

There are four RCT that compared PRP versus corticosteroid injections. Peerbooms et al. published positive results at 6 and 12 months [81]. In an extension of the former study, Gosens et al. [82] confirmed those results 24 months after treatment. One-hundred patients with symptoms for 6 months were randomly assigned in the PRP group or the corticosteroid group. The injections were performed in two steps. First, one of 1 mL of PRP or corticosteroids with 0.5 % bupivacaine with epinephrine and, second, the remaining PRP with corticosteroids. Twelve weeks after the procedure, the VAS and Disabilities of the Arm, Shoulder, and Hand (DASH) scores were better in PRP than in corticosteroid group. Moreover, at the sixth month, the difference was already statistically significant [81], and the effects kept stable over a 2-year follow-up time [82].

In contrast, there are two other studies that did not find significant differences at 6 weeks or 3 months after treatment. In the first, the blinding system was not specified, the number of patients was 30, it was conducted for only 6 weeks, and they used the VAS and DASH scores [85]. The second was double blinded, the number of patients was 60, and it was randomized to receive PRP, saline, or glucocorticoid. The validated score was the Patient-Rated Tennis Elbow Evaluation (PRTEE) [86].

Interestingly, Kohl et al. [86] found that a single injection with either PRP or glucocorticoid was not significantly superior to a saline injection.

The PRP used in all these trials was L-PRP. The type of activation was unactivated in three papers and unknown in one [85]. Lastly all of them only used a single injection. Of these four studies only in Krogh's study the injection was under ultrasound control.

PRP Versus Autologous Whole Blood (AWB)

Three RCT compared L-PRP with autologous blood injections for refractory lateral epicondylitis. Creaney et al. [83] conducted a RCT of 150 patients, 80 receiving monthly US-guided two injections of PRP and 70 patients injected with autologous blood in the same fashion. Improvement was seen in PRTEE score for both arms of the study at 6 months, but it was no statistically different.

Thanasas et al. [84] divided 24 patients equally into two groups, one treated with a single 3-mL injection of AWB and a second one with 3 mL of L-PRP, both under ultrasound guidance. VAS scale and Liverpool Elbow Score were used for the evaluation. PRP group had a significantly greater improvement in VAS scores than AWB group only at 6 weeks. This significant difference was not seen at 3 and 6 month controls.

In 2014 Raeissadat et al. [88] randomized 40 patients with duration of symptoms more than 3 months and VAS score of a minimum of 5. Group 1 was treated with a single injection of 2 mL of L-PRP and Group 2 with 2 mL of autologous blood. Pain and functional improvements were assessed with VAS scale, modified Mayo Clinic performance index for the elbow, and pressure pain threshold at baseline and 4 and 8 weeks. No statistically significant difference was noted between groups, and they concluded that both treatments are effective to treat LE with a slight superiority of PRP in 8-week follow-up.

The use of injections of PRP to treat LE has been seen to have an excellent safety profile [80–88].

Currently four controlled trials (comparing PRP to lidocaine, AWB, dry needle tendon fenestration, saline injection, and no injection) are being conducted as registered in clincaltrials.gov. So far, research comparing both L-PRP and P-PRP is lacking, and it should be the aim of the medical community in order to clarify if the presence of WBCs is beneficial for the tendon healing.

Conclusions

Since we know that depending on the presence of leucocytes, the amount of platelets from the baseline, and the type of activation we can categorize different types of PRP, the results from the studies and clinical trials performed with one of the described PRP cannot be extended to the others.

Thus, we should tend to standardize not only the PRP type but also the number of injections, the use of ultrasound to ensure the site of injection, the method of injection itself, the rehabilitation protocols, and even the patient outcome measure scores for this pathology.

In conclusion, there is currently insufficient evidence to support the use of PRP therapy for treating LE, due to the fact that the results of the different studies are controversial, given the heterogeneity in formulations and application protocols.

Therefore more research and an effort in standardization of PRP preparation methods and their applications protocol are still needed to establish the real role of PRP in the conservative treatment of LE.

10.5.2.3 PRP Protocol for LE [57]

In our group's treatment protocol, a patient complaining of chronic (more than 3 months) lateral elbow pain with the diagnosis of lateral epicondylitis should be advised to avoid the cause of the injury and start a individualized program of rehabilitation. In case of acute pain, some analgesics could be added.

In those patients with no improvement of the pain and with a physical examination that excludes other causes of lateral pain, a treatment program and ultrasound-guided PRP injections (in a sterile fashion), not only of the injured area of the tendon but also of the healthy both side extremes of the tendon and within the elbow joint, will be offered. The basis to inject in the surrounding healthy tissue is to activate the mesenchymal cells that are located there. So they can differentiate into tenocytes and migrate to the degenerate site. This phenomenon is called chemotaxis.

First of all, an ultrasound exploration of the lateral elbow is conducted. Then, once the ultrasound probe has been longitudinally located along the injured tendon, we insert the needle from distal to proximal, in a parallel track to the collagen fascicles; PRP is injected (shortly after CaCl2 addition) within the site of altered tendon substance using a 21-G needle attached to a Luer Lock syringe. The intention is to inject the maximum volume that can be confined within the area of degeneration, commonly between 3 and 5 mL (depending on the specific tendon and clinical case). Next, at some point during the extraction of the needle, additional PRP is delivered to the healthy tendon. We also inject plasma around the tendon between the tendon and the paratenon, and finally, a smaller volume is delivered into the associated fat and another 2–3 mL into the elbow joint.

Cold therapy is applied for approximately 10 min after the PRP injection in order to control pain. Local anesthetic and corticoids should be avoided due to the fact that they inactivate the PRP products. After the injection, the patients are instructed to limit physical activities for 24 h and to use cold therapy two to three times during the day. Only pain killers are allowed. NSAIDs should be avoided because they may interact in the healing process (Table 10.1).

In general, we perform two or three PRP injections separated 1 week each on an outpatient basis.

These criteria are largely arbitrary and are based on our clinical experience. Moreover, because PRP therapies promote early healing, 1 week may be adequate for monitoring individual outcomes and making decisions about further plasma injections. Ultrasonographic monitoring and symptoms drive our clinical decision regarding whether to perform additional PRP injections.

We do not change rehabilitation protocols after the PRP injection, and these include eccentric strengthening exercises, which are always personalized to the patient's condition. The only change is that we tend to move into different rehabilitation phases sooner.

Table 10.1 Suggested PRP injection protocol for LE

Sterile fashion
NO local anesthetics neither corticosteroids
US exploration and localization of painful area/tendon (longitudinal axis)
Outpatient basis ultrasound guided: 2–3 PRP injection (3–5 mL), weekly revaluation
Standard physical therapy protocol (eccentric exercises)

Pitfalls of Treatment

- In every sport-related injury, the balance between the rest needed for the treatment and the expectancy of sport practice is many times difficult to achieve.
- There are many types of PRP products, different protocols, and no consensus about the way the PRP therapies should be applied for LE.
- The PRPs used in the clinical studies until date for this chronic and histologically degenerative condition have been L-PRP in the majority, applied a single time, without image control.
- The use of US-guided injection implies collaboration with the radiology department and expertise learned by the physician in charge of the patient.
- The use of local anesthesia or corticosteroids mixed with the PRP product may alter the effect of PRP.
- Despite advances in PRP science, there is a lack of level I studies to ensure that PRP therapies are definitively useful in LE.

Pearls of Treatment

The key to lateral epicondylitis treatment could be summarized as below:

- A good anamnesis and workup of the injured elbow.
- Any other cause of lateral elbow pain should be ruled out.
- Initially a "wait and see" policy with or without analgesic makes sense.
- Try to avoid injections of glucocorticoids, unless there is a huge inflammation component.
- Consider PRP therapies in chronic cases, always before surgical treatment.
- Perform the injections in a sterile fashion, under ultrasound control, without local anesthesia, and think about evaluating the patient the next week and repeating the injection depending on the sonographic findings, believing that a single injection is not enough for a degenerative tissue to heal.

Clinical Case

Borja is a 31-year-old paddle tennis player. He is a former Spanish National Team member and actually playing in the Professional Tour. He is left handed. He came to our clinic complaining of progressive lateral elbow pain that limited his performance, and that was only temporary relieved by physiotherapy and one corticoid injection. Physical examination showed pain on palpation and resisted contraction of ECR muscles, without signs of tendon rupture in the US scan. A thorough review of the possible causes of the pain onset revealed that his sponsors had changed his racquet design for the new season, and he had been playing with the new one for some two months before symptoms arouse. After discussing the treatment options with the patient, we decided that he should return to his previous racket model (although it represented a minor problem with his sponsors, we solved by painting the old model with the new one's decoration), and that an orthobiological treatment would be better than more corticoid injections. Leukocyte-poor PRP (Mishra's type 4-B) was injected following our standard protocol for epicondylitis: under ultrasound control, only the growth-rich fraction (3 cc) was used, injecting it into the ECRB tendon origin, and also in the surrounding tissue; no local anesthesia was used, and the elbow was kept in a sling for the next 48 h. After the injection pain resolved, he was allowed to gradually return to training. One month later, he played his first competition match without pain, and symptoms have not recurred.

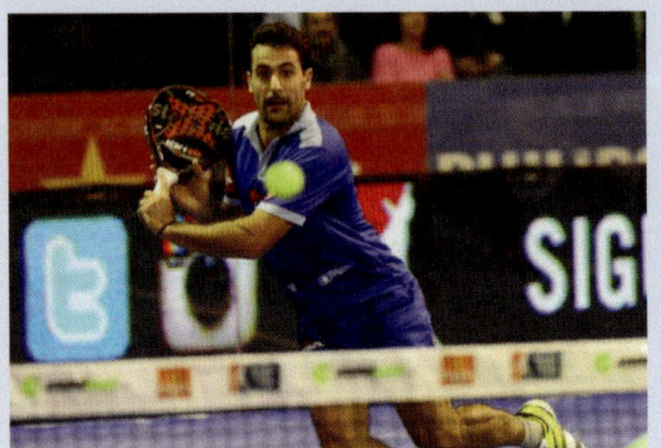

References

1. Runge F. Zur Genese und Behandlung des schreibe Kranfes. Bed Klin Worchenschr. 1873;10:245–8 (in German).
2. Major HP. Lawn-tennis elbow. BMJ. 1883;2:557. letter.
3. Luk J, Tsang R, Leung HB. Lateral epicondylalgia: midlife crisis of a tendón. Hong Kong Med J. 2014;20:145–51.
4. Nirschl RP. Tennis elbow. Orthop Clin North Am. 1973;4:787–800.
5. Nirschl RP. Elbow tendinosis/tennis elbow. Clin Sports Med. 1992;11:851–70.
6. Bishai SK, Plancher KD. The basic science of lateral epicondylosis: update for the future. Technol Orthop. 2006;21:250–5.
7. Kannus P, Józsa L. Histopathological changes preceding spontaneous rupture of a tendon: a controlled study of 891 patients. J Bone Joint Surg Am. 1991;73-A:1507–25.
8. Kraushaar BS, Nirschl RP. Tendinosis of the elbow (tennis elbow). Clinical features and findings of histological, immunohistochemical, and electron microscopy studies. J Bone Joint Surg Am. 1999;81:259–78.
9. Baker CL, Nirschl RP. Lateral tendon injury: open and arthroscopic treatment. In: Altchek DW, Andrews JR, editors. The Athlete's elbow. Philadelphia: Lippincott Williams & Wilkins; 2001. p. 91–103.
10. Schulze-Tanzil G, Al-Sadi O, Wiegand E, Ertel W, Busch C, Kohl B, Pufe T. The role of pro- inflammatory and immunoregulatory cytokines in tendon healing and rupture: new insights. Scand J Med Sci Sports. 2011;21(3):337–51.
11. Rees JD, et al. Tendons – time to revisit inflammation. Br J Sports Med. 2014;48:1553–7.
12. Cyriax JH. The pathology and treatment of tennis elbow. J Bone Joint Surg. 1936;18:921–40.
13. Walker-Bone K, Palmer KT, Reading I, Coggon D, Cooper C. Prevalence and impact of musculoskeletal disorders of the upper limb in the general population. Arthritis Rheum. 2004;51:642–51.
14. Sanders TL et al. The epidemiology and health care burden of tennis elbow. A population- based study. Am J Sports Med. 2015; pii: 0363546514568087. [Epub ahead of print].
15. Shiri R, Viikari-Juntara E. Lateral and medial epicondylitis: role of occupational factors. Best Pract Res Clin Rheumatol. 2011;25:43–57.
16. Shiri R, Viikari-Juntura E, Varonen H, et al. Prevalence and determinants of lateral and medial epicondylitis: a population study. Am J Epidemiol. 2006;164:1065–74.
17. Shiri R, Varonen H, Heliövaara M, Viikari-Juntura E. Hand dominance in upper extremity musculoskeletal disorders. J Rheumatol. 2007;34(5):1076–82.
18. Hamilton PG. The prevalence of humeral epicondylitis: a survey in general practice. J R Coll Gen Pract. 1986;36(291):464–5.
19. Boyer MI, Hastings II H. Lateral tennis elbow: "Is there any science out there?". J Shoulder Elbow Surg. 1999;8:481–91.

20. Priest JD, Braden V, Gerberich JG. The elbow and tennis. Part 1. Phys Sports Med. 1980;8:80.
21. Fichez O. Epicondylite: histoire naturelle et etude critique des differents traitements. J Traumatol Sport. 1998;15(3):163–72.
22. De Smedt T, de Jong A, Leemput WV, et al. Lateral epicondylitis in tennis: update on aetiology, biomechanics, and treatment. Br J Sports Med. 2007;41:816–9.
23. Eygendaal D, Rahussen FTG, Diercks RL. Biomechanics of the elbow joint in tennis players and relation to pathology. Br J Sports Med. 2007;41:820–3.
24. Tosti R, Jennings J, Sewards JM. Lateral epicondylitis of the elbow. Am J Med. 2013;126(357):357. e1-357.e6.
25. Hume PA, Reid D, Edwards T. Epicondylar injury in sport. Epidemiology, type, mechanisms, assessment, management and prevention. Sports Med. 2006;36(2):151–70.
26. Sánchez M, Anitua E. A new biological approach to orthopedic surgery and sports medicine. 1st ed. Vitoria: Team Work Media; 2013. Chapter 144–58.
27. Behzad H, Sharma A, Mousavizadeh R, et al. Mast cells exert pro-inflammatory effects of relevance to the pathophysiology of tendinopathy. Arthritis Res Ther. 2013;15(6):R184.
28. Sharma P, Maffulli N. Tendon injury and tendinopathy: healing and repair. J Bone Joint Surg Am. 2005;87:187–202.
29. Alfredson H, Bjur D, Thorsen K, Lorentzon R, Sandstrom P. High intratendinous lactate levels in painful chronic Achilles tendinosis. An investigation using microdialysis technique. J Orthop Res. 2002;20:934–8.
30. Alfredson H, Ohberg L. Sclerosing injections to areas of neo-vascularisation reduce pain in chronic Achilles tendinopathy: a double blind randomised controlled trial. Knee Surg Sports Traumatol Arthrosc. 2005;13:338–44.
31. Goldie I. Epicondylitis lateralis humeri (epicondylagia or tennis elbow). A pathogenetical study. Acta Chir Scand Suppl. 1964;57 suppl 339:1.
32. Coonrad RW, Hooper WR. Tennis elbow: its courses, natural history, conservative and surgical management. J Bone Joint Surg Am. 1973;55:1177–82.
33. Ahmad Z. Lateral epicondylitis. A review of pathology and management. Bone Joint J. 2013;95-B:1158–64.
34. Chen J, Wang A, Xu J, et al. In chronic lateral epicondylitis, apoptosis and autophagic cell death occur in the extensor carpi radialis brevis tendon. J Shoulder Elbow Surg. 2010;19:355–62.
35. Nirschl RP, Pettrone FA. Tennis elbow. The surgical treatment of lateral epicondylitis. J Bone Joint Surg Am. 1979;61(6A):832–9.
36. Brummel J, et al. Epicondylitis: lateral. Sports Med Arthrosc Rev. 2014;22:e1–6.
37. Connell D, Burke F, Coombes P, et al. Sonographic examination of lateral epicondylitis. Am J Roentgenol. 2001;176:777–82.
38. Van Hofwegen C, Baker 3rd CL, Baker Jr CL. Epicondylitis in the athlete's elbow. Clin Sports Med. 2010;29:577–97.
39. Buckup K. Clinical tests for the musculoskeletal system: examinations-sign-phenomena. 2nd ed. Stuttgart: Thieme; 2008. p. 129–33.
40. Gardner RC. Tennis elbow: diagnosis, pathology and treatment: nine severe cases treated by a new reconstructive operation. Clin Orthop. 1970;72:248–53.
41. Edelson G, Kunos CA, Vigder F, Obed E. Bony changes at the lateral epicondyle of possible significance in tennis elbow syndrome. J Shoulder Elbow Surg. 2001;10:158–63.
42. Miller TT, Shapiro MA, Schultz E, et al. Comparison of sonography and MRI for diagnosing epicondylitis. J Clin Ultrasound. 2002;30:193–202.
43. Naam NH, Nemani S. Radial tunnel syndrome. Orthop Clin North Am. 2012;43:529–36.
44. Rajeev A, Pooley J. Lateral compartment cartilage changes and lateral elbow pain. Acta Orthop Belg. 2009;75:37–40.
45. Smidt N, Lewis M, van der Windt DAWM, Hay EM, Bouter LM, Croft P. Lateral epicondylitis in general practice: course and prognostic indicators of outcome. J Rheumatol. 2006;33:2053–9.
46. Sayegh ET, Strauch RJ. Does nonsurgical treatment improve longitudinal outcomes of lateral epicondylitis over no treatment? A meta-analysis. Clin Orthop Relat Res. 2015;473:1093–107.
47. Bisset L, et al. Mobilisation with movement and exercise, corticosteroid injection, or wait and see for tennis elbow: randomised trial. BMJ. 2006. doi:10.1136/bmj.38961.584653.AE.
48. Coombes BK, et al. Effect of corticosteroid injection, physiotherapy, or both on clinical outcomes in patients with unilateral lateral epicondylalgia a randomized controlled trial. JAMA. 2013;309(5):461–9.
49. Mardani-Kivi M, Karimi-Mobarakeh M, Karimi A, et al. The effects of corticosteroid injection versus local anesthetic injection in the treatment of lateral epicondylitis: a randomized single-blinded clinical trial. Arch Orthop Trauma Surg. 2013;133:757–63.
50. Buchbinder R, Johnston RV, Barnsley L, Assendelft WJ, Bell SN, Smidt N. Surgery for lateral elbow pain. Cochrane Database Syst Rev. 2011;3:CD003525.
51. Hall MP, Band PA, Meislin RJ, Jazrawi LM, Cardone DA. Platelet-rich plasma: current concepts and application in sports medicine. J Am Acad Orthop Surg. 2009;17(10):602–8.
52. Sánchez M, Azofra J, Anitua E, et al. Plasma rich in growth factors to treat an articular cartilage avulsion: a case report. Med Sci Sports Exerc. 2003;35:1648–52.
53. Sánchez M, Anitua E, Orive G, et al. Platelet-rich therapies in the treatment of orthopaedic sport injuries. Sports Med. 2009;39:345–54.
54. Mishra A, Harmon K, Woodall Jr J, Vieira A. Sports medicine applications of platelet rich plasma. Curr Pharm Biotechnol. 2012;13(7):1185–95.
55. Hsu WK, Mishra A, Rodeo SR, et al. Platelet-rich plasma in orthopaedic applications: evidence-based recommendations for treatment. J Am Acad Orthop Surg. 2013;21(12):739–48.
56. Sánchez M, Albillos J, Angulo F, et al. Platelet-rich plasma in muscle and tendon healing. Oper Technol Orthop. 2012;22:16–24.
57. Dohan Ehrenfest DM, Rasmusson L, Albrektsson T. Classification of platelet concentrates: from pure platelet-rich plasma (P-PRP) to leucocyte- and platelet-rich fibrin (L-PRF). Trends Biotechnol. 2009;27:158–67.
58. DeLong JM, Russell RP, Mazzocca AD. Platelet-rich plasma: the PAW classification system. Arthroscopy. 2012;28(7):998–1009.

59. Mastrangelo AN, Vavken P, Fleming BC, et al. Reduced platelet concentration does not harm PRP effectiveness for ACL repair in a porcine in vivo model. J Orthop Res. 2011;29:1002–7.
60. Wiegerinck JI, Reilingh ML, de Jonge MC, et al. Injection techniques of platelet-rich plasma into and around the Achilles tendon: a cadaveric study. Am J Sports Med. 2011;39:1681–168.
61. Dragoo JL, Braun HJ, Durham JL, et al. Comparison of the acute inflammatory response of two commercial platelet-rich plasma systems in healthy rabbit tendons. Am J Sports Med. 2012;40:1274–81.
62. Sundman EA, Cole BJ, Fortier LA. Growth factor and catabolic cytokine concentrations are influenced by the cellular composition of platelet-rich plasma. Am J Sports Med. 2011;39:2135–40.
63. Filardo G, Kon E, Pereira Ruiz MT, Vaccaro F, Guitaldi R, Di Martino A, Cenacchi A, Fornasari PM, Marcacci M. Platelet-rich plasma intra-articular injections for cartilage degeneration and osteoarthritis: single- versus double-spinning approach. Knee Surg Sports Traumatol Arthrosc. 2012;20:2082–91.
64. Carofino B, et al. Corticosteroids and local anesthetics decrease positive effects of platelet-rich plasma: an in vitro study on human tendon cells. Arthroscopy. 2012;28(5):711–9.
65. Martin JI, et al. Platelet-rich plasma (PRP) in chronic epicondylitis: study protocol for a randomized controlled trial. Trials. 2013;14:410.
66. Anitua E, Alkhraisat MH, Orive G. Perspectives and challenges in regenerative medicine using plasma rich in growth factors. J Control Release. 2012;157:29–38.
67. Anitua E, Sanchez M, Orive G. Potential of endogenous regenerative technology for in situ regenerative medicine. Adv Drug Deliv Rev. 2010;62(7–8):741–52.
68. Nurden AT. Platelets, inflammation and tissue regeneration. Thromb Haemost. 2011;105(Suppl1):S13–33.
69. Discher DE, Mooney DJ, Zandstra PW. Growth factors, matrices, and forces combine and control stem cells. Science. 2009;324(5935):1673–7.
70. Martino MM, Briquez PS, Ranga A, et al. Heparin-binding domain of fibrin(ogen) binds growth factors and promotes tissue repair when incorporated within a synthetic matrix. Proc Natl Acad Sci U S A. 2013;110(12):4563–8.
71. Anitua E, Zalduendo M, Prado R, et al. Morphogen and pro-inflammatory cytokine release kinetics from PRGF-Endoret fibrin scaffolds: evaluation of the effect of leukocyte inclusion. J Biomed Mater Res A. 2015;103(3):1011–20.
72. Anitua E, Orive G. Endogenous regenerative technology using plasma- and platelet-derived growth factors. J Control Release. 2012;157(3):317–20.
73. Zhang J, Wang JHC. Platelet–rich plasma releasate promotes differentiation of tendon stem cells into active tenocytes. Am J Sports Med. 2010;38:2477–86.
74. Schnabel LV, Mohammed HO, Miller BJ, et al. Platelet rich plasma (PRP) enhances the anabolic gene expression pattern in flexor digitorum superficialis tendons. J Orthop Res. 2007;25:230–40.
75. Anitua E, Sanchez M, Zalduendo MM, et al. Fibroblastic response to treatment with different preparations rich in growth factors. Cell Prolif. 2009;41:162–70.
76. Anitua E, Sanchez M, De la Fuente M, et al. Plasma rich in growth factors (PRGF-Endoret) stimulates tendon and synovial fibroblasts migration and improves the biological properties of hyaluronic acid. Knee Surg Sports Traumatol Arthrosc. 2012;20:1657–65.
77. Anitua E, Sánchez M, Nurden AT, et al. Autologous fibrin matrices: a potential source of biological mediators that modulate tendon cell activities. J Biomed Mater Res. 2006;77:285–93.
78. Mishra A, Pavelko T. Treatment of chronic elbow tendinosis with buffered platelet rich plasma. Am J Sports Med. 2006;34:1774–8.
79. Peerbooms JC, Sluimer J, Bruijn DJ, Gosens T. Positive effect of an autologous platelet concentrate in lateral epicondylitis in a double-blind randomized controlled trial: Platelet-rich plasma versus corticosteroid injection with a 1-year follow-up. Am J Sports Med. 2010;38:255–62.
80. Gosens T, Peerbooms JC, van Laar W, den Oudsten BL. Ongoing positive effect of platelet-rich plasma versus corticosteroid injection in lateral epicondylitis: a double- blind randomized controlled trial with 2-year follow-up. Am J Sports Med. 2011;39:1200–8.
81. Creaney L, Walla A, Curtis M, Connell D. Growth factor- based therapies provide additional benefit beyond physical therapy in resistant elbow tendinopathy: a prospective, double-blind, randomised trial of autologous blood injections versus platelet-rich plasma injections. Br J Sports Med. 2011;45:966–71.
82. Thanasas C, Papadimitriou G, Charalambidis C, Paraskevopoulos I, Papanikolaou A. Platelet- rich plasma versus autologous whole blood for the treatment of chronic lateral elbow epicondylitis: a randomized controlled clinical trial. Am J Sports Med. 2011;39:2130–4.
83. Omar Aziza S, Maha EI, Amal SA, Mahmoud S. Local injection of autologous platelet rich plasma and corticosteroid in treatment of lateral epicondylitis and plantar fasciitis: randomized clinical trial. Egypt Rheumatol. 2012;34:43–9.
84. Krogh TP, Fredberg U, Stengaard-Pedersen K, et al. Treatment of lateral epicondylitis with platelet-rich plasma, glucocorticoid, or saline: a randomized, double-blind, placebo-controlled trial. Am J Sports Med. 2013;41:625–35.
85. Mishra AK, Skrepnik NV, Edwards SG, et al. Efficacy of platelet-rich plasma for chronic tennis elbow: a double- blind, prospective, multicenter, randomized controlled trial of 230 patients. Am J Sports Med. 2014;42:463–71.
86. Raeissadat SA, Rayegani SM, Hassanabadi H, et al. Is platelet-rich plasma superior to whole blood in the management of chronic tennis elbow: one year randomized clinical trial. BMC Sports Sci Med Rehabil. 2014;6:12.
87. Chaudhury S, de La Lama M, Adler RS, et al. Platelet-rich plasma for the treatment of lateral epicondylitis: sonographic assessment of tendon morphology and vascularity (pilot study). Skeletal Radiol. 2013; 42:91–7.
88. Hechtman KS, Uribe JW, Botto-vanDemden A, Kiebzak GM. Platelet-rich plasma injection reduces pain in patients with recalcitrant epicondylitis. Orthopedics. 2011;34:92.

11 Conservative Treatment in Lateral Elbow Pain

Renée Keijsers and Denise Eygendaal

11.1 Introduction

There are many synonyms to denote lateral elbow pain, such as tennis elbow, lateral epicondylitis, epicondylalgia, tendinitis, tendinopathy, or tendinosis of the common extensor origin. To create uniformity, lateral elbow pain is considered a general term to clarify the terminology [1]. Lateral elbow pain is a common disorder with a prevalence of 1–3 % in the general population. The incidence seems independent of sex and ethnical background [2–4]. Only age influences the incidence with the highest incidence between 45 and 54 years. It is a disorder that is associated with patients in working age from the age of 20 up to 65 years. The exact etiology of lateral elbow pain is not completely understood. High physical demands, smoking, and obesity are strong determinants of lateral elbow pain [5–7]. It is also a common sports injury. Fifty percent of all tennis players will get an episode of lateral elbow pain during their career, but that contributes in only 5 % of all cases [8]. The current consensus is that repetitive trauma results in lesions and an abnormal vascular reaction in the common extensor tendon. The tendinous origin of the extensor carpi radialis brevis is usually involved. Microscopic evaluation of involved tissue shows proliferation of fibroblasts and ingrowth of new blood vessels [11–13].

11.2 Treatment Options

Lateral elbow pain is basically a self-limiting condition; a wait-and-see with avoidance of aggravating activities shows 80 % resolution after 6 months and 90 % resolution after 1 year [6, 9, 10]. The duration of symptoms cannot be predicted, but certain characteristics have a poorer prognosis. The prognosis for recovery in the long term is worse when the patient experiences more pain, when the duration of the symptoms lasts longer, and with recurrent symptoms [6, 9, 14]. This also means that 10 % of the patients have persistent symptoms despite prolonged watchful waiting. The goal of treatment is to reduce pain or to shorten duration of symptoms, restore function with return to work and resuming sports, and thereby improve quality of life. This goal should be achieved with conservative or minimally invasive interventions and with attention to possible side effects of treatment. A lot of different treatment options are available; however, there is still no consensus on the optimal treatment of lateral elbow pain.

R. Keijsers, MD • D. Eygendaal, MD, PhD (✉)
Upper Limb Unit of the Amphia Hospital Breda, Breda, The Netherlands

Department of Orthopedic Surgery, Academic Medical Centre, Amsterdam, The Netherlands
e-mail: denise@eygendaal.nl

L.A. Pederzini et al. (eds.), *Elbow and Sport*, DOI 10.1007/978-3-662-48742-6_11

11.3 Physiotherapy

In physical therapy, there are several interventions for lateral elbow pain, such as deep transverse friction massage, exercises (e.g., eccentric exercises, concentric exercises, and stretching), extracorporeal shock wave therapy (ESWT), and mobilizing and manipulative techniques. Usually a combination of different methods of treatment is used. Deep transverse friction massage was first demonstrated in the 1930s. The goal of treatment is to prevent abnormal fibrous adhesions and abnormal scarring. The Cochrane review on deep transverse friction massage for treating lateral elbow tendinitis states that there is no sufficient evidence to determine the effects of deep transverse friction on pain, improvement in grip strength, and functional status, as no evidence of clinically important benefits was found. Pain relief of 30 % or greater, quality of life, patient global assessment, adverse events, and withdrawals due to adverse events were not assessed or reported [20].

A systematic review and meta-analysis of Bisset et al. [25] stated that there is a lack of evidence for the long-term benefit of physical interventions in general. However, there is evidence for the effectiveness of manipulative techniques of the elbow on the short term. Further research with long-term follow-up into manipulation and exercise as treatments is indicated [25, 27].

After this review, more studies on the effect of exercises have been published with variable results. Studies on the effectiveness of concentric and eccentric strengthening found no significant differences in outcome measures [26, 27]. This is contradicted by another study that concludes that isokinetic exercises are effective compared to the non-strengthening control group, on reduction of pain intensity, mainly after 1 month of treatment, an absence of strength deficit on the involved side through bilateral comparison for the forearm supinator and wrist extensor muscles, decreasing thickness and a recovered homogenous tendon structure, and a more marked improvement in disability status during occupational, spare time, and sports activities [28].

Further research is indicated on the effect of exercise therapy in the treatment of lateral elbow pain, but based on results with patellar and Achilles tendinopathy, strengthening exercises are recommended.

11.4 Shock Wave (ESWT)

Acoustic waves have been used to treat chronic lateral elbow pain. The evidence suggests that extracorporeal shock wave therapy is not beneficial in the treatment of lateral elbow pain, with no significant short-term or long-term effects. Besides this, the treatment is generally uncomfortable with transient adverse effect as pain, nausea, and reddening [23, 25].

11.5 Orthotic Devices

Many different types of braces and other orthotic devices such as splints, casts, bands, or straps are available for treating lateral elbow pain. The underlying theory is that immobilization should completely limit expansion and no force can be made by the extensor muscles. Binding the muscle may also limit expansion of muscle and decrease the contribution of muscle fibers proximal to the band. The Cochrane review on the effect of orthotic devices found no clear evidence of effectiveness of the device and states that more well-designed and well-conducted RCTs are warranted despite the common use of the devices [24]. A systematic review from Borkholder et al. [34] found early positive, but not conclusive, support for the effectiveness of splinting lateral epicondylitis [34].

11.6 Medication

To reduce the lateral elbow pain, painkillers as paracetamol and nonsteroidal anti-inflammatory drugs (NSAIDs) are frequently used. The Cochrane review on the effect of NSAIDs, in which 15 trials (involving 759 participants) were included, concludes that topical NSAIDs (applied to the skin in a gel) may improve treatment success. However, the quality of the evidence is low and it may result in a skin rash [21].

No definite conclusion regarding the effectiveness of NSAIDs taken orally can be drawn, due to the low quality of the evidence. Possible side effects of NSAIDs are stomach, kidney, or heart problems [21].

11.7 Injection Therapy

Currently, different injectables are used in the treatment of lateral elbow pain without proper scientific evidence. A recent meta-analysis by Krogh et al. [13] confirmed this statement and found a paucity of evidence from unbiased trials on which to base treatment recommendations. One of the problems in the comparison of the different injectables is the variation in injection technique; the number and depth of perforations varies widely, as well as the amount of fluid injected [17]. A recent cadaver study by the authors, in which experienced orthopedic surgeons were asked to inject dye in the ECRB tendon in a cadaver elbow, showed that only one-third of the surgeons actually injected the dye into the ECRB tendon and 60 % of all injections were intra-articularly located as well. So even in experienced hands, blind injection in the ECRB is not accurate, which makes comparison of different injectables impossible without a standardized, ultrasound-guided technique.

Below an overview of the most common injection therapies and the current evidence of their effectiveness is given.

11.7.1 Steroid Injections

Injections for lateral elbow pain with corticosteroids have been used since the 1950s. Several studies report no long-term benefits of a steroid injection. In fact, on the long term the results of steroid injections are worse than wait-and-see, with seven out of ten patients pain-free compared to eight to nine out of ten with wait-and-see [15–19]. On the short term eight to nine out of ten patients are pain-free after 2–6 weeks, compared to three out of ten with a wait-and-see policy [18].

In addition to the limited treatment outcomes, various side effects have been reported after injecting steroids. An increase in pain during 1–3 days is reported in 10–50 % of the treated patients. As rare side effects of corticosteroid injections, hot flashes, hypopigmentation, and subcutaneous necrosis can occur [18, 19, 29].

In the treatment of lateral elbow pain, there is no place for steroid injections. However, when a quick relief of pain is required, for example, in athletes who have to play an important match, a steroid injection could be considered. The poorer prognosis in the long term should be taken into account.

11.7.2 Autologous Whole Blood Injections

Autologous blood contains platelets with growth factors that may help in the healing process of chronic injuries. These platelet growth factors stimulate the healing process and lead to partial modification of the damaged tissue. The hypothesis is that these growth factors stimulate angiogenesis and cell proliferation and increase the recruitment of repair cells and tensile strength [28].

A review by Vos et al. on the effects of autologous blood injections in the management of tendinopathies showed no benefit of autologous whole blood injections in three high-quality RCTs compared with a control group [35].

11.7.3 Platelet-Rich Plasma (PRP)

The review by Vos et al. mentioned above also reviewed the effect of PRP in the management of tendinopathies in general. They stated that there were no high-quality studies on PRP treatment. There is also a lot of variation in the amount and mixture of growth factors combined with using different cell separating systems [36]. Thereby it is uncertain whether platelet activation prior to injection is necessary. There is limited evidence to support the use of injections with PRP in the management of chronic tendinopathy. Further research is needed [35].

The Cochrane review on the effect of PRP injections in the treatment of lateral elbow pain states that there is currently insufficient evidence to support the use of PRP for treating musculoskeletal soft tissue injuries. There is a need for standardization of PRP preparation methods [33]. See Chap. 11 for more detailed information on PRPs.

11.7.4 Hyaluronic Acid Injections

Hyaluronic acid is a biological substance distributed throughout the body; this high molecular weight polysaccharide is a major component of synovial fluid and surrounding structures of the joints. Periarticular efficacy and safety have been reported for soft tissue use in acute ankle sprain [37]. A first randomized controlled trial on the effect of hyaluronic acid compared to saline injections in the treatment of lateral elbow pain shows promising results [38].

11.7.5 Dextrose Injections

Injection therapy with application of dextrose is a common treatment in chronic musculoskeletal pain, including lateral epicondylitis. Animal model studies suggest that the treatment by perforation with application of dextrose may enlarge and strengthen ligament and tendon insertions. However, the precise mechanism is unclear [39].

A double-blind pilot RCT of 24 patients comparing the effect of dextrose versus saline shows a beneficial effect after 52 weeks. However, it is a pilot study, and therefore the sample size is too small to draw conclusions on the efficacy; further research is needed [40].

11.7.6 Botulinum Toxin

Since 1997, botulin toxin injections were used in the treatment of lateral elbow pain [30]. Botulinum toxin reduces muscular activity and causes muscle paralysis, by irreversibly blocking the presynaptic release of acetylcholine at the neuromuscular junction. The muscle relaxation will last for 12–16 weeks [31]. It is thought that the relaxation of the extensor muscles causes a reduced tension on the tendons, but the exact mechanism of action remains unclear. Besides the paralysis, botulinum toxin might also have some analgesic properties [32].

A few randomized controlled trials have assessed the effectiveness of botulinum toxin injection for lateral elbow pain, with conflicting results [41–44]. A meta-analysis of four RCTs showed that botulinum toxin was found to be marginally superior to placebo, but all the trials were at high risk of bias. All trials reported temporary side effects with paresis/weakness in the extension of the wrist and the third and fourth finger [17].

In the current literature, the main obstacle in the comparison of the different injection therapies is the variation in injection technique. Most injections are manually performed, without ultrasound guidance, and it is therefore difficult to determine the exact location of the injection site. To compare the different techniques, it is recommended to perform future studies in a standardized manner with ultrasound guidance.

11.7.7 Acupuncture

Acupuncture has long been used to treat lateral elbow pain in China and in Western countries; it originated in China approximately 2,000 years ago and is one of the oldest medical procedures in the world. The word "acupuncture" is derived from the Latin words "acus" (needle) and "punctura" (penetration). The Cochrane study on the effect of acupuncture (including 4 small RCTs, with 48 to 93 participants) stated that there is insufficient evidence to either support or refute the use of acupuncture (either needle or laser) in the treatment of lateral elbow pain. On the short term needle acupuncture is of benefit with respect to pain, but this effect only lasts up to 24 h. Further research is needed before conclusions can be drawn regarding the effect of acupuncture on lateral elbow pain [22].

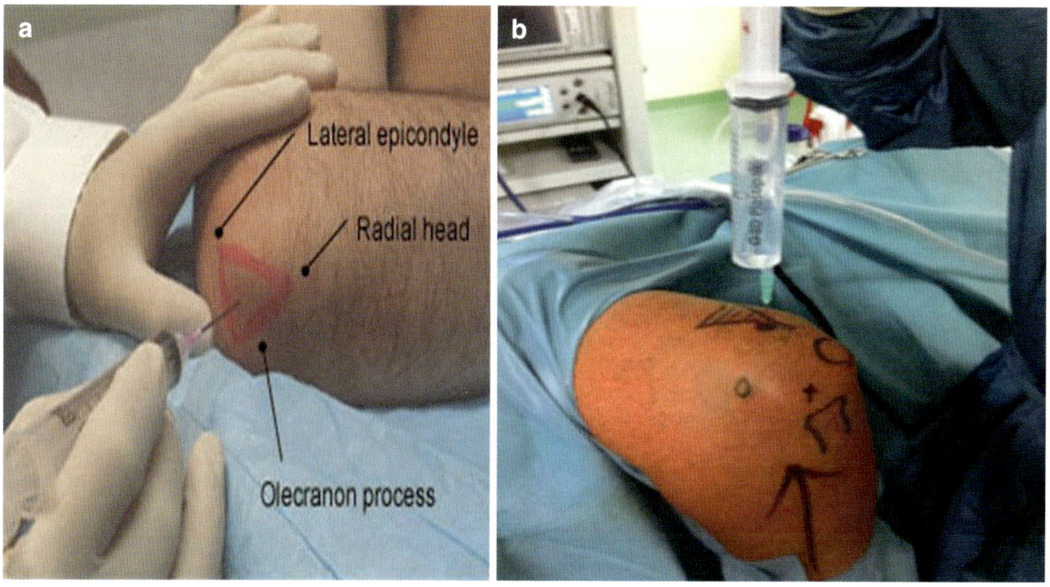

Fig. 11.1 Anatomic landmarks and technique of Injections for postero-lateral soft-spot approach (**a**) and posterior trans-triceps approach (**b**)

Pearls

If a patient suffers from both an ECRB tendinopathy and articular elbow pathology, intra-articular injections can be added to the above treatment options of the ECRB tendinopathy. In most textbooks injections into the elbow joint are advocated through the posterolateral soft spot between the radial head, olecranon, and capitellum. Van Wagenberg et al. proposed a posterior transtriceps approach, with a flexed elbow, right in the olecranon fossa. This is an easy and safe technique for intra-articular injections of the elbow [45] Figs. 11.1 and 11.2.

Pitfalls

Blind injection in the ECRB is not accurate, which makes comparison of different injectables impossible without a standardized, ultrasound-guided technique. New randomized trials should use an ultrasound-guided technique, with standardization of the number and depth of perforations, as well as the amount of fluid injected for proper comparison of different injectables.

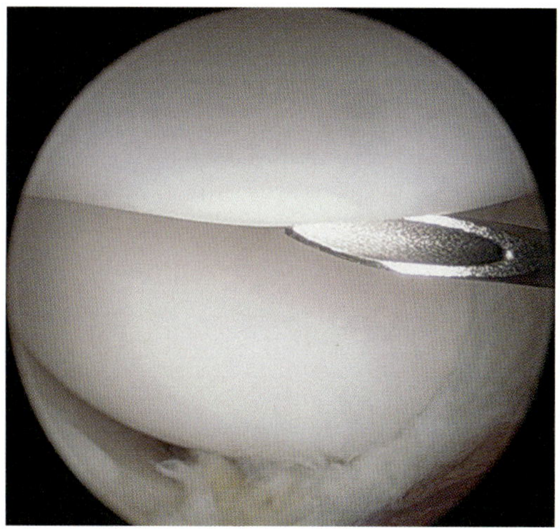

Fig. 11.2 Arthroscopic view of the needle inside the joint

References

1. Silagy M, O'Bryan E, Johnston RV, Buchbinder R. Autologous blood and platelet rich plasma injection therapy for lateral elbow pain. Cochrane Database SystRev. 2014;(2):CD010951.doi:10.1002/14651858.CD010951.
2. Hamilton PG. The prevalence of humeral epicondylitis: a survey in general practice. J R Coll Gen Pract. 1986;36:464–5.
3. Verhaar JA. Tennis elbow: anatomical, epidemiological and therapeutic aspects. Int Orthop. 1994;18:263–7.

4. Walker-Bone K, Palmer KT, Reading I. Prevalence and impact of musculoskeletal disorders of the upper limb in the general population. Arthritis Rheum. 2004;51:642–51.
5. Shiri R, Viikari-Juntura E, Varonen H, Heliövaara M. Prevalence and determinants of lateral and medial epicondylitis: a population study. Am J Epidemiol. 2006;164(11):1065.
6. Haahr JP, Andersen JH. Physical and psychosocial risk factors for lateral epicondylitis: a population based case-referent study. Occup Environ Med. 2003;60:322–9.
7. Leclerc A, Landre MF, Chastang JF. Upper-limb disorders in repetitive work. Scand J Work Environ Health. 2001;27:268–78.
8. Pluim BM, Fuller CW, Batt ME, Chase L, Hainline B, Miller S, Montalvan B, Renström P, Stroia KA, Weber K, Wood TO. Consensus statement on epidemiological studies of medical conditions in tennis, April 2009. Br J Sports Med. 2009;43(12):893–7. doi:10.1136/bjsm.2009.064915.
9. Kraushaar BS, Nirschl RP. Tendinosis of the elbow (tennis elbow). Clinical features and findings of histological, immunohistochemical, and electron microscopy studies. J Bone Joint Surg Am. 1999;81:259–78.
10. Haahr JP, Andersen JH. Prognostic factors in lateral epicondylitis: a randomized trial with one-year follow-up in 266 new cases treated with minimal occupational intervention or the usual approach in general practice. Rheumatology (Oxford). 2003;42:1216–25.
11. Krogh TP, Fredberg U, Stengaard-Pedersen K, Christensen R, Jensen P, Ellingsen T. Treatment of lateral epicondylitis with platelet-rich plasma, glucocorticoid, or saline: a randomized, double-blind, placebo-controlled trial. Am J Sports Med. 2013;41(3):625–35. doi:10.1177/0363546512472975. Epub 2013 Jan 17.
12. Assendelft WJ, Hay EM, Adshead R, Bouter LM. Corticosteroid injections for lateral epicondylitis: a systematic overview. Br J Gen Pract. 1996;46:209–16.
13. Krogh TP, Bartels EM, Ellingsen T, Stengaard-Pedersen K, Buchbinder R, Fredberg U, Bliddal H, Christensen R. Comparative effectiveness of injection therapies in lateral epicondylitis: a systematic review and network meta- analysis of randomized controlled trials. Am J Sports Med. 2013;41(6):1435–46. doi: 10.1177/0363546512458237.
14. Smidt N, Van der Windt DA, Assendelft WJ, Deville WL, Korthals-de BI, Bouter LM. Corticosteroid injections, physiotherapy, or a wait-and-see policy for lateral epicondylitis: a randomised controlled trial. Lancet. 2002;359:657.
15. Bot SD, van der Waal JM, Terwee CB, van der Windt DA, Bouter LM, Dekker J. Course and prognosis of elbow complaints: a cohort study in general practice. Ann Rheum Dis. 2005;64(9):1331–6. Epub 2005 Feb 11.
16. Keefe FJ, Rumble ME, Scipio CD, Giordano LA, Perri LM. Psychological aspects of persistent pain: current state of the science. J Pain. 2004;5:195–211.
17. Nirschl RP, Ashman ES. Elbow tendinopathy: tennis elbow. Clin Sports Med. 2003;22:813–36.
18. Potter HG, Hannafin JA, Morwessel RM, DiCarlo EF, O'Brien SJ, Altchek DW. Lateral epicondylitis: correlation of MR imaging, surgical, and histopathologic findings. Radiology. 1995;196(1):43–6.
19. Bisset L, Beller E, Jull G, Brooks P, Darnell R, Vicenzino B. Mobilisation with movement and exercise, corticosteroid injection, or wait and see for tennis elbow: randomised trial. BMJ. 2006; 333:939.
20. Loew LM, Brosseau L, Tugwell P, Wells GA, Welch V, Shea B, Poitras S, De Angelis G, Rahman P. Deep transverse friction massage for treating lateral elbow or lateral knee tendinitis. Cochrane Database Syst Rev. 2014;(11):CD003528. doi:10.1002/14651858.CD003528.pub2.
21. Pattanittum P, Turner T, Green S, Buchbinder R. Non-steroidal anti- inflammatory drugs (NSAIDs) for treating lateral elbow pain in adults. Cochrane Database Syst Rev. 2013;(5):CD003686. doi:10.1002/14651858.CD003686.pub2.
22. Green S, Buchbinder R, Barnsley L, Hall S, White M, Smidt N, Assendelft WJJ. Acupuncture for lateral elbow pain. Cochrane Database Syst Rev. 2002;(1):CD003527. doi:10.1002/14651858.CD003527.
23. Buchbinder R, Green S, Youd JM, Assendelft WJJ, Barnsley L, Smidt N. Shock wave therapy for lateral elbow pain. Cochrane Database Syst Rev. 2005;(4):CD003524. doi:10.1002/14651858.CD003524.pub2.
24. Struijs PAA, Smidt N, Arola H, van Dijk CN, Buchbinder R, Assendelft WJJ. Orthotic devices for the treatment of tennis elbow. Cochrane Database Syst Rev. 2002;(1):CD001821. doi:10.1002/14651858.CD001821.
25. Bisset L, Paungmali A, Vicenzino B, Beller E. A systematic review and meta- analysis of clinical trials on physical interventions for lateral epicondylalgia. Br J Sports Med. 2005;39:411–22.
26. Martinez-Silvestrini JA, Newcomer KL, Gay RE, Schaefer MP, Kortebein P, Arendt KW. Chronic lateral epicondylitis: comparative effectiveness of a home exercise program including stretching alone versus stretching supplemented with eccentric or concentric strengthening. J Hand Ther. 2005;18(4):411–9, quiz 420.
27. Luginbühl R, Brunner F, Schneeberger AG. No effect of forearm band and extensor strengthening exercises for the treatment of tennis elbow: a prospective randomised study. Chir Organi Mov. 2008;91(1):35–40. doi:10.1007/s12306-007-0006-3. Epub 2008 Feb 10.
28. Croisier JL, Foidart-Dessalle M, Tinant F, Crielaard JM, Forthomme B. An isokinetic eccentric programme for the management of chronic lateral epicondylar tendinopathy. Br J Sports Med. 2007;41(4):269–75. Epub 2007 Jan 15. doi: 10.1136/bjsm.2006.033324.
29. Smidt N, Assendelft WJ, van der Windt DA, Hay EM, Buchbinder R, Bouter LM. Corticosteroid injections

for lateral epicondylitis: a systematic review. Pain. 2002;96(1–2):23–40.
30. Morre HH, Keizer SB. Treatment of chronic tennis elbow with botulinum toxin. Lancet. 1997;349:1746.
31. Ramachandran M, Eastwood DM. Botulinum toxin and its orthopaedic applications. J Bone Joint Surg Br Vol. 2006;88-B:981–7. doi: 10.1302/0301-620X.88B8.18041.
32. Smidt N, Dingjan RA, Buchbinder R, Assendelft WJJ. Botulinum toxin injection for tennis elbow (Protocol). Cochrane Database Syst Rev. 2011;(1):CD008961. doi:10.1002/14651858.CD008961.
33. Moraes VY, Lenza M, Tamaoki MJ, Faloppa F, Belloti JC. Platelet-rich therapies for musculoskeletal soft tissue injuries. Cochrane Database Syst Rev. 2014;(4):CD010071. doi:10.1002/14651858.CD010071.pub3.
34. Borkholder CD, Hill VA, Fess EE. The efficacy of splinting for lateral epicondylitis: a systematic review. J Hand Ther. 2004;17(2):181–99.
35. de Vos RJ, van Veldhoven PL, Moen MH, Weir A, Tol JL, Maffulli N. Autologous growth factor injections in chronic tendinopathy: a systematic review. Br Med Bull. 2010;95:63–77. doi:10.1093/bmb/ldq006. Epub 2010 Mar 2.
36. Dohan Ehrenfest DM, Rasmusson L, Albrektsson T. Classification of platelet concentrates: from pure platelet-rich plasma (P-PRP) to leucocyte- and platelet- rich fibrin (L-PRF). Trends Biotechnol. 2009;27(3):158–67. doi: 10.1016/j.tibtech.2008.11.009.
37. Petrella RJ, Petrella MJ, Cogliano A. Periarticular hyaluronic acid in acute ankle sprain. Clin J Sport Med. 2007;17(4):251–7. doi: 10.1097/JSM.0b013e3180f6169f.
38. Petrella RJ, Cogliano A, Decaria J, Mohamed N, Lee R. Management of tennis elbow with sodium hyaluronate periarticular injections. Sports Med Arthrosc Rehabil Ther Technol. 2010;2:4. doi: 10.1186/1758-2555-2-4.
39. Placzek R, Drescher W, Deuretzbacher G, Hempfing A, Meiss AL. Treatment of chronic radial epicondylitis with botulinum toxin a: a double-blind, placebo-controlled, randomized multicenter study. J Bone Joint Surg Am. 2007;89:255–60. http://dx.doi.org/10.2106/JBJS.F.00401.
40. Hayton MJ, Santini AJ, Hughes PJ, Frostick SP, Trail IA, Stanley JK. Botulinum toxin injection in the treatment of tennis elbow: a double-blind, randomized, controlled, pilot study. J Bone Joint Surg Am. 2005;87:503–7.
41. Rabago D, Best T, Beamsly M, et al. A systematic review of prolotherapy for chronic musculoskeletal pain. Clin J Sports Med. 2005;15(5):376–80.
42. Scarpone M, Rabago DP, Zgierska A, Arbogast G, Snell E. The efficacy of prolotherapy for lateral epicondylosis: a pilot study. Clin J Sport Med. 2008;18:248–54. doi: 10.1097/JSM.0b013e318170fc87.
43. Espandar R, Heidari P, Rasouli MR, et al. Use of anatomic measurement to guide injection of botulinum toxin for the management of chronic lateral epicondylitis: a randomized controlled trial. CMAJ. 2010;182:768–73 doi: 10.1503/cmaj.090906.
44. Lin YC, Tu YK, Chen SS, Lin IL, Chen SC, Guo HR. Comparison between botulinum toxin and corticosteroid injection in the treatment of acute and subacute tennis elbow a prospective, randomized, double- blind, active drug-controlled pilot study. Am J Phys Med Rehabil. 2010;89:653–9. doi: 10.1097/PHM.0b013e3181cf564d.
45. Wagenberg JM, Turkenburg JL, Rahusen FT, Eygendaal D. The posterior transtriceps approach for intra-articular elbow diagnostics, definitely not forgotten. Skeletal Radiol. 2013;42:55–9. doi:10.1007/s00256-012-1430-5.

Degenerative Elbow in Sportsmen 12

Luigi Adriano Pederzini and Emanuele Tripoli

12.1 Introduction

Elbow pathologies are very common and may limit participation in sports and occupational endeavours, as well as activities of daily living [11]. Many sports competitions involve the elbow joint. Throwing, pushing, opposing and gripping are frequent in different sports. These activities can all lead to significant elbow stress. Acute traumas or repeated microtraumas can affect the joint surfaces, ligaments and muscles, determining a loss of function. Overuse syndromes are the most common aetiologic factors in athletes producing early joint degeneration. Javelin and baseball throwers, boxers, weightlifters and tennis players often present typical degenerative elbows [12, 30]. In particular, repetitive overhead throwing imparts high valgus and extension loads to the athlete's elbow, often leading to either acute or chronic injury or progressive structural changes.

In recent decades, there has been a sharp rise in the number of participants in overhead-throwing sports. These sports are not limited to baseball but also include softball, football, tennis, squash, golf, volleyball and javelin. The increase in participation has brought a concurrent increase in the incidence of injury to the upper extremity [7, 14].

Common injuries encountered in the throwing elbow include ulnar collateral ligament tears, ulnar neuritis, flexor-pronator strain, lateral epicondylitis, medial epicondyle apophysitis or avulsion, valgus extension overload syndrome with olecranon osteophytes, olecranon stress fractures, osteochondritis dissecans (OCD) of the capitellum and loose bodies [7, 30].

The spectrum of the elbow lesions encountered in the throwing athlete can best be explained by examining the forces at the elbow joint during the throwing motion. For example, baseball throwing generates large valgus and extension forces. The combination of large valgus loads with rapid elbow extension produces tensile stress along the medial compartment restraints (ulnar collateral ligament, flexor-pronator mass, medial epicondyle apophysis and ulnar nerve) and shear stress in the posterior compartment (posteromedial tip of the olecranon and trochlea), and compression stress is produced laterally. This phenomenon has been termed "valgus extension overload syndrome" and forms the basic pathophysiologic model behind the most common elbow injuries in the throwing athlete [7].

Repetitive near-tensile failure loads applied during throwing result in microtrauma to the anterior band of the ulnar collateral ligament and may eventually lead to ligament attenuation or failure. Continued valgus and extension forces may produce olecranon tip osteophytes, loose

L.A. Pederzini
Orthopaedic and Traumatologic Unit,
Nuovo Ospedale di Sassuolo, Sassuolo, Italy
e-mail: gigiped@hotmail.com

E. Tripoli
Orthopaedic and Traumatologic Unit, Nuovo
Ospedale di Sassuolo, Sassuolo, Italy

L.A. Pederzini et al. (eds.), *Elbow and Sport*, DOI 10.1007/978-3-662-48742-6_12

bodies in the posterior or radiocapitellar compartment and a kissing lesion (articular damage on the posteromedial trochlea caused by the olecranon osteophyte) or chondromalacia on the posteromedial and posterolateral aspects of the humerus.

As a result of valgus extension overload forces, lesions of the posterior compartment, including olecranon osteophytes and loose bodies, have been reported as the most common diagnoses that require surgery in throwing athletes [7, 14].

A posterior elbow impingement results from mechanical abutment of the bone and soft tissue caused by pathologic processes such as fibrous tissue deposit in the olecranon fossa, chondral injury, osteophytes and loose bodies [12].

12.2 Patient Evaluation

12.2.1 History and Physical Examination

A detailed history and a thorough physical examination are mandatory in order to evaluate the athletes' elbow. Information regarding time or changes in training regimens as well as previous injuries may help us to better understand the patient's current condition. Pain, stiffness and instability of the elbow should be accurately investigated.

While posttraumatic stiff elbow is strictly connected to a recent trauma (1 year), degenerative stiff elbow pictures can be determined by overuse syndromes, primary osteoarthritic changes or sequelae of not recent (more than 1 year) traumatic event.

Every single decrease of the elbow ROM can be considered as a stiff elbow depending from the work, sport activity and functional requests of the patient. Clinical evaluation must consider sex, dominant arm, etiopathogenesis, preoperative MEPI (pain, ROM, balance and function) and radiological and clinical findings [22]. Generally pain throughout the entire arc of motion indicates a joint with a damaged bearing surface and advanced degenerative changes. This can be associated with night pain, effusions and progressive stiffness. The elbow should be examined for deformity, swelling, crepitus and previous surgical incisions. Vascular and neurologic evaluation should include assessment of the ulnar nerve that can involve irritability, subluxation and sensory or motor function deficit. Finally muscle strength and collateral ligament stability are evaluated [6, 28]. An accurate characterisation of normal and pathologic elbow structures is important to guide treatment planning.

12.2.2 Radiologic Imaging

Conventional radiographs, consisting of two orthogonal views of the elbow (AP, lateral), are the standard initial evaluation for osseous deformity and then completed with axial and oblique views of the affected side. Comparison views of the opposite elbow may be done if necessary.

If medial instability is suspected, stress AP radiographs can be performed with the use of a valgus stress radiography machine. Radiographs are evaluated for the presence of olecranon osteophytes, calcification within the ulnar collateral ligament, osteochondral damage to the capitellum or loose bodies [7, 28].

CT scan is more accurate and has greater interobserver agreement than conventional radiography in detecting osteophytes and loose bodies. CT scan also can be helpful for detecting stress fractures of the olecranon, and it may be preferable for identifying the fracture line and the typical sclerotic bone signifying stress reaction.

3D reconstruction CT has gained popularity as a tool for visualising osteophyte distribution and assessing complex deformity patterns when planning surgical debridement [28] (Fig. 12.1).

The accuracy of the method of diagnostic imaging of the soft tissue structures around the elbow continues to raise considerable debate. MRI can be useful to diagnose collateral ligament injuries but also in the evaluation of loose bodies, osteochondral lesions, olecranon osteophytes and neurologic complaints [11].

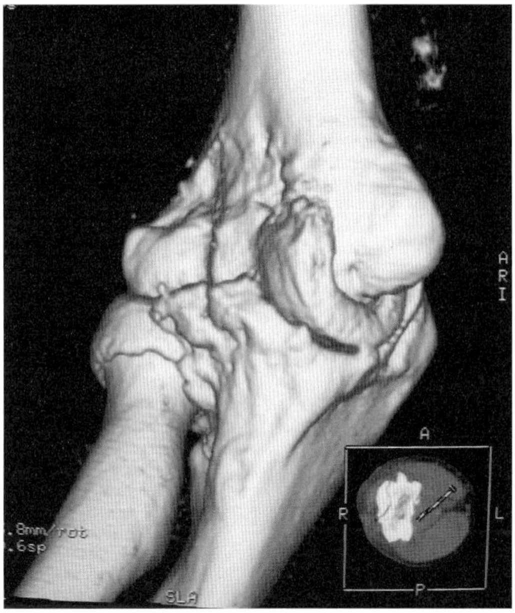

Fig. 12.1 3D reconstruction CT is important in order to visualise osteophyte distribution and assess complex deformity patterns when planning surgical debridement

12.3 Management in Degenerative Elbow

The mainstay of early treatment of the young patient with posttraumatic arthritis consists of maintaining joint mobility and reducing activities that place stress across the elbow such as weight-bearing or repetitive motions. Nonsteroidal anti-inflammatory drugs and selective intraarticular corticosteroid injections can control pain and facilitate daily use of the degenerative elbow.

After considering 6-month failure of conservative treatment (mobilisation, splinting and physical therapy), intact articular space, absence or mild anatomical incongruency, ROM reduction and sport- and occupation-related disability, a patient can be a candidate for an arthroscopic arthrolysis [21, 28]. On the other hand, arthroscopic technique can be useful in association with open surgery in order to avoid large surgical approaches. Sometimes removal of a columnar plate or screws can be associated with an arthroscopic arthrolysis.

The presence of osteophytes, synovitis and loose bodies is also an anatomo-pathological finding in the course of repetitive microtrauma in which the altered joint mechanism allows to develop an early degenerative picture [21, 28].

12.4 Osteochondritis Dissecans Lesions

Osteochondritis dissecans occurs most commonly in overhead-throwing athletes and in gymnasts between the ages of 13 and 16 years [8, 12]. It typically affects the young adolescent athlete involved in high-demand, repetitive overhead or weight-bearing activities. The most commonly associated sports are baseball, gymnastics, racquet sports, football and weightlifting [3, 8].

OCD can be a cause of painful elbow with limited ROM. These young patients, usually athletes complaining pain and dysfunction, limit their activity becoming unable to participate in sport. Although lesions have been reported in the trochlea, radial head and olecranon, the most common site of OCD of the elbow is in the capitellum [3, 8, 12].

Radiographs reveal rarefaction, radiolucency or fragmentation of the anterolateral capitellum. MRI has become the standard imaging modality to identify OCD, and it can provide an accurate assessment of the size, extent and stability of the lesion.

Determination of lesion stability and the integrity of the articular cartilage cap are really important regarding the decision to prescribe nonoperative treatment or proceed with the surgery [8].

Panner's disease, most common between 4 and 8 years of age, should not be confused with true OCD because it involves the entire ossification centre, while only the anterolateral capitellum is involved in osteochondritis dissecans of the capitellum [3, 8].

Treatment for stable, early stage OCD lesions consists in avoiding repetitive stress of the elbow and observation. If the lesion has not resolved in 3–6 months, then consideration of surgical management is made.

Surgical management is the treatment of choice for unstable lesions, lesions that have failed nonoperative management and loose bodies. Lesions that are unstable have a tendency to remain symptomatic even if no loose body is present, therefore leading to surgery [8].

Multiple operative procedures have been described for treating OCD. Surgical treatments include drilling of the lesion, fragment removal with or without curettage of the residual defect, fragment fixation by a variety of methods (pull-out wiring, Herbert's screw, bone peg grafting, etc.), reconstruction with osteochondral autograft and autologous chondrocyte implantation [3].

In the literature, several studies report different results with open procedure, but more recently arthroscopy has been employed with encouraging scores in the treatment of capitellar OCD [3, 8, 22].

Baumgarten and colleagues report excellent results in a group of 17 patients whose elbows were treated with arthroscopic debridement with a complete return to sport activities at the pre-injury level in 82 % of cases [3, 5, 8].

Reports of arthroscopic treatment of OCD of the capitellum with removal of loose bodies, debridement and abrasion chondroplasty describe overall improvements in pain and range of motions with variable return to pre-injury level of sporting activity [3, 22].

A grading system based on absent, partial or total detachment of the bone plug has been developed by Baumgarten et al. to aid in decision-making during elbow arthroscopy. The recommendation presented for Grade 1 lesions is either observation or arthroscopic drilling of the lesion. Grade 2 lesions were treated with debridement of the cartilage to healthy tissue. Grade 3 lesions were treated with loosening of the fragment to create a Grade 4 lesion, which was then resected. Grade 5 lesions were treated with a diligent search for the loose bodies [5, 8].

In our patients we prefer arthroscopic evaluation and treatment for lesions requiring operative management. Removal of the bone plug and microfracture is mandatory in order to eliminate catching and popping, while it is still controversial the possibility to bone graft the lesion [22].

In some cases we have been performed an arthroscopic mosaicplasty taking the graft from the homolateral knee putting the patient in lateral decubitus and extrarotating the hip performing knee arthroscopy. The 6.5 mm cylinder graft token from the lateral knee trochlea was inserted in the elbow lesioned area carefully checking the angle of the drilling and of the insertion of the bony cartilaginous cylinder. Arthroscopically the perpendicular insertion of the cylinder allows a complete coverage of the OCD area. Four months later MRI shows a nice bone incorporation of the graft. Post-operatively the CPM started in day 2 and passive exercises in day 4 post-op. Patients were back to normal activity in 4 months [22] (Figs. 12.2, 12.3 and 12.4).

12.5 Arthroscopic Technique in Degenerative Elbow

Arthroscopy is increasingly used to diagnose and treat elbow pathologies although the elbow has always been considered a difficult joint to be endoscopically explored. Arthroscopy knowledge increase and technology breakthrough in the last few years have allowed a standardisation of techniques and a better definition of indications. In the 1980s, Andrews J. R. and Carson W, G, [2], Hempfling H. [10] and Lindenfeld T. N. [15] published the first indications, techniques and notions on elbow arthroscopy. In 1981, on the basis of their observations, Morrey et al. determined that the elbow functional motion ranged from 30 to 130° of flexion [17]; however, a lot of daily activities performed at work or while doing physical exercise require an extension above 30°. As a matter of fact, for sportsmen and manual workers even a small decrease in ROM, together with slight symptoms of pain and inability to perform specific tasks, can be unacceptable and, hence, interfere with their daily work or sport activities. For this reason, there has been an extension of indications concerning stiff elbows treatment [16].

In 1992, O'Driscoll and Morrey presented 72 cases of elbow arthroscopy [19], and in 2001 they published a review of 473 cases in which they analysed the complications related to this procedure [13]. In the previous year, Reddy A. S. et al. [24] had published a review of 172 cases in which

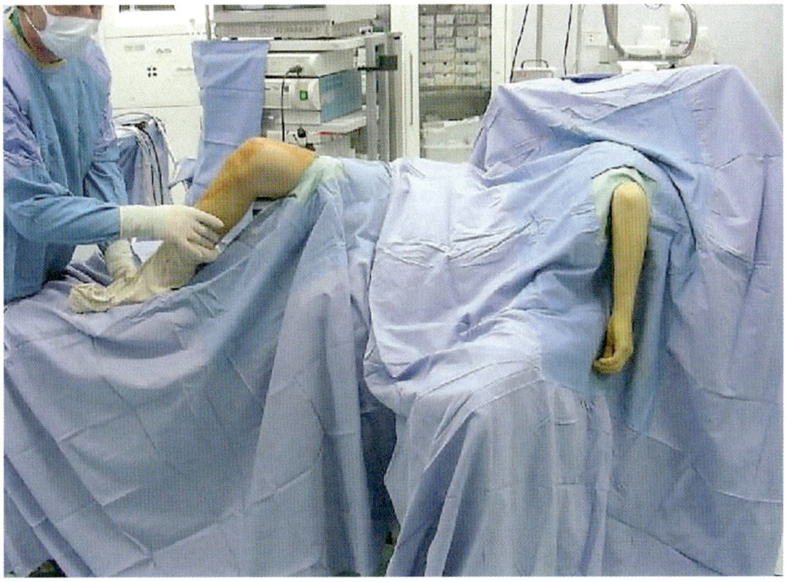

Fig. 12.2 The mosaicplasty from the knee to the elbow is performed on lateral decubitus positioning and the hip in extrarotation to allow knee arthroscopy for taking the graft from the lateral trochlea

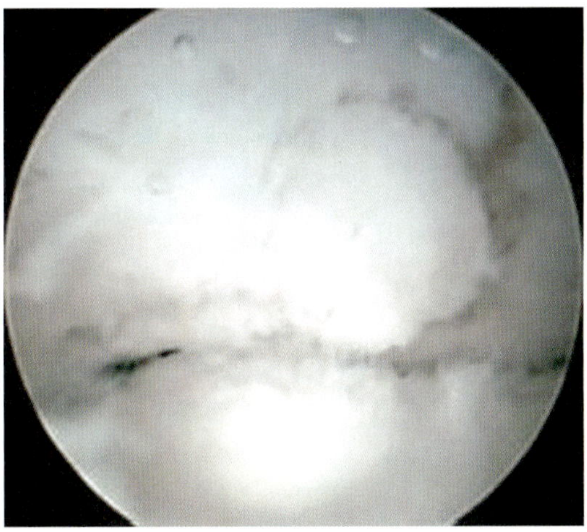

Fig. 12.3 The graft is positioned on the lateral humeral condyle to fill the OCD gap

patients had undergone arthroscopic elbow surgery with a 7-year follow-up. The list of indications for elbow arthroscopy has grown over the past years, and today it includes osteochondritis dissecans (OCD), plica syndrome, synovectomy in R.A. and other synovitis, lateral epicondylitis, loose bodies removal [23, 29] and stiff elbows related to degenerative or posttraumatic causes [6, 16]. Recently, Conso C. [9] as well as Shubert T. [27] and Salini V. [26] have published the results obtained by comparing, respectively, 32, 24 and 15 arthroscopic cases presenting a moderate stiffness of the elbow and other pathologies, with those obtained with open techniques. There

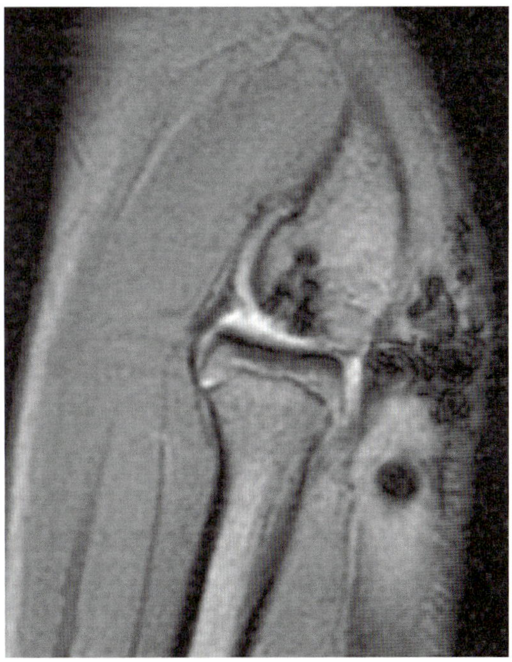

Fig. 12.4 Four-month control MRI shows a good bone incorporation of the osteochondral cylinder

are several studies regarding this subject in the literature, but all of them are based on a small number of patients with a variety of pathologies treated with different surgical techniques [1, 4, 18, 20, 25, 30].

Anaesthetist identifies nerve trunks by applying electrostimulation and places a catheter without injecting the anaesthetic. Patients then undergo general anaesthesia. When they wake up, only after a neurological evaluation, peripheral block is performed. After the induction of anaesthesia, ROM is carefully assessed and a complete ligamentous balancing is carried out. The tourniquet is inflated to 250 mmHg. The patient is then placed prone, with the shoulder abducted 90°, the elbow flexed to 90° and the arm held up by an arm holder secured to the operating table. Sterile field is set up and elbow joint landmarks are drawn by a dermographic pen (medial and lateral epicondyle, ulnar nerve, radial head, posterior soft spot). Soft spot posterior portals, supero-antero medial portals and supero-antero lateral portals are marked. Ulnar nerve neurolysis has always been performed by making a 2 cm skin incision, except in full ROM cases (full ROM painful elbows, occasionally decreased ROM). An 18-gauge needle is inserted in the elbow through the "soft spot" in the middle of the triangular area delimited by the epicondyle, the radial head and the olecranon, while the joint is distended by injecting 20 ml of normal saline solution to introduce the trocar while shifting neurovascular anterior structures away. Five portals, three posterior and two anterior, are always used. After the incision is made, soft tissues are retracted by using a fine haemostat. Posterior compartment arthroscopy is firstly performed by introducing a 4,5 mm 30° arthroscope through the posterolateral portal (soft spot). Then a second portal is established, 1,5 cm proximal to the latter. These two portals allow to use the scope and the shaver at the same level of the posterior portion of the radial head. Joint distension is achieved by a pump set at 35–50 mmHg. Once we get a good and complete view of the proximal radio-ulnar joint (posteriorly), a third posterior portal is placed in the olecranon fossa, close to the triceps medial border and oriented 2–3 cm proximal to the olecranon tip. A complete olecranon fossa and its lateral wall debridement can be performed as well as, if present, a lateral olecranon and humerus loose bodies removal to allow a better sliding of the articular surfaces. We use a different approach related to osteophyte dimension and ulnar nerve presence on the medial side. After inserting the arthroscope through the most proximal portal, we evaluate osteophyte dimensions; if they are small, we protect the ulnar nerve by positioning a retractor in an accessory portal slightly posterior to the ulnar nerve, and we resect the osteophytes arthroscopically. If they are large, we prefer to remove the osteophytes by performing a small arthrotomy at the end of the procedure, thus avoiding fluid extravasation during arthroscopy. The medial approach is always used after ulnar nerve neurolysis, which is the first surgical step of the procedure. This is necessary to prevent the overstretching of the nerve testing flexion and extension during elbow arthroscopy. The scope is then introduced in the anterior compartment through the supero-antero medial portal, 2 cm proximal and 1 cm anterior to the epitrochlea. In the stiff elbow the medial approach is preferable because it allows to locate the ulnar nerve by palpation, which is not possible on the lateral side. The anterolateral portal is created using an inside-out technique and placing a Wissinger rod 2 cm proximal and 1 cm anterior to the lateral epicondyle. A plastic cannula is introduced on the rod, and, subsequently after having the rod removed, a shaver can be positioned and the anterior debridement carried out (removal of loose bodies, anterior osteophytes and synovectomy). In several cases, in the presence of a thick capsule (posttraumatic causes), an anterior capsulectomy may be required. We start trimming the proximal humeral capsule by a shaver, but the real anterior capsulectomy is performed by a basket forceps, at about 1 cm proximally to the apex of the coronoid, firstly in a lateral-medial and then in a medial-lateral direction. After arthroscopy, ROM is assessed. One or two suction drainages are positioned into the joint, arthroscopic accesses are sutured and a splint holding the joint in full extension is applied to correct the articular loss of extension. On post-op day 1, patients start a 20 min continuous passive motion (CPM) four times a day, together with an assisted physiokinesis therapy, at least 60 min per day. On day 2 they start a self-assisted active and passive mobilisation in flexion-extension. On day 3 drains are removed and we continue with the rehabilitative programme. Indomethacin 50 mg three times per day is somministrated for 15 days. At the time of discharge from the hospital, patients are taught of the exercises they need to practise at home. They continue the same programme with a therapist for 3 months.

12.6 Discussion

Throwing, pushing, opposing and gripping are frequent in different sports and all can lead to significant elbow stress. In many sportsmen acute traumas or repeated microtraumas can affect the joint surfaces, ligaments and muscles, determining a loss of function.

If nonsurgical treatment has failed, the type of surgical treatment required depends on the extent of degenerative changes. When degenerative changes are absent or mild, soft tissue release offers reliable increases in elbow motion and pain release. When moderate degenerative changes exist within the joint, débridement arthroplasty of osteophytes and soft tissue has shown some success with increase in joint motion. With advanced degenerative changes, the therapeutic options are more limited [28].

In the last 15 years, elbow arthroscopy has been studied by different authors to reduce frequent complications described in previous authors' publications [13, 24].

The use of different portals, the ulnar nerve isolation, the use of arthroscopic retractors and the avoidance of an excessive intraarticular joint pressure are all fundamental elements for an accurate elbow arthroscopy. In other words it is important to achieve a clear arthroscopic vision, avoiding nerves and vessel injuries risks. Once established this, it will be easier to understand pathologies and their treatments. Posttraumatic and degenerative arthroscopic cases have different features. In posttraumatic cases, the articular space is smaller, fibrosis is higher and capsule consistency, when removed by basket forceps, is harder. In degenerative cases, articular space is larger, fibrosis is lower and capsule consistency is weaker. Indications for stiffness arthroscopic treatment are still, in many cases, surgeon dependant [21].

In 2000 Reddy et al. presented a review of a large number of patients operated by several different surgeons, in different decubitus and by different techniques reporting low rate of minor complications but a complete lesion of the ulnar nerve. As Reddy described, we obtain the same low rate of complications using the technique previously presented in a large series of patients (212 patients) operated by the same surgeon in 5 years (2004–2008) with an average follow-up of 58 months with 1.8 % of neurological complications and 10.8 % of minor complications [21].

In 2001, Morrey et al. reported extensive case studies in which they analysed complications following arthroscopic surgery [13]. In some cases, other authors report limited case studies where they compare the outcomes achieved by open techniques with arthroscopic ones [1, 4, 18, 20, 25, 30].

In case of articular congruence damage, posttraumatic anatomical alterations or previous surgical outcome, arthroscopic indication is not common, while open surgery can be useful and decisive. On the other hand, arthroscopy is used in case of hypertrophy of the olecranon caused by long-standing instability, radial head osteophytes connected to a previous fracture and hypertrophy of the coronoid caused by an intense physical or manual activity. The use of five portals (three posterior and two anterior) allows a clear and complete joint view. In our opinion, a complete view of the anterior and posterior compartments is mandatory in any case, even if the pathology involves only one of the compartments. Even if the joint limitation affects only one of the two compartments, the lack of range of motion can lead to anatomo-pathological changes also in the other compartment, in the long run. The use of retractors is important in every stage of the surgery because it minimises any risk of damage to vascular and nervous structures. During posterior debridement, the medial olecranon osteophyte

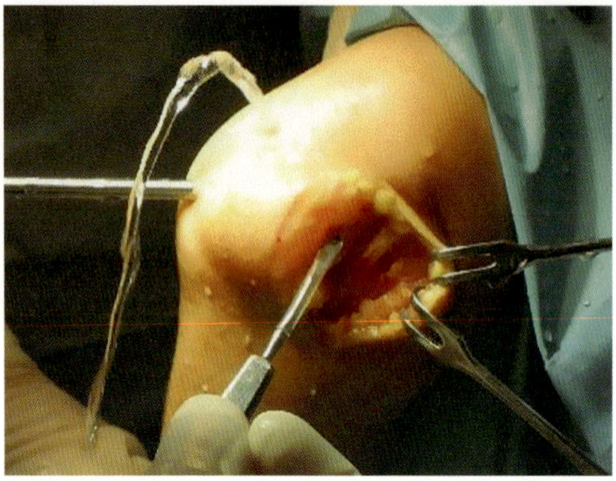

Fig. 12.5 After ulnar nerve release, the scope is positioned in the soft spot and an accessory portal is performed in the subcutaneous tissue in order to protect the ulnar nerve intraarticularly

removal should be carefully considered: a retractor can help, but in some cases due to big osteophytes proximity to the ulnar nerve, arthroscopic surgery is not recommended (Fig. 12.5).

The previous isolation of the ulnar nerve enables open surgery, avoiding risks. Posterior debridement and olecranon osteophyte removal allow an extension improvement that, together with the surgical procedures above-mentioned, increases total ROM. Also anterior capsulectomy allows an extension improvement. On the contrary, flexion is favoured by posterior capsulectomy and removal of anterior hypertrophic coronoid or humeral osteophytes. During anterior capsulectomy, it is important to pay attention to the brachialis muscle, which is visible once the capsule is removed and can be very thin as consequence of the stiffness. This is necessary not only because of the proximity of the humeral artery but also to avoid muscle bleeding, which can lead to possible calcifications.

Only when ROM is almost complete and neurological disorders nearly absent, neurolysis is not performed (removal of one to two loose bodies). Neurolysis of the ulnar nerve is nearly always recommended in cases of severe stiffness and where there is a marked ROM recovery.

The results reported in the literature are extremely encouraging [1, 4, 17, 21, 23, 27] allowing an increase ROM in degenerative cases.

Post-operative functional rehabilitation should be immediate to keep the intraoperative obtained ROM, thus reducing the inevitable risk of adhesion formation that can significantly limit the movement recovery. The suggested rehabilitation protocol can obviously be modified relatively to patient's needs in terms of more or less rehabilitation activity.

From the complication analysis, it is clear how common the presence of synovial fistulas is. These are related to the intense flexion-extension mobilisation, which causes a synovial fluid leakage throughout surgical portals (locus minoris resistentiae) and prevents healing. During arthroscopy, the precaution of isolating the ulnar nerve before arthroscope introduction turned out to be extremely useful if compared to adverse outcomes when it was not performed.

Conclusions

The elbow joint is involved in several sport activities like throwing, pushing, opposing and gripping. Previous acute trauma or overuse syndromes can determine problems in the joint surface, ligaments and muscles determining elbow's damage and loss of functions. Bony lesions are represented by osteophytes, spurs, loose bodies and osteochondral defects. Soft tissue lesions are represented by capsular adhesions with increased thickness in the anterior and posterior aspects of the capsule. These anatomical pictures involving the elbow joint basically determine the clinical picture of the degenerative stiff elbow. In the last 10 years, elbow arthroscopy has become the choice method in treating these pathologies. The arthroscopic technique has been developed in order to have a safe procedure. The opportunity to arthroscopically release a stiff elbow or remove loose bodies or treat OCD by microfracture or more recently by arthroscopic mosaicplasty seems to confirm the quality of the arthroscopic option. Longer follow-up and a better evaluation of the level of the return to sport must be depicted in the future to confirm these impressions.

References

1. Adams JE, Wolff 3rd LH, Merten SM, Steinmann SP. Osteoarthritis of the elbow: results of arthroscopic osteophyte resection and capsulectomy. J Should Elb Surg. 2008;17(1):126–31.
2. Andrews JR, Carson WG. Arthroscopy of the elbow. Arthroscopy. 1985;1(2):97–107.
3. Baker CL, Romeo AA. Osteochondritis dissecans of the capitellum. Am J Sport Med. 2010;38:1917–28.
4. Ball CM, Meunier M, Galatz LM, Calfee R, Yamaguchi K. Arthroscopic treatment of post-traumatic elbow contracture. J Should Elb Surg. 2002;11(6):624–9.
5. Baumgarten TE, Andrews JR, Satterwhite YE. The arthroscopic classification and treatment of osteochondritis dissecans of the capitellum. Am J Sport Med. 1998;26(4):520–3.
6. Bruno RJ, Lee ML, Strauch RJ, Rosenwasser MP. Posttraumatic elbow stiffness: evaluation and management. J Am Acad Orthop Surg. 2002;10(2):106–16.
7. Cain EL, Dugas JR, Wolf RS, Andrews JR. Elbow injuries in throwing athletes: a current concepts review. Am J Sport Med. 2003;31:621–34.
8. Coates KE, Poehling G. Osteochondritis Dissecans lesions and loose bodies of the elbow. Elb Arthrosc. 2013;3:25–33. ed Springer.
9. Conso C, Bleton R. Arthroscopy in stiff elbow: report of 32 cases. Rev Chir Orthop Reparatrice Appar Mot. 2007;93(4):333–8.
10. Hempfling H. Endoscopic examination of the elbow joint from the dorsoradial approach. Z Orthop Ihre Grenzgeb. 1983;121(3):331–2.
11. Ho CP. Sports and occupational injuries of the elbow: MR imaging findings. AJR. 1995;164:1465–71.
12. Kandemir U, Fu FH, Mc Mahon P. Elbow injuries. Curr Opin Rheumatol. 2002;14:160–7.
13. Kelly EW, Morrey BF, O'Driscoll SW. Complications of elbow arthroscopy. J Bone Joint Surg Am. 2001;83- A(1):25–34.
14. Kibler WB. Clinical biomechanics of the elbow in tennis: implications for evaluation and diagnosis. J Am Coll Sport Med. 1994;26:1203–6.
15. Lindenfeld TN. Medial approach in elbow arthroscopy. Am J Sports Med. 1990;18(4):413–7.
16. Morrey BF. The posttraumatic stiff elbow. Clin Orthop Relat Res. 2005;431:26–35.
17. Morrey BF, Askew LJ, Chao EY. A biomechanical study of normal functional elbow motion. J Bone Joint Surg Am. 1981;63(6):872–7.
18. Nguyen D, Proper SI, MacDermid JC, King GJ, Faber KJ. Functional outcomes of arthroscopic capsular release of the elbow. Arthroscopy. 2006;22(8):842–9.
19. O'Driscoll SW, Morrey BF. Arthroscopy of the elbow. Diagnostic and therapeutic benefits and hazards. J Bone Joint Surg Am. 1992;74(1):84–94.
20. Ogilvie-Harris DJ, Schemitsch E. Arthroscopy of the elbow for removal of loose bodies. Arthroscopy. 1993;9:5–8.
21. Pederzini LA, Nicoletta F, Tosi M, Prandini M, Tripoli E, Cossio A. Elbow arthroscopy in stiff elbow. Knee Surg Sports Traumatol Arthrosc KSSTA. 2014;22: 467–73. Ed. Springer.
22. Pederzini LA, Tripoli E, Tosi M, Nicoletta F, Scuccimarra T. Tricks in elbow arthroscopy. Sport Inj. 2014. pp. 1–14 (online doi: 10.1007/978-3-642-36801-1_48-1).
23. Rahusen FT, Brinkman JM, Eygendaal D. Results of arthroscopic debridement for osteochondritis dissecans of the elbow. Br J Sports Med. 2006; 40(12):966–9.
24. Reddy AS, Kvitne RS, Yocum LA, ElAttrache NS, Glousman RE, Jobe FW. Arthroscopy of the elbow: a long-term clinical review. Arthroscopy. 2000;16(6): 588–94.
25. Rupp S, Tempelhof S. Arthroscopic surgery of the elbow: therapeutic benefits and hazards. Clin Orthop. 1995;4:140–5.
26. Salini V, Palmieri D, Colucci C, Croce G, Castellani ML, Orso CA. Arthroscopic treatment of post- traumatic elbow stiffness. J Sports Med Phys Fitness. 2006;46(1):99–103.
27. Schubert T, Dubuc JE, Barbier O. A review of 24 cases of elbow arthroscopy using the DASH questionnaire. Acta Orthop Belg. 2007;73(6):700–3.
28. Sears BW, Puskas GJ, Morrey ME, Sanchez-Sotelo J, Morrey BF. Posttraumatic elbow arthritis in the young adult: evaluation and management. J Am Acad Orthop Surg. 2012;11:704–14.
29. Steinmann SP, King GJ, Savoie III FH. Arthroscopic treatment of the arthritic elbow. Instr Course Lect. 2006;55:109–17.
30. Ward WG, Anderson TE. Elbow arthroscopy in a mostly athletic population. J Hand Surg [Am]. 1993;18:220–4.

Biceps Tendon Pathology

13

Gregory Bain, Joideep Phadnis, and Hani Saeed

13.1 Introduction

Distal biceps tendon rupture is a rare injury, making up 3–12 % of all biceps injuries [15] with an incidence of 1.2 per 100,000 people [8]. Rupture results from explosive eccentric contracture against resistance, resulting in significant flexion and supination strength and endurance deficit [20]. It most commonly affects male patients between 30 and 60 [1], with other risk factors including smoking [8], anabolic steroid use [10] and weight lifting [15].

Partial distal biceps tears are far less common, may go undiagnosed for some time [14] and cause considerable anterior elbow pain during activity. There is a paucity of evidence regarding their optimal treatment; however, endoscopy is especially useful for these tears as an accurate diagnosis of the degree of tearing, tendinosis and footprint coverage can be made. Chronic tears pose a surgical challenge due to tendon retraction or pseudotendon formation but have been successfully treated by fixation in extreme flexion or by grafts.

G. Bain, MBBS, FRACS, FA (Ortho)A, PhD (✉)
J. Phadnis, MBChB, MRCS, Dip SportsMed, FRCS
H. Saeed, MD, BPharm
Department of Orthopaedic Surgery and Trauma, Flinders University, Adelaide, SA, Australia

Department of Orthopaedic Surgery and Trauma, Flinders Medical Centre, Adelaide, SA, Australia
e-mail: greg@gregbain.com.au

Distal biceps repair reliably restores function regardless of technique and approach, although debate remains regarding whether to use a single- or double-incision technique and which technique is most effective. Cortical buttons, suture anchors, transosseous tunnels and interference screws have all been used with satisfactory results.

13.2 Surgical Anatomy

The distal biceps tendon can be divided into three zones: (i) pre-aponeurosis (musculotendinous junction), (ii) aponeurosis, where the lacertus fibrosus arises and (iii) post-aponeurosis, where the tendons of the short head and the long head are connected by loose connective tissue [14].

The tendon externally rotates 90° as it travels from its musculotendinous junction to its insertion at the ulna surface of the radial tuberosity. The short head passes anterior to the long head to insert in a fan-like manner into the distal portion of the radial tuberosity. The long head has an oval footprint and inserts proximally and more posteriorly to the short head, occupying most of the tuberosity [18, 23]. Therefore, in full supination, the long head of biceps tendon drapes around the radial tuberosity.

The teardrop-shaped bicipitoradial bursa completely encompasses both parts of the tendon and is more adherent to the ulna aspect of the distal biceps than the radial aspect. It lies between the

L.A. Pederzini et al. (eds.), *Elbow and Sport*, DOI 10.1007/978-3-662-48742-6_13

groove in the brachialis muscle and the distal biceps tendon with the elbow extended and between the proximal radius and the biceps tendon during pronation (Fig. 13.1).

The tendon footprint is located at the posteromedial margin of the radial tuberosity, 25–30° posterior to the frontal plane. It measures a mean length of 21 mm, with a width of 7 mm, and has footprint of 108 mm [12, 15].

Both partial and complete ruptures occur at the tendon-bone interface. Considering that the biceps tendon insertion has a lever of approximately 1 cm relative to the rotational axis of the radius, at least 3.0–3.5 cm of distal biceps tendon is needed to wrap around the proximal radius during its rotation from 90° supination to 90° pronation [27].

13.3 Presentation and Investigations

13.3.1 History

There is usually a history of sudden and sharp extension load to an elbow flexed at 90° with the biceps in a contracted state. This is followed by sharp pain, typically in the antecubital fossa, but sometimes felt in the posterolateral elbow. These may be associated with an audible "pop" [1].

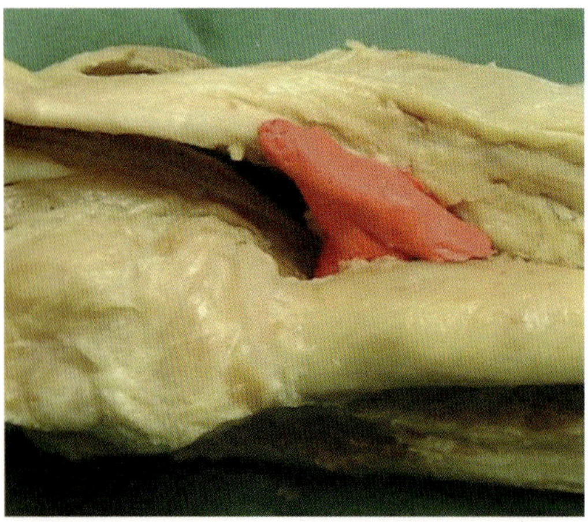

Fig. 13.1 Location of the bicipitoradial bursa between the distal biceps tendon and the radius (proximal, *left*; distal, *right*) (Used with permission from [5])

Partial tears tend to be more painful than complete tears and patients tend to remain symptomatic or progress despite non-surgical treatment [17, 18].

Those with distal biceps tendonitis/tendinosis or bicipitoradial bursitis often present with deep-seated anterior elbow pain, generally exacerbated by repetitive use. The condition is atraumatic but patients often relate their symptoms to a vague inciting event. Uncommonly for distal biceps pathology, these patients tend to be female often with co-morbidities that predispose to tendon degeneration such as diabetes, renal disease and immunosuppressive therapy.

An unrepaired rupture leads to a deficit of 27 % in supination and 47 % loss of supination endurance when compared with the normal contralateral arm. Flexion strength and endurance are decreased by 21 % [2]. Freeman et al. (2009) found a mean 25 % reduction in supination strength but only a statistically non-significant 7 % loss of flexion when compared with the normal contralateral arm.

13.3.2 Examination

In any tear, there may be ecchymosis over the antecubital fossa, palpable gap in biceps tendon and/or tenderness on palpation over the radial tuberosity. Weakness of supination against resistance tends to be more marked than flexion as brachialis compensates for weakness of flexion.

The signs of partial tears are subtle and diagnosis is difficult owing to unreliable clinical examination. There may be crepitus or grinding on passive rotation of the forearm [4] and weakness of resisted supination. A direct tuberosity compression test has been described where the examiner palpates the lateral aspect of the fully supinated radium 2.5 cm distal to the radiocapitellar joint. The patient is then asked to rotate the forearm. If this elicits more pain than the normal contralateral side, the test is considered positive [11].

Several clinical tests to aid in the diagnosis of complete rupture have been described [28], described the hook sign (Table 13.1), where the patient is asked to actively supinate and flex the elbow to 90°. The examiner then hooks their finger under the distal biceps tendon from the lateral aspect of the elbow. In the case of a complete distal biceps tendon rupture, the hook test is thought to be the most useful test in making the diagnosis, as the examiner is unable to satisfactorily hook their finger under the tendon. However, it can be unclear when the biceps tendon sheath remains attached distally despite retraction of the tendon or when a pseudotendon develops to bridge the gap in a chronic tear. The hook test is also unclear in partial or single head ruptures. In Table 13.2, the features of the hook test have been correlated with pathologies in which they might appear.

Table 13.1 Clinical assessment using the hook test

Hook test finding	Grade	Features of tendon
Normal	N	Taut, unyielding and symmetric with contralateral arm
Abnormal	A1	Taut, but yielding and asymmetric with contralateral arm
Abnormal	A2	Lax and asymmetric
Abnormal	A3	Absent cord

13.3.3 Imaging

Plain radiographs are not particularly helpful in the diagnosis of tendon rupture, but AP and lateral X-rays should be sought for preoperative planning.

A new *ultrasound* technique involving a medial approach through the pronator window has been adopted to diagnose distal biceps tears. This technique has resulted in more complete

Table 13.2 Classification, clinical findings and management of distal biceps pathologies

Grade	Injury	Clinical	Hook test	MRI	Recommended management
0	Tendinosis, bursitis	Atraumatic, tender, swollen	N	Bursitis, effusion, tendinosis	Nonoperative, bursectomy, biopsy
1A	Low-grade partial tear (<50 % footprint detachment)	Pain and weakness against resistance	N, A1	Bursitis, effusion, footprint irregularity	Endoscopic debridement
1B	Isolated head rupture	Weakness against resistance	A1	Isolated head avulsion	Repair isolated head
1C	High-grade partial tear (>50 % footprint detachment)	Pain and weakness against resistance	A1	Incomplete footprint detachment	Complete and repair
2	Complete tendon rupture, lacertus intact	Tendon medialised by intact lacertus, marked weakness	A2	Complete footprint detachment, tendon within sheath	Repair
3	Complete tendon and lacertus rupture with retraction	Retracted muscle, marked weakness	A3	Complete footprint detachment, retracted tendon and muscle	Repair
4A	Chronic rupture	Tendon medialised by intact lacertus, marked weakness	A1, A2	Complete detachment and contracted tendon within sheath (A2). A pseudotendon may bridge the native tendon to the footprint (A1)	Repair
4B	Chronic retracted rupture	Retracted muscle, marked weakness	A3	Complete footprint detachment, retracted tendon within fibrous cocoon	Repair in flexion or use tendon graft

visualisation of the ulnarly facing radial tuberosity and distal biceps insertion [30] but remains less reliable than magnetic resonance imaging (MRI).

MRI has been shown to depict the level and nature of the tear (Table 13.2). A FABS view (flexed, abducted and supinated views) has been described to allow a longitudinal view of the tendon to be obtained in one slice [6], allowing easier recognition of pathology. However, MRI has a sensitivity of 59 % for partial ruptures and cannot distinguish between those that require repair and those that do not [19].

13.3.4 Indication for Endoscopy

Endoscopy can provide both diagnostic and therapeutic implications in distal biceps pathology and has become the gold standard for diagnosis in our practice. It is particularly useful in assessing and diagnosing suspected partial or complete tears, extent of the tear and quality of residual tendon to allow for repairs in the acute setting. In chronic cases, endoscopy allows for identification and debridement of the pseudotendon and any scar tissue that extends to the footprint on the radial tuberosity and facilitates retrieval of chronically retracted tendons.

However, endoscopy is relatively contraindicated in patients with pre-existing abnormal anatomy, such as from previous injury or surgery at the elbow and antecubital fossa. Additionally, endoscopic repairs should only be attempted after a considerable number of open repairs have been performed and familiarity with diagnostic endoscopy has been developed.

13.3.5 Classification

Distal biceps pathology can be classified according to degree (partial or complete), temporally (acute or chronic) or anatomically into the three zones described above. Most injuries occur in zone 3 (tendon-bone interface). In this chapter, tendon pathology at zone three has been graded on a scale from 0 to 4 (Table 13.2). Each grade has distinct clinical, radiological and operative findings. The hook test, as described above, should be interpreted carefully in certain grades.

13.4 Surgical Techniques

13.4.1 Two-Incision Technique

The two-incision technique of distal biceps tenodesis was initially described by Boyd and Anderson [3] and modified by Morrey, leading to lower rates of heterotopic ossification and synostosis.

Anteriorly, a 3–4 cm transverse incision over the antecubital fossa is made and tendon is secured using a grasping stitch. The forearm is then fully supinated and a blunt artery forceps is passed through the dorsolateral aspect of the forearm, along the medial border of the radius, until it visibly tents the skin. At this point, it is crucial that the tip of the forceps passes along the radius only and does not breach the periosteum of the ulna to minimise the risk of radioulnar synostosis. An incision is then made on the dorsolateral aspect of the forearm over the tip of the forceps and blunt dissection is performed down to the radius.

The forearm is pronated to bring the radial tuberosity into view and placing the posterior interosseous nerve (PIN) away from the operative field. The surface of the tuberosity is burred and drill holes are made. Using forceps, the sutures attached to the proximal portion of the tendon are passed through the radius to the dorsolateral incision and tied over bone. Aggressive use of lavage may minimise the risk of heterotopic ossification and synostosis [24].

13.4.2 Single Anterior Incision

Multiple single anterior approaches have been described, utilising suture anchors, Endobuttons and Biotenodesis interference screws or combinations of cortical button and interference screw fixations [22] with good results. Endoscopically assisted procedures with anchors [21] as well as the Endobutton technique have also been published [9].

The senior author developed the Endobutton technique in 1994, altering the technique to optimise the anatomic restoration of the biceps footprint. A single longitudinal anterior incision is made distal to the antecubital fossa and dissection is continued through the deep fascia. The proximal portion of the torn tendon is retrieved and two braided number 2 nonabsorbable sutures are anchored to the distal biceps tendon using a Bunnell stitch, leaving trailing sutures exiting the distal end of the tendon. The radial tuberosity is then exposed with blunt digital dissection using the biceps tendon tract as a guide. The forearm is then fully supinated and right angle retractors used to aid exposure.

For anatomical biceps restoration, the tendon should not be attached to the radius from anterior to posterior, but more medial to lateral. This position makes repair using a single anterior incision technically difficult, as the biceps tuberosity lies in an ulnar position when the arm is in full supination. The senior author currently pronates the arm approximately 70° to place two drill holes from the radial cortex starting immediately opposite the tuberosity and drilling anterolaterally to posteromedially towards and through the radial tuberosity. The sutures from the distal biceps tendon are passed through the holes in an anterograde fashion from tuberosity to opposite cortex using a suture passer. They are then threaded through the Endobutton, tensioned and tied so that the button lies against the opposite cortex. The drill is aimed away from the PIN [13] and the Endobutton is placed under direct vision, preventing entrapment and minimising risk of synostosis and proximal radius fractures associated with large burr holes.

13.4.3 Endoscopic Repair

A 2.5 cm longitudinal incision over the palpable biceps tendon, 2 cm distal to the anterior elbow crease, is made as the standard viewing portal for the endoscopy and instruments. The lateral cutaneous nerve of the forearm is identified and protected as the distal biceps tendon and its bursa are identified. A small, transverse portal is then made on the radial side at the apex of the bursa for introduction of the scope (Fig. 13.2). At this stage, it is important to stay lateral to the biceps tendon to avoid the median nerve and brachial artery.

Endoscopic repair should not be attempted unless a clear plan of the proposed procedure is in place (Fig. 13.3) [7, 31]. Dry endoscopy is used as the bursa, proximal radius and distal biceps tendon are inspected to allow clear identification of tissue planes. The tendon is examined dynamically through forearm rotation and with traction around the tendon for evidence of fraying, delamination, synovitis and partial tear. Using a Wissinger rod, a posterior working portal can be created, to allow the shaver to come from a different direction (Fig. 13.4). If present, tenosynovitis and low-grade fraying is debrided without suction using a full-radius resector without teeth. The aperture should be in full view whenever the resector is active to minimise the risk of soft tissue being caught.

If the partial tendon rupture is to be completed, a hooked monopolar cautery device is used for division of the remaining tendon insertion [17]. If the tendon is completely torn, a chondrotome is used to debride the natural footprint. A 2.5 mm drill is advanced from the anterior cortex of the radius exiting just posterior to the footprint. A suture on a straight needle is advanced backwards through this drill hole and

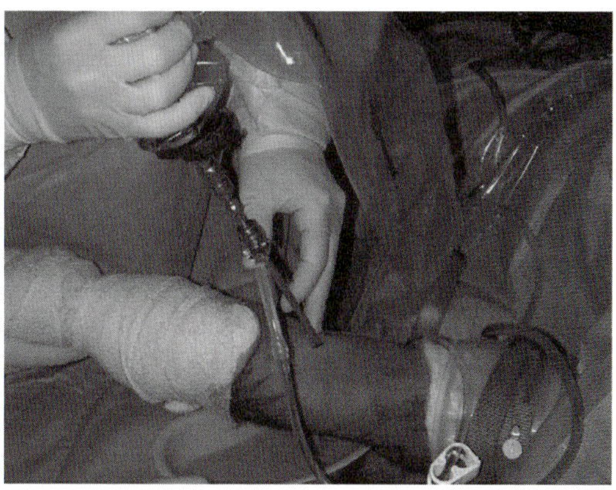

Fig. 13.2 Orientation of the surgeon and the scope during distal biceps tendon endoscopy in the left elbow (Used with permission from Eames and Bain [5])

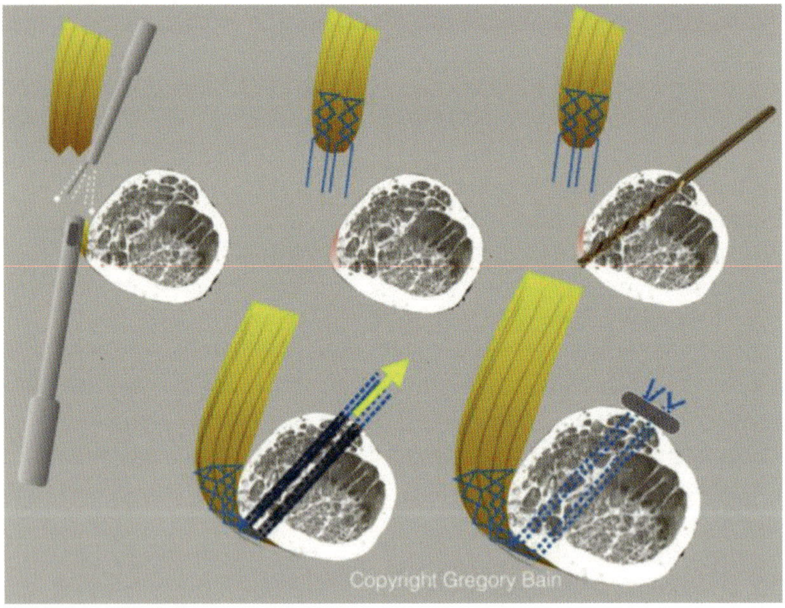

Fig. 13.3 Distal biceps endoscopic-assisted repair. (**a**) Endoscopic debridement of the torn biceps tendon stump. (**b**) Whipstitch of the torn tendon with nonabsorbable suture. (**c**) Two oblique drill holes made in the radial tuberosity aiming to exit on the dorsal ulnar surface. (**d**) Sutures shuttled through drill holes. (**e**) Sutures tied over Endobutton restoring the tendon to its footprint on the ulnar aspect of the tuberosity

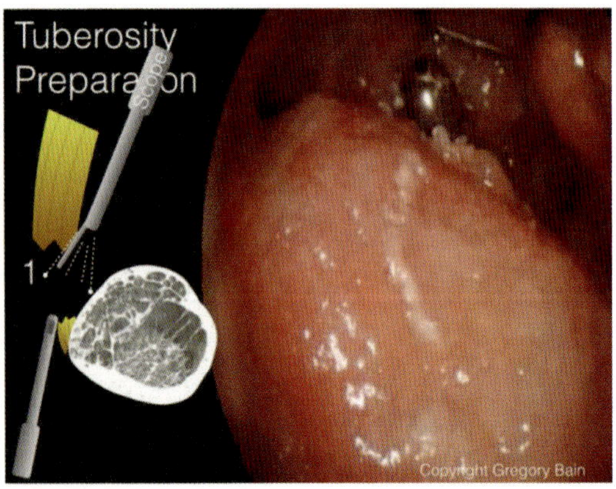

Fig. 13.4 Posterior working portal created using Wissinger rod. Scope in the front and the resector is coming over the horizon of the radius. Note the clarity of the dry endoscopy

the loop is retrieved (Fig. 13.5). This is used to shuttle the preplaced whipstitch in the distal biceps tendon. The sutures are threaded through an Endobutton and tied firmly to the anterior aspect of the proximal radius. This accurately recreates the biceps footprint and provides transosseous Endobutton fixation (Fig. 13.6a, b) [7]. A similar non endoscopic footprint technique has also been previously described [32].

13.4.4 Chronic Biceps Tendon Rupture

Management of chronic distal biceps tendon tear can be challenging owing to tendon retraction and scarring and the location of major neurovascular structures in the cubital fossa. If the patient has a low demand or is a high surgical risk, nonoperative treatment is mainstay. Surgery requires a more extensive approach and reattachment may not be possible with retraction greater than 4 cm, although good results have been reported for repair in extreme flexion [26]. Endoscopy, in this setting, can be useful to identify a pseudotendon and the level of the retracted tendon. If the lacertus fibrosis is still intact, the tendon can usually be directly repaired, although it will be tight and there will be a fixed flexion deformity. The senior author releases the lacertus from the tendon, repairs the tendon to the tuberosity and lastly repairs the lacertus. This ensures it does not deform the line of the tendon and does not compress the median nerve and the brachial artery beneath the lacertus. It is our experience that even a 70° flexion deformity repaired with an Endobutton will correct over the period of about 1 month, with gentle active mobilisation. In severe cases, tendon grafts such as semitendinosus autograft or tendon allograft may be used to bridge the deficient tendon.

13.5 Outcomes

Post-repair, those with grade 0 and grade 1A are encouraged to mobilise and strengthen the arm with physiotherapist. In those with grade 1B to grade 4 injuries, a sling is provided and the patient is encouraged to mobilise as tolerated with no resisted supination or flexion for 6 weeks. The outcome of surgical repair for distal biceps tendon rupture is good. The largest reported series using single incision technique found that 96 % were satisfied or very satisfied with the outcome of surgical repair at an average of 29 months after surgery [25]. In a series of 27 patients, Dillon et al. [16] found that the Endobutton gave return of 101 % of flexion strength and 99 % supination strength with no loss of motion. This group included patients with a chronic tear that was primarily repaired without tendon augmentation. Peeters et al. [29] demonstrated mean flexion strength of 80 % and supination strength of 91 % in 26 patients reviewed who had a mean of 16-month follow-up.

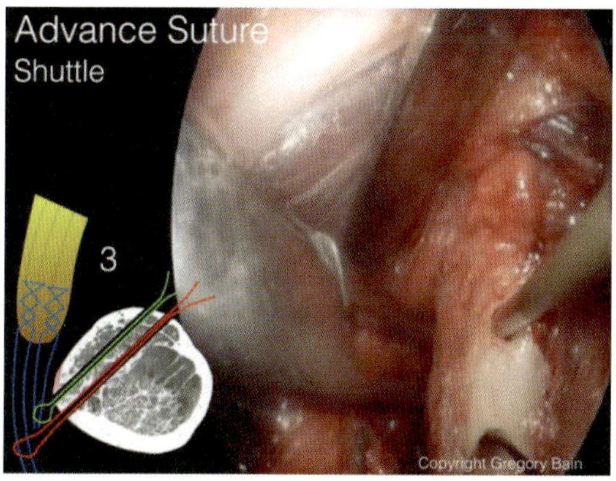

Fig. 13.5 Advancing the suture – the Tuohy needle is advanced through the drill hole and grasped on the posterior aspect of the radius

13.6 Complications

Reported complications include failure of repair, infection, haematoma, nerve palsies and fracture through drill holes in the proximal radial radius. Nerve palsies are usually transient and contributed to by aggressive retraction. Injuries may involve the lateral cutaneous nerve of the forearm, superficial branch of the radial nerve and posterior interosseous nerve and, rarely, the median nerve [21]. The PIN recovered spontaneously and radial neck fractures healed with internal fixation and bone graft. Rare complications

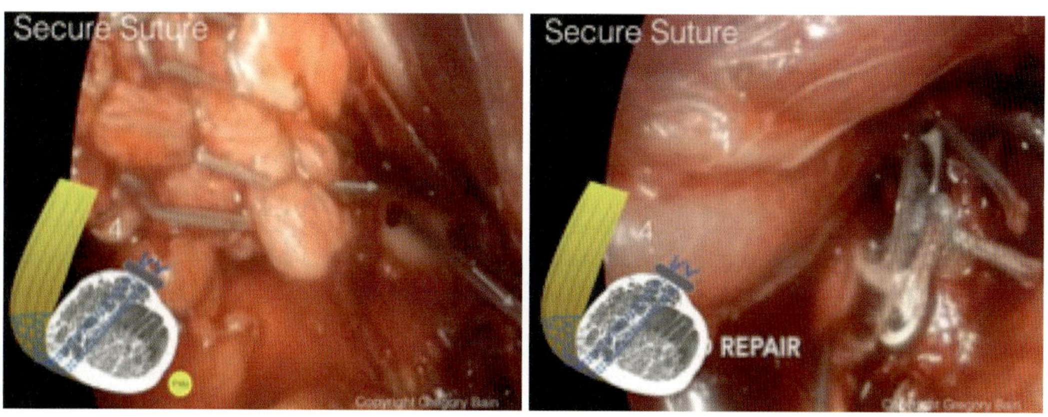

Fig. 13.6 Fixation of the tendon to the radial tuberosity. (**a**) The suture is used to advance the tendon onto the footprint. (**b**) The final position with the tendon advanced onto the footprint and the Endobutton on the anterior radius

Technical Tips for Procedures About the Elbow

1. Preoperatively and intraoperatively ensure that the patient is accurately classified, as this will direct treatment.
2. Enter the bicipitoradial bursa on the radial side under direct vision to avoid damage to neurovascular structures.
3. Use dry endoscopy to improve visualisation and prevent soft tissue swelling.
4. Use a full-radius resector without teeth and without suction to avoid entrapping soft tissues.
5. Reinsert the tendon onto its anatomic footprint on the posterior rim of the tuberosity.

include heterotopic ossification and radioulnar synostosis. Complication rates are higher for chronic injuries and revisions.

References

1. Ramsey ML. Distal biceps tendon injuries: diagnosis and management. J Am Acad Orthop Surg. 1999;7(3):199–207.
2. Baker BE, Bierwagen D. Rupture of the distal tendon of the biceps brachii. Operative versus non-operative treatment. J Bone Joint Surg Am. 1985;67(414):7.
3. Boyd HB, Anderson LD. A method for reinsertion of the distal biceps brachii tendon. J Bone Joint Surg Am. 1961;43:1041–3.
4. Dellaero DT, Mallon WJ. Surgical treatment of partial biceps tendon ruptures at the elbow. J Should Elbow Surg. 2006;15(2):215–7.
5. Eames MHA, Bain GI. Distal biceps tendon endoscopy and anterior elbow arthroscopy portal. Tech Should Elbow Surg. 2006;7(3):139–42.
6. Giuffre BM, Moss MJ. Optimal positioning for MRI of the distal biceps brachii tendon: flexed abducted supinated view. AJR Am J Roentgenol. 2004;182(4):944–6.
7. Phadnis J, Bain G. Endoscopic-assisted Distal Biceps Footprint Repair. Tech Hand Up Extrem Surg. 2015 Jun;19(2):55–9.doi: 10.1097/BTH.0000000000000078.
8. Safran MR, Graham SM. Distal biceps tendon ruptures: incidence, demographics, and the effect of smoking. Clin Orthop Relat Res. 2002;404:275–83.
9. Sharma S, MacKay G. Endoscopic repair of distal biceps tendon using an EndoButton. Arthroscopy. 2005;21(7):897.
10. Visuri T, Lindholm H. Bilateral distal biceps tendon avulsions with use of anabolic steroids. Med Sci Sports Exerc. 1994;26(8):941–4.
11. Abboud JA, Ricchetti ET, Tjoumakaris FP, Bartolozzi AR, Hsu JE. The direct radial tuberosity compression test: a sensitive method for diagnosing partial distal biceps tendon ruptures. Curr Orthop Pract. 2011;22(1):76.
12. Athwal GS, Steinmann SP, Rispoli DM. The distal biceps tendon: footprint and relevant clinical anatomy. J Hand Surg [Am]. 2007;32(8):1225–9.
13. Bain GI, Prem H, Heptinstall RJ, Verhellen R, Paix D. Repair of distal biceps tendon rupture: a new technique using the Endobutton. J Should Elbow Surg. 2000;9(2):120–6.
14. Bain GI, Johnson LJ, Turner PC. Treatment of partial distal biceps tendon tears. Sports Med Arthrosc. 2008;16(3):154–61.
15. D'Alessandro DF, Shields Jr CL, Tibone JE, Chandler RW. Repair of distal biceps tendon ruptures in athletes. Am J Sports Med. 1993;21(1):114–9.
16. Dillon MT, Bollier MJ, King JC. Repair of acute and chronic distal biceps tendon ruptures using the EndoButton. Hand (N Y). 2011;6(1):39–46.
17. Durr HR, Stabler A, Pfahler M, Matzko M, Refior HJ. Partial rupture of the distal biceps tendon. Clin Orthop Relat Res. 2000;(374):195-200.
18. Eames MHA, Bain GI, Fogg QA, van Riet RP. Distal biceps tendon anatomy: a cadaveric study. J Bone Joint Surg Am. 2007;89(5):1044–9.
19. Festa A, Mulieri PJ, Newman JS, Spitz DJ, Leslie BM. Effectiveness of magnetic resonance imaging in detecting partial and complete distal biceps tendon rupture. J Hand Surg [Am]. 2010;35(1):77–83.
20. Freeman CR, McCormick KR, Mahoney D, Baratz M, Lubahn JD. Nonoperative treatment of distal biceps tendon ruptures compared with a historical control group. J Bone Joint Surg Am. 2009;91(10):2329–34.
21. Grégory T, Roure P, Fontès D. Repair of distal biceps tendon rupture using a suture anchor. Am J Sports Med. 2009;37(3):506–11.
22. Heinzelmann AD, Savoie FH, Ramsay JR, Field LD, Mazzocca AD. A combined technique for distal biceps repair using a soft tissue button and biotenodesis interference screw. Am J Sports Med. 2009;37(5):989–94.
23. Jarrett CD, Weir DM, Stuffmann ES, Jain S, Miller MC, Schmidt CC. Anatomic and biomechanical analysis of the short and long head components of the distal biceps tendon. J Should Elbow Surg. 2012; 21(7):942–8.
24. Mazzocca AD, Spang JT, Arciero RA. Distal biceps rupture. Orthop Clin N Am. 2008;39(2):237–49. vii.
25. McKee MD, Hirji R, Schemitsch EH, Wild LM, Waddell JP. Patient-oriented functional outcome after repair of distal biceps tendon ruptures using a single-incision technique. J Should Elbow Surg. 2005;14(3):302–6.

26. Morrey ME, Abdel MP, Sanchez-Sotelo J, Morrey BF. Primary repair of retracted distal biceps tendon ruptures in extreme flexion. J Should Elbow Surg. 2014;23(5):679–85.
27. Nesterenko S, Domire ZJ, Morrey BF, Sanchez-Sotelo J. Elbow strength and endurance in patients with a ruptured distal biceps tendon. J Should Elbow Surg. 2010;19(2):184–9.
28. O'Driscoll SW, Goncalves LB, Dietz P. The hook test for distal biceps tendon avulsion. Am J Sports Med. 2007;35(11):1865–9.
29. Peeters T, Ching-Soon NG, Jansen N, Sneyers C, Declerg G, Verstreken F. Functional outcome after repair of distal biceps tendon ruptures using the endobutton technique. J Should Elbow Surg. 2009;18(2):283–7.
30. Smith J, Finnoff JT, O'Driscoll SW, Lai JK. Sonographic evaluation of the distal biceps tendon using a medial approach. J Ultrasound Med. 2010;29(5):861–5.
31. Walschot LHB, Phadnis J, Bain GI. Endoscopic distal biceps repair, the elbow and wrist: AANA Advanced Arthroscopic Surgical Techniques. Publisher Slack, In Press.
32. Tanner C, Johnson T, Muradov P, Husak L. Single incision power optimizing cost-effective (SPOC) distal biceps repair. J Shoulder Elbow Surg. 2013;22(3):305-11. doi: 10.1016/j.jse.2012.10.044

14 Triceps Tendon Pathology

Melanie Vandenberghe and Roger van Riet

14.1 Introduction and Scope of the Problem

Triceps tendon ruptures are rare [9]. Triceps brachii tendon ruptures are associated with a variety of sports. Overuse is the most common cause of injury in athletes [10]. Bodybuilders and weight lifters are specifically at risk because of possible anabolic steroid abuse, errors in technique, and sometimes skeletal immaturity [21]. A specific group that is prone to overuse of the triceps are wheelchair athletes. Direct trauma or a fall on the outstretched hand may cause a triceps tendon rupture [4], placing contact athletes at risk, as well as, for example, cyclists and motorcycle riders prone to falling on the outstretched hand causing high-energy eccentric loading on the triceps. Ruptures of the distal triceps represent less than 1 % of all tendon ruptures [9]. There is no data on the incidence in athletes, but in the normal population, the male to female ratio is 7:1 and in 60 %, the dominant arm is affected [10]. The average age is 47 years old and consistent with other tendon ruptures. Tendon avulsion from the bone is seen in most cases although musculotendinous ruptures have also been described [11]. Intramuscular rupture of the triceps brachii muscle is extremely rare. We have treated only two cases of intramuscular ruptures. In one patient, there was a blunt trauma from a windsurfing accident, causing a transverse rupture of the muscle belly. The other patient was a professional field hockey player with a longitudinal triceps muscle tear, very similar to more common hamstring tears in athletes.

14.2 History and Physical Examination

Triceps tendon injuries are often missed, leading to a delay in diagnosis. A thorough exam should avoid this delay in diagnosis and eventual treatment.

General medical history should include predisposing factors, such as age, type of sports, and previous medical and surgical history [5]. Renal failure [2], diabetes, and COPD are less likely in athletes, but olecranon bursitis [1, 3], local steroid injections, trauma to the elbow leading to posttraumatic arthritis, and previous surgery all increase the risk of a triceps tendon injury. Chronic tendonitis with pain may have been present for a long time before the rupture occurred and will give an indication on the quality of the tendon.

The mechanism leading to the tendon rupture will often be very suggestive. Patients will typically remember a specific incident. Bodybuilders

M. Vandenberghe, MD • R. van Riet, MD, PhD
Department of Orthopedic Surgery and Traumatology, AZ Monica,
Stevenslei 20, Antwerp 2100, Belgium
e-mail: drrogervanriet@azmonica.be; rogervanriet@hotmail.com

L.A. Pederzini et al. (eds.), *Elbow and Sport*, DOI 10.1007/978-3-662-48742-6_14

and weight lifters will usually feel a crack during bench press or other chest or triceps exercises. A thorough history of uses and abuses is important in this group as low-energy trauma may be sufficient to rupture the tendon in this group. The quality of the tendon is likely to be decreased and this will affect the decision on whether to repair or reconstruct the tendon as well as the postoperative protocol.

A second group of patients will report a higher energy trauma, such as a fall from a motorbike resulting in an eccentric load on the triceps with the elbow in mid-flexion, or a blunt or penetrating blow to the posterior side of the elbow. Associated lesions, such as a fracture, may complicate the clinical examination in these patients and a triceps tendon rupture may therefore be missed (Fig. 14.1). In these patients, a thorough neurological examination should also be conducted, as ulnar palsy or tunnel syndrome may complicate triceps tendon ruptures [7, 8].

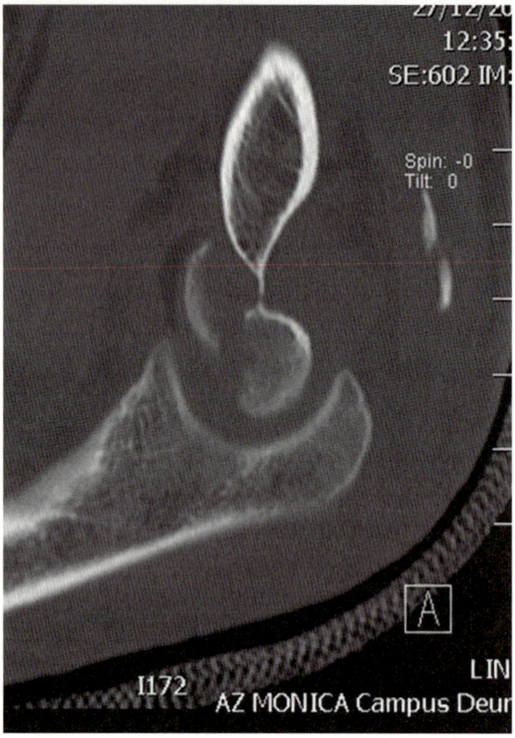

Fig. 14.1 CT scan showing a rare injury pattern with a capitellar shear fracture and complete triceps tendon rupture from a snowboarding accident (Courtesy of MoRe Foundation)

Partial ruptures are underdiagnosed for different reasons. Not all patients seek medical care as pain may be tolerable or intermittent and there is no obvious deformity. A delayed presentation is typical as these patients will often have good elbow function and range of motion with the sole symptom being pain on resisted extension. These patients may not seek medical advice for months or even years after the index injury and some may not be seen until a full rupture occurs [4].

The clinical examination is important and will typically vary with the extent of the rupture, possible associated lesions, and the time from the index injury. In acute ruptures, a posterior swelling, bruising, or ecchymosis can be seen on inspection. In chronic, complete ruptures, two problems are apparent. Besides decreased extension strength, these patients often complain of the asymmetrical appearance of both arms from atrophy or retraction of the muscle belly. Especially in muscular patients, this deformity may be pronounced.

The physical exam of the elbow starts with a general examination of the elbow. Range of motion will, in the absence of associated trauma, typically be normal. Passive flexion is often painful as the ruptured tendon in acute lesions will get stretched with increasing flexion. Extension is typically decreased bilaterally in weight lifters due to biceps hypertrophy.

In a complete rupture, it will be difficult or impossible for the patient to extent the arm against gravity or against resistance. In most cases, the lateral and/or medial triceps expansions will still be intact and the patient will have at least some extension force. It is important to compare both sides as some patients may still have considerable extension strength even with a full-thickness tear. This is especially the case in chronic ruptures.

Triceps strength is tested by extending the arm. This leads to weakness in resistance compared to the other side. It is important to start with the elbow fully flexed (flexion beyond 90°) as this will detect an isolated rupture of the deep triceps insertion.

A modified Thompson test has been described, where the muscle belly is squeezed and no resultant extension of the forearm results [6].

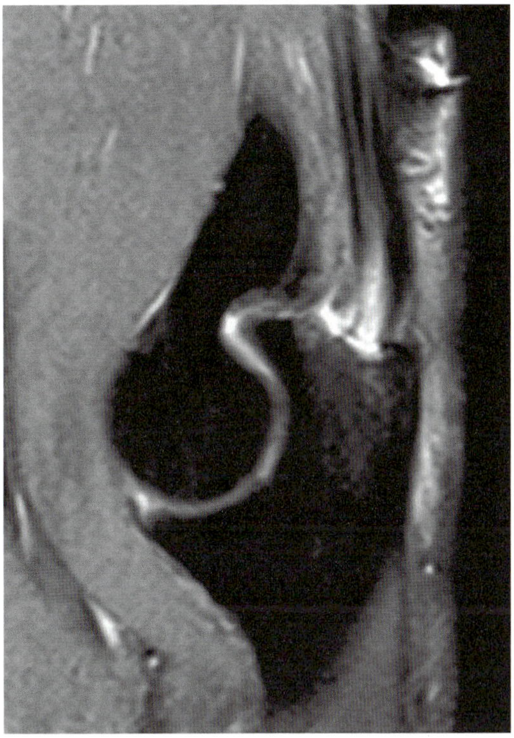

Fig. 14.2 MRI scan showing a partial rupture at the deep layer of the triceps tendon (Courtesy of MoRe Foundation)

Palpation should always be performed with the triceps both relaxed and contracted. Sometimes, there is a palpable gap in the tendon, especially in complete, full-thickness ruptures of the tendon proper. However, palpation will be painful and the patient may not tolerate deep palpation. A hematoma may fill the gap and this may falsely feel like a soft tissue swelling rather than a ruptured tendon.

In a partial tear, no gap may be palpable as superficial fibers will still be intact and cover the defect (Fig. 14.2). In chronic lesions, even in complete ruptures, the gap in the tendon will often have filled with scar tissue (Fig. 14.3).

14.3 Imaging

Plain radiographs can show the presence of flecks of avulsed bone from the olecranon. This is pathognomonic for this lesion and is called the "flake sign" (Fig. 14.4). Radiographs are also

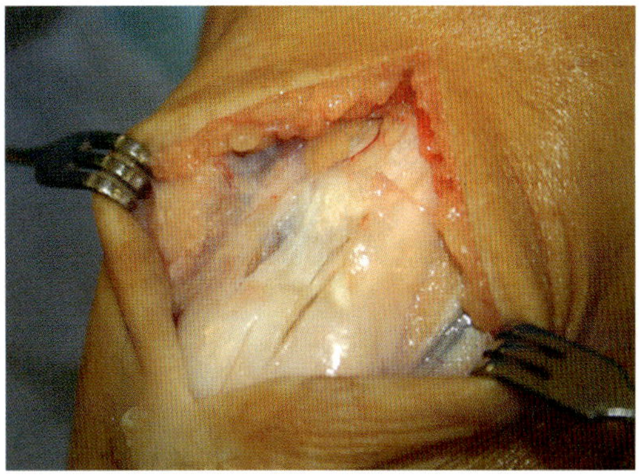

Fig. 14.3 Intraoperative view of a chronic triceps tendon rupture. Notice how the gap is filled by scar tissue in an attempt to heal the tear (Courtesy of MoRe Foundation)

used to rule out associated lesions or signs of chronic triceps tendon overuse, such as the commonly found traction spur (Fig. 14.5). Bony associated lesions can further be examined using a CT scan, but this is not necessary for isolated triceps tendon lesions (Fig. 14.1).

An ultrasound (Fig. 14.6) can confirm the diagnosis if a triceps tendon rupture is suspected [12].

Magnetic resonance imaging (MRI; Fig. 14.7) is often not necessary to confirm the diagnosis, but in chronic cases or partial ruptures (Fig. 14.2), MRI is of value in the diagnosis and localization of the tear [13, 14]. It is also used to quantify the extent of the tear and is very helpful in the possible need for triceps repair at the preoperative planning. Classically, on the MRI, a fluid-filled gap can be seen where the muscle is retracted. The triceps muscle belly may not have the tendency to migrate proximally as the lateral and/or medial triceps expansions are often intact, despite a full-thickness rupture of the tendon proper.

14.4 Treatment Options

Treatment of triceps tendon ruptures depends on different criteria such as the extent of the rupture and/or the activity level of the patient [22].

Ruptures involving greater than 50 % of the tendon, as shown on MRI, are recommended for early surgical repair to prevent late functional

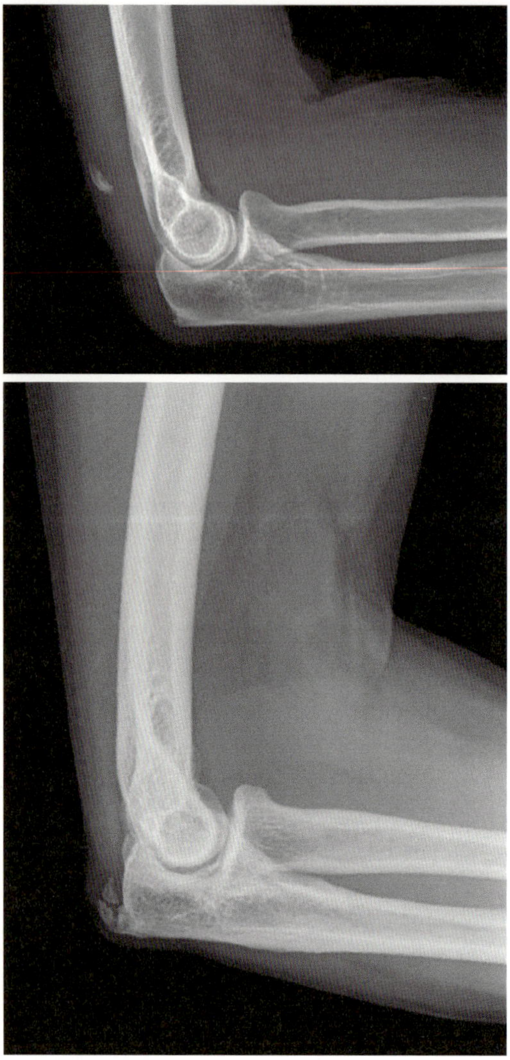

Fig. 14.4 Plain radiograph showing the flake sign. This is pathognomonic for an acute triceps tendon avulsion (Courtesy of MoRe Foundation)

disability [10, 23]. With partial ruptures up to 50 % of the tendon and in the absence of an extension lag, surgical repair is controversial [24] and depends mainly on the functional impairment to the patient. If an extension lag is present, surgical repair is recommended [25–28].

Results of conservative treatment are unclear and often unpredictable. Nonoperative treatment may involve splinting with elbow immobilization for 3–6 weeks at 30° of flexion [29] followed by a training program specifically tailored to the athlete.

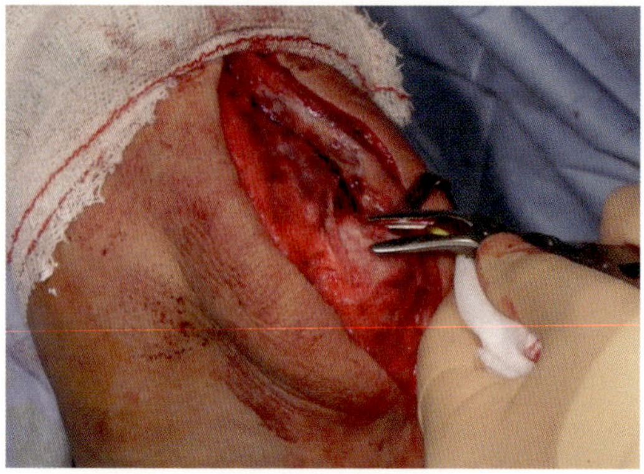

Fig. 14.5 Signs of chronic triceps tendon overuse. (**a**) A traction spur is commonly found in chronic overuse of the triceps tendon (Courtesy of MoRe Foundation). (**b**) Clear calcification of the triceps tendon insertion leading to a high-grade partial rupture (Courtesy of MoRe Foundation)

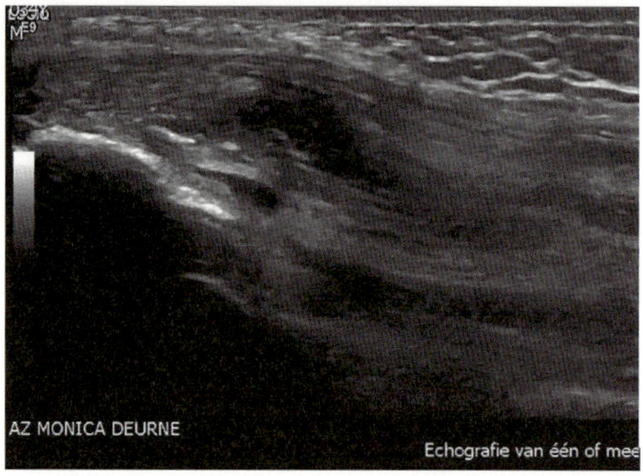

Fig. 14.6 Ultrasound scan showing a partial triceps tendon tear (Courtesy of MoRe Foundation)

Even with a partial rupture, a surgical procedure can be proposed. This to avoid the evolution to complete rupture and functional degradation but other factors also play a role, such as the timing in the season or remaining goals in the athlete's career.

When the triceps rupture is associated with fracture of the radial head, or rupture of the medial collateral ligament, surgery is indicated [6].

14.5 Surgical Technique

Anesthesia can be general or regional with a supraclavicular block. The patient is placed in prone position or lateral decubitus, with the arm

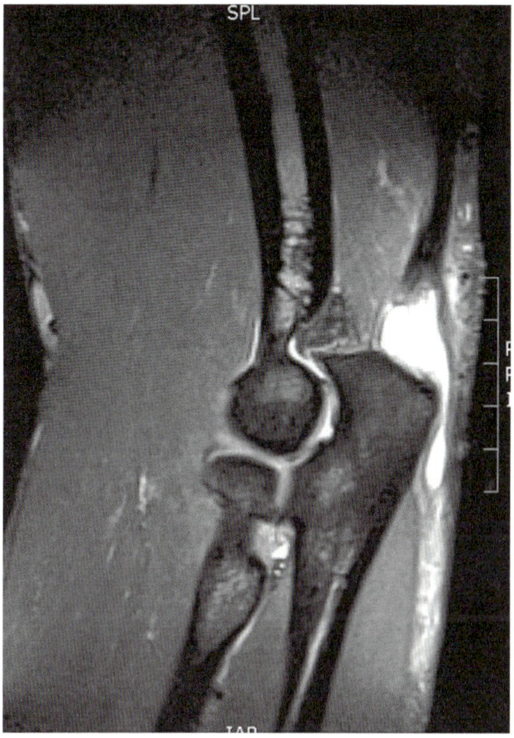

Fig. 14.7 MRI scan showing a complete full-thickness rupture of the triceps tendon with moderate retraction (Courtesy of MoRe Foundation)

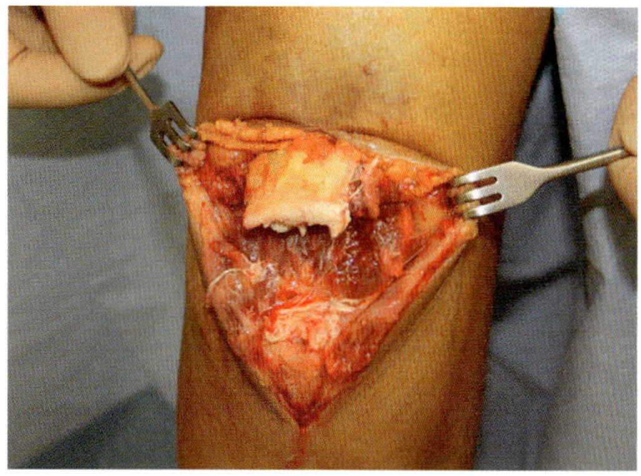

Fig. 14.8 Intraoperative view of an acute triceps tendon rupture (Courtesy of MoRe Foundation)

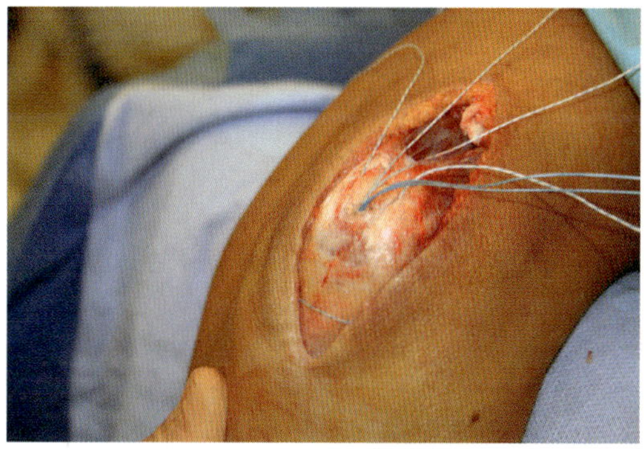

Fig. 14.9 Hybrid fixation of a full-thickness triceps tendon tear, using bone tunnels and anchors

over a support. A tourniquet can be installed but is often not inflated in order to increase the chance of reducing the tendon back to its insertion on the bone.

A posterior incision is made, centered over the olecranon. The length of the incision depends on the retracted position of the tendon. The olecranon is debrided of any residual tendon tissue, scar tissue, or fibrosis to create a bleeding surface in order to promote healing of the tendon to the bone interface (Fig. 14.8). A non-resorbable no. 2 suture is used to securely suture the tendon on both the lateral and medial sides. A 2.5 mm drill is used to create bone tunnels in the proximal ulna. A suture retriever can be used to shuttle the sutures through the bone and the sutures are tied proximally, taking care to bury the knot and not to leave it directly on the subcutaneous border of the ulna, as this may cause pain. Alternatively or additionally (Fig. 14.9), one or multiple strong bone anchors can be used [30], depending on the preference of the surgeon. In this case, a knotless repair [31] can be done or the sutures are tied proximally and buried in the triceps muscle, to avoid irritation.

Once the repair has been done, it is important to test the tension-free mobility of the elbow and the integrity and strength of the repair (Fig. 14.10). Gapping may occur with further flexion of the elbow and the surgeon should decide if reinforcement of the repair is necessary at this stage or if the elbow needs to be protected by restricting the amount of flexion for a period of time postoperatively.

In chronic cases, a direct repair may be possible and is the preferred technique [10]. The incision and approach to the tendon are not different in the chronic setting. Usually, there is no clear palpable or visible gap between the olecranon

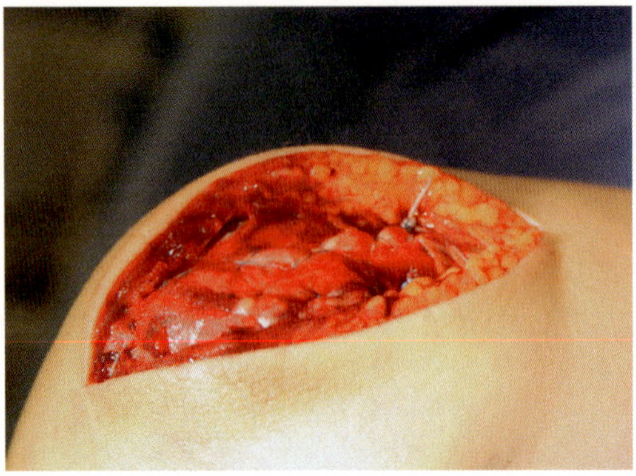

Fig. 14.10 Intraoperative testing of the strength of the fixation will determine the immediate postoperative protocol. No gapping was found in this patient and the patient was allowed to mobilize the elbow as tolerated in a compressive bandage to protect the wound (Courtesy of MoRe Foundation)

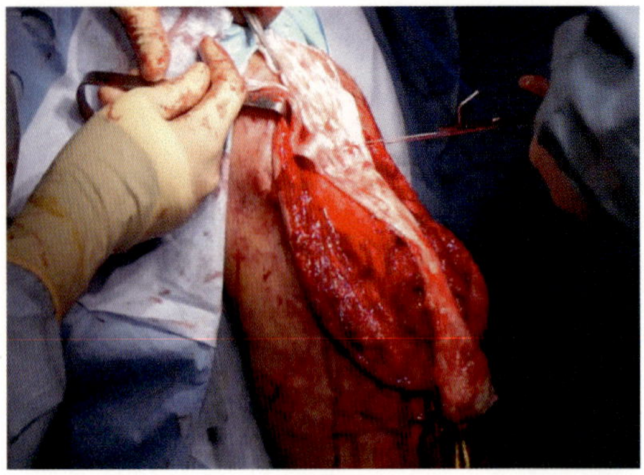

Fig. 14.11 An Achilles tendon was used to augment the repair of this chronic triceps tendon tear, nearly 5 years after the initial injury in a professional bodybuilder (Courtesy of MoRe Foundation)

and the triceps stump, as it is filled with scar tissue. It may be difficult to determine the demarcation between scar tissue and viable triceps tendon. Careful debridement of scar tissue is necessary to obtain healthy tendon for repair. The tendon is mobilized and the elbow is positioned in extension to facilitate the primary repair. The tendon is then repaired to bone, as described above. If it is not possible to bring the retracted tendon back to bone or if too much tension is needed or failure of the repair occurs when the elbow is tested from extension to flexion, the repair is augmented with a graft. Both auto- and allograft tendons [32–34], as well as synthetic grafts [35], have been used to augment the repair. A hamstring or palmaris longus graft can be used and woven through the triceps stump and attached to the proximal ulna [32, 33].

Our preference is to use an Achilles tendon allograft [10]. The advantage of this graft is that the fan-shaped graft resembles the anatomy of the triceps tendon (Fig. 14.11). The Achilles tendon can cover the defect that may remain after maximal mobilization of the triceps tendon stump. The elbow is held in extension and the triceps is temporarily fixed as close as possible to the olecranon, in order to tension the muscle. The graft is then placed over the triceps muscle, musculotendinous junction, and the tendon. The graft covers the remaining defect between the triceps stump and the olecranon and is draped over the proximal ulna. Non-resorbable no. 2 sutures are used to suture the graft to the triceps. We use medial, central, and lateral rows of sutures. It is important not only to make sure that the graft is securely fixed for the strength of the repair but also to avoid hematoma or seroma formation between the graft and the tendon, jeopardizing ingrowth of the graft. There are essentially two different methods to fix the Achilles tendon distally to the olecranon. The calcaneal bone block at the distal end of the graft can be shaped to fit over the proximal ulna and can be fixed with cerclage wires. This has the advantage of bone-to-bone contact, which may offer a stronger fixation. Unfortunately, even with an excellent fit, the bone graft is quite bulky and may cause problems, due to its direct subcutaneous position. We reserve this option for patients with poor bone stock or bone loss, such as rheumatoid patients or following arthroplasty of the elbow, and have not used this method in athletes. In most traumatic triceps tendon ruptures in this group, the bone of the proximal ulna is of sufficient quality to allow for fixation of the graft through bone tunnels or with bone anchors, as previously described. Reconstructions or augmented repairs have been shown to be stronger than direct repairs in a cadaveric study [36] and can lead to a good clinical outcome in the general population, despite the poor quality of the chronically ruptured tendon and the potential for residual elbow stiffness [10]. However, better peak strength and a shorter time to recovery have been reported in repairs compared to reconstructions and are certainly preferable in this group of high-demand patients [10].

14.6 Rehabilitation

During surgery, the initial rehabilitation program will be determined. The tension that is necessary for a strong repair will determine if the repair needs to be protected. In acute cases, direct repair on the olecranon is often tension-free and full range of motion is permitted immediately. So, if the elbow can be moved freely and no gapping is seen through a full range of motion, only a protective bandage will be used. The patient is allowed to flex the elbow actively. Passive flexion exercises are not permitted in the first 6 weeks. Passive and gravity-assisted extensions are encouraged immediately.

After 6 weeks, progressive stretching will be initiated, as well as active and resisted extension exercises.

When the tendon repair or reconstruction needs to be protected, we will immobilize the elbow in varying degrees of extension. This is depending on the tension and strength of the repair. A dynamic elbow brace [37, 38] is fitted and flexion will be blocked at 30° for 2 weeks with full extension permitted. Gradually, flexion is increased with 30° intervals every 2 weeks or slower when necessary. Normally, full flexion is permitted after 6 weeks and further rehabilitation will be done as noted above. Return to sports is highly dependent on the type of sport but is typically allowed between 3 and 6 months post surgery.

14.7 Complications

Reruptures are very uncommon [10, 39]. A loss in the range of motion is expected, approximately 10° loss of flexion and extension on average. Peak strength will return to 92 % of normal for acute repairs, but only to 66 % of normal in chronic reconstructions [10], an important reason not to delay surgery or further diagnostics in this patient group.

Infection, wound problems, and nerve pathology have to be prevented. Resulting from the sutures, an olecranon bursitis may arise due to irritation of the sutures or from the operative insult. There have been no reports of an olecranon fracture.

Pearl

Reruptures are very uncommon after fixation of a ruptured triceps tendon and the results are generally good. A loss in the range of motion is expected, approximately 10 degrees loss of flexion and extension on average. Peak strength will return to 92 % of normal for acute repairs, but only to 66 % of normal in chronic reconstructions.

Pitfall: Corticosteroid Use

Derivatives of testosterone are used for the purpose of improving performance among competitive and power athletes. They have attained a highly controversial position despite increased controls in competitive sports [15].

Short-term administration of these drugs has a *positive influence* on strength and bodyweight. Strength gains about 5–20 % and the athlete gains about 2–5 kg bodyweight, attributed to an increase of the lean body mass.

Possible *side effects* of anabolic steroids are related to metabolic dysfunction and abnormal structure of connective tissue. Both systemic steroids and local injections may predispose tendon injury or to rupture [19].

Scientific and medical literature addressing this concern is rare and additional investigation is warranted. Consideration should be given to potential tendon alteration and ruptures among the side effects of steroid abuse [20].

Electron microscopy has been used to study tendon collagen fibrils, after treatment with an anabolic steroid hormone. The occurrence of dysplastic, ruptured, and dissociated collagen fibrils has been reported [16]. However, another study did not show changes in the appearance of fibril diameter or shape [17].

Marqueti found impaired tissue remodeling in the Achilles tendons of animals treated with anabolic steroids and undergoing physical exercise. This created down-regulating of the matrix metallopeptidase activity, thus increasing the potential for tendon injury [18].

The combination of anabolic use with physical overload will probably create the increased risk of injury in high-level athletes.

Pearls

- Although often missed, a thorough clinical exam should be sufficient to diagnose a triceps tendon rupture.
- Ultrasound and MRI can aid the diagnosis.
- MRI is the gold standard for evaluating partially or chronic triceps tendon ruptures.
- Conservative treatment can be successful in the smaller partial ruptures with limited to no functional impairment.
- A direct repair of the tendon to the olecranon is preferable, even in chronic cases.
- Examine the strength of the repair during surgery.
- An augmentation of the repair can be done, using a variety of grafts, if a direct repair is not possible or if fixation is not strong enough.
- Strength and tension of the repair or reconstruction during surgery will guide the initial rehabilitation period.
- A hinged brace can be used to progressively allow flexion of the elbow.

Pitfalls

- Pain and swelling can obscure a triceps tendon rupture in the acute phase.
- Even in full-thickness tears, resisted extension strength can still be high in athletes if the lateral or medial triceps extensions are still intact.
- Delayed presentation and therapy will lead to a prolonged rehabilitation period and decreased final peak strength.
- Suture knots may be painful and should be buried.
- Failure to test tension-free range of motion may put the repair at risk.
- A hematoma between a graft and the tendon will impair healing.

References

1. Lambers K, Ring D. Elbow fracture-dislocation with triceps avulsion: report of 2 cases. J Hand Surg [Am]. 2011;36(4):625–7.
2. Gupta RR, Murthi AM. Distal humeral fracture with associated triceps tendon avulsion in a renal transplant recipient. Orthopedics. 2010;33(3). Epub.
3. Tatebe M, Horii E, Nakamura R. Chronically ruptured triceps tendon with avulsion of the medial collateral ligament: a report of 2 cases. J Should Elb Surg. 2007;16(1):e5–7.
4. Bennet BS. Triceps tendon rupture. J Bone Joint Surg Am. 1962;44:741–4.
5. Celli A, Arash A, Adams RA, Morrey BF. Triceps insufficiency following total elbow arthroplasty. J Bone Joint Surg Am. 2005;87(9):1957–64.
6. Viegas SF. Avulsion of the triceps tendon. Orthop Rev. 1990;19(6):533–6.
7. Herrick RT, Herrick S. Ruptured triceps in powerlifter presenting as cubital tunnel syndrome. A case report. Am J Sports Med. 1987;15:514–6.
8. Duchow J, Kelm J, Kohn D. Acute ulnar nerve compression syndrome in a powerlifter with triceps tendon rupture: a case report. Int J Sports Med. 2000;21:308–10.
9. Anzel SH, Covey KW, Weiner AD, Lipscomb PR. Disruption of muscles and tendons. An analysis of 1,014 cases. Surgery. 1959;45:406–14.
10. van Riet RP, Morrey BF, Ho E, O'Driscoll SW. Surgical treatment of distal triceps ruptures. J Bone Joint Surg Am. 2003;85(10):1961–7.
11. Wagner JR, Cooney WP. Rupture of the triceps muscle at the musculotendinous junction: a case report. J Hand Surg [Am]. 1997;22:341–3.

12. Tagliafico A, Gandolfo N, Michaud J, Perez MM, Palmieri F, Martinoli C. Ultrasound demonstration of distal triceps tendon tears. Eur J Radiol. 2012;81(6):1207–10.
13. Gaines ST, Durbin RA, Marsalka DS. The use of magnetic resonance imaging in the diagnosis of triceps tendon ruptures. Contemp Orthop. 1990;20:607–11.
14. Tiger E, Mayer DP, Glazer R. Complete avulsion of the triceps tendon: MRI diagnosis. Comput Med Imaging Graph. 1993;17:51–4.
15. Hartgens F, Kuipers H. Effects of androgenic-anabolic steroids in athletes. Sports Med. 2004;34(8):513–54.
16. Michna H. Virchows Arch B Cell Pathol Incl Mol Pathol. 1986;52(1):75–86.
17. Inhofe PD, Grana WA, Egle D, Min KW, Tomasek J. The effects of anabolic steroids on rat tendon. An ultrastructural, biomechanical, and biochemical analysis. Am J Sports Med. 1995;23(2):227–32.
18. Marqueti RC, Parizotto NA, Chriguer RS, Perez SE, Selistre-de-Araujo HS. Androgenic-anabolic steroids associated with mechanical loading inhibit matrix metallopeptidase activity and affect the remodeling of the achilles tendon in rats. Am J Sports Med. 2006;34(8):1274–80.
19. Stannard JP, Bucknell AL. Rupture of the triceps tendon associated with steroid injections. Am J Sports Med. 1993;21(3):482–5.
20. Laseter JT, Russell JA. Anabolic steroid-induced tendon pathology: a review of the literature. Med Sci Sports Exerc. 1991;23(1):1–3.
21. Sollender JL, Rayan GM, Barden GA. Triceps tendon rupture in weight lifters. J Should Elb Surg. 1998;7(2):151–3.
22. Strauch RJ. Biceps and triceps injuries of the elbow. Orthop Clin N Am. 1999;30(1):95–107.
23. Pina A, Garcia I, Sabater M. Traumatic avulsion of the triceps brachii. J Orthop Trauma. 2002;16(4):273–6.
24. Inhofe PD, Moneim MS. Late presentation of triceps rupture. A case report and review of the literature. Am J Orthop (Belle Mead NJ). 1996;25(11):790–2. Review.
25. Morrey BF. Rupture of the triceps tendon. In: The elbow and its disorders. 3rd ed. Philadelphia: WB Saunders; 2000
26. Mair SD, Isbell WM, Gill TJ, Schlegel TF, Hawkins RJ. Triceps tendon ruptures in professional football players. Am J Sports Med. 2004;32(2):431–4.
27. Blackmore SM, Jander RM, Culp RW. Management of distal biceps and triceps ruptures. J Hand Ther. 2006;19(2):154–68.
28. Vidal AF, Drakos MC, Allen AA. Biceps tendon and triceps tendon injuries. Clin Sports Med. 2004;23(4):707–22.
29. Farrar 3rd EL, Lippert 3rd FG. Avulsion of the triceps tendon. Clin Orthop Relat Res. 1981;161:242–6.
30. Bava ED, Barber FA, Lund ER. Clinical outcome after suture anchor repair for complete traumatic rupture of the distal triceps tendon. Arthroscopy. 2012;28(8):1058–63.
31. Clark J, Obopilwe E, Rizzi A, Komatsu DE, Singh H, Mazzocca AD, Paci JM. Distal triceps knotless anatomic footprint repair is superior to transosseous cruciate repair: a biomechanical comparison. Arthroscopy. 2014;30(10):1254–60.
32. Dos Remedios C, Brosset T, Chantelot C, Fontaine C. Repair of a triceps tendon rupture using autogenous semi-tendinous and gracilis tendons. A case report and retrospective chart review. Chir Main. 2007;26(3):154–8.
33. Scolaro JA, Blake MH, Huffman GR. Triceps tendon reconstruction using ipsilateral Palmaris longus autograft in unrecognized chronic tears. Orthopedics. 2013;36(1):e117–20.
34. Sanchez-Sotelo J, Morrey BF. Surgical techniques for reconstruction of chronic insufficiency of the triceps. Rotation flap using anconeus and tendo achilles allograft. J Bone Joint Surg (Br). 2002;84(8):1116–20.
35. Nikolaidou ME, Banke IJ, Laios T, Petsogiannis K, Mourikis A. Synthetic augmented suture anchor reconstruction for a complete traumatic distal triceps tendon rupture in a male professional bodybuilder with postoperative biomechanical assessment. Case Rep Orthop. 2014;2014:962930.
36. Petre BM, Grutter PW, Rose DM, Belkoff SM, McFarland EG, Petersen SA. Triceps tendons: a biomechanical comparison of intact and repaired strength. J Should Elb Surg. 2011;20(2):213–8.
37. Greer MA, Miklos-Essenberg ME. Early mobilization using dynamic splinting with acute triceps tendon avulsion. J Hand Ther. 2005;18(3):365–71.
38. Monasterio M, Longsworth KA, Viegas S. Dynamic hinged orthosis following a surgical reattachment and therapy protocol of a distal triceps tendon avulsion. J Hand Ther. 2014;27(4):330–4.
39. Weistroffer JK, Mills WJ, Shin AY. Recurrent rupture of the triceps tendon repaired with hamstring tendon autograft augmentation: a case report and repair technique. J Should Elb Surg. 2003;12:193–6.

Triceps Repair

15

Giuseppe Giannicola, Gianluca Bullitta,
Federico Maria Sacchetti, Marco Scacchi,
Giovanni Merolla, and Giuseppe Porcellini

15.1 Introduction

The triceps brachii is the main extensor muscle of the elbow and as such plays a key role in normal upper extremity function. Distal rupture of the triceps tendon is a relatively uncommon injury. In their review of 1,014 tendon ruptures, Anzel et al. reported a prevalence of 0.8 %, while Mair et al. recorded only 21 cases of triceps rupture in the National USA Football League over a 6-year period [1, 2]. However, Koplas et al. recently found a high prevalence of triceps tendon tears (3.8 %) upon MRI examination, suggesting that the number of triceps tendon injuries is underestimated in imaging studies and in the orthopedic literature and that this type of lesion is frequently misdiagnosed [3].

Distal triceps tendon tears are more common in men, particularly in professional sports players. Although the average age of occurrence is about 35 years, tears have been reported in every age group, from children to elderly patients [4–7].

To assist the orthopedic sports physician in the evaluation and treatment of triceps tendon injuries, this chapter considers the anatomy, etiology, clinical presentation, diagnostic protocols, conservative and operative treatments, and outcomes for partial and complete ruptures.

15.2 Anatomy and Function

The triceps brachii is a pennate muscle whose name derives from its tripartite origin, consisting of the lateral, long, and medial heads. The triceps, which runs the entire length of the posterior humerus, is the only muscle in the posterior compartment of the arm. As Gray described, the lateral head originates from three sites, which are the posterior humerus between the teres minor insertion and the superior aspect of the spiral groove, the lateral border of the humerus, and the lateral intermuscular septum [8]; the long head originates at the infraglenoid tuberosity, where the scapula joins the shoulder capsule. The medial (or deep) head originates from the posterior humerus distal to the spiral groove, medial humerus, and medial intermuscular septum. Therefore, each head originates distal to the other, with increasingly larger areas of origin. The long and lateral heads are superficial to the deep medial head and blend in the midline of the humerus to form a common tendon, or intermuscular septum, which is covered by the triceps aponeurosis (Fig. 15.1); in some cases the latter structure is absent

G. Giannicola, MD, PhD (✉) • G. Bullitta, MD
F.M. Sacchetti, MD • M. Scacchi, MD
Orthopedics and Traumatology, "Sapienza"
University of Rome, Rome, Italy
e-mail: giannicola.giuseppe@gmail.com;
gbullitta@alice.it

G. Merolla, • G. Porcellini
Unit of Shoulder and Elbow Surgery, D. Cervesi
Hospital, Cattolica –AUSL della Romagna Ambito
Territoriale di Rimini, Cattolica, Italy
e-mail: giovannimerolla@hotmail.com;
giovanni.merolla@auslrn.net

L.A. Pederzini et al. (eds.), *Elbow and Sport*, DOI 10.1007/978-3-662-48742-6_15

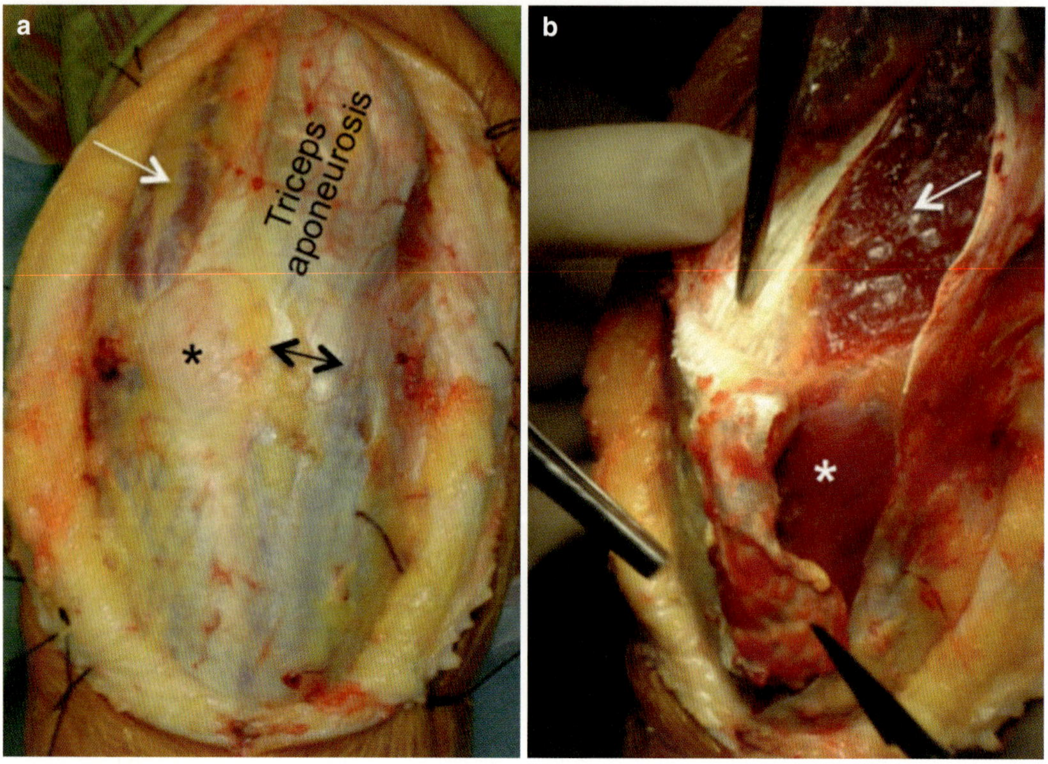

Fig. 15.1 (**a**) Posterior aspect of the elbow, showing the triceps brachii muscle and a clearly represented triceps aponeurosis. The *asterisk* indicates the olecranon whereas the *double-headed arrow* shows the lateral expansion of the aponeurosis. The *white arrow* points at the long head of the triceps (**b**); the triceps aponeurosis was detached and reflected (surgical blade) and the common tendon was revealed, as indicated by the surgical clamp. The *arrow* indicates the lateral head of the triceps, whereas the *asterisk* indicates the anconeus muscle. The *finger* indicates the long head of the triceps brachii, which is located medially to the tendon

(Fig. 15.2). The mean length of the superficial tendon is 15.2 cm (range, 13.3–17.1) measured from the tip of the olecranon to the most proximal extent of the tendon medially [9].

The triceps insertion is a wide area or footprint rather than a focal point on the olecranon. In a cadaveric study, the triceps footprint was found to cover a large area of the supero-posterior aspect of the olecranon, with a mean surface ranging from 466 to 646 mm^2; moreover, it was found to start 12 mm distal to the tip of the olecranon and to overlap with the posterior capsule [10]. The tendon width at the insertion was greater than that of the olecranon, which indicates that the distal triceps does not end at a specific insertion point, but extends well distal to the olecranon tip and includes the medial, lateral, and posterior borders of the olecranon.

The extensor mechanism of the elbow comprises two components: the triceps tendon itself (the confluence of the tendon from all three heads inserting on the olecranon) and the lateral and medial triceps expansions. The mean length and width of the distal tendon at the level of insertion are reported to be 20.52 mm (SD 2.02) and 22.65 mm (SD 2.40), respectively [10]. The lateral triceps expansion fans out laterally from fibers of the triceps and blends into the fascia of the anconeus muscle, the extensor carpi ulnaris muscle, and the posterior border of the ulna; the triceps expansion also inserts on the antebrachial fascia of the forearm distally [11]. The expansion length from a line between both epicondyles to its insertion is 4.02 cm (range 2.3–6.0 cm) [12]. Owing to its wide lateral insertion, the triceps expansion often needs to be concomitantly repaired in cases of triceps rupture. Although the triceps seems to be able to compensate for injuries to the triceps expansion (e.g., by sacrificing the triceps expansion in the classic intra-articular olecranon osteotomy expo-

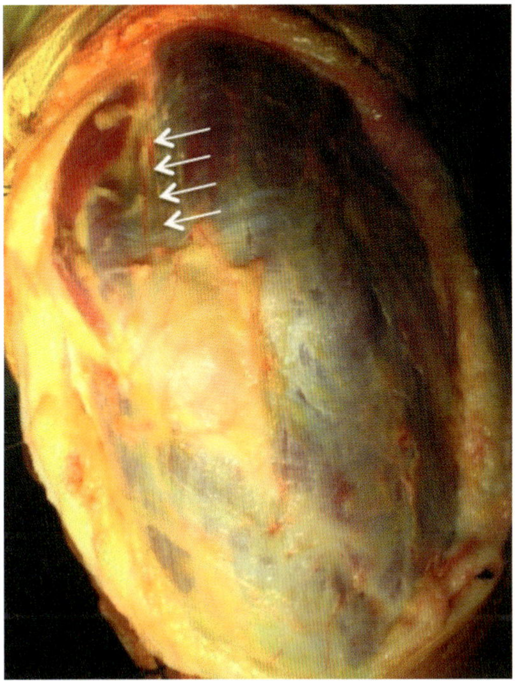

Fig. 15.2 Posterior aspect of the elbow showing absence of the triceps aponeurosis. The superficial muscle fibers of the lateral and long head are easily distinguishable. The *arrows* indicate the site of the common tendon of the triceps, covered by the muscle fibers

sure), the triceps expansion does not fully compensate for injuries to the triceps (e.g., triceps avulsion). The insertion of the medial aspect of the triceps expansion is located on the posterior crest of the ulna, adjacent to the medial head [13]. Hypertrophy of the medial head of the triceps muscle may cause ulnar nerve impingement, a condition occasionally observed in weightlifters [13]. The distal portion of the medial head has a distinct muscle belly, while the deep insertion is muscular with a small amount of tendon [11]. Upon gross examination, the tendon of the medial head of the triceps is smaller and deeper to the tendon of long and lateral heads. There is invariably a thin fascial layer that separates the long and lateral heads from the deeper medial head. This fascial plane has been clearly defined, and dissection can easily be accomplished. The deep tendon is readily identifiable after the overlying conjoined tendon of the long and lateral heads of the triceps has been divided longitudinally. However, upon histological analysis, no separation between the deep and superficial tendons is observed at their insertion on the olecranon [11].

The triceps is innervated by the radial nerve (C6–C8). The main function of the triceps is to extend the forearm at the ulno-humeral joint. However, since it originates at the infraglenoid tuberosity, the long head of the triceps is also believed to contribute to arm adduction and extension. The overall muscle-tendon length of the triceps is critical to its motor function; indeed, a biomechanical study has shown that a 2 cm length reduction between its origin and insertion may result in a 40 % loss in extension strength [14]. Gerbeaux et al. investigated the lever arm of the triceps muscle in cadaveric specimens [15]. Adopting the long head of the triceps as their model, they showed that the lever arm value of the triceps ranged from a maximum of about 0.5 radians (45°) to a minimum of about 2 radians (180°). This finding suggests that the triceps lever arm is greatest when the elbow is fully flexed. Although in this cadaveric model the triceps was fixed, it is noteworthy that the scapular insertion of the long head of the triceps provides a greater degree of freedom, producing a potentially more dynamic system in vivo. The length of the triceps lever arm suggests that it exerts the greatest strength in flexion, though it should be borne in mind that the separation of individual sarcomeric units substantially weakens the triceps when it is stretched; the triceps thus exerts more power when the elbow is closer to full extension [8].

15.3 Etiology and Mechanism of Injury

Considerable force is required before a normal triceps tendon ruptures. Direct posterior force on the elbow and weightlifting are two common mechanisms [4, 16–20]. Other documented causes include swinging a baseball bat, motor vehicle accidents, seizures, pitching, volleyball serving, punching, and hammering [21–28]. If direct trauma is excluded, the biomechanics of injury are similar in each of these mechanisms. Uncoordinated contraction of the triceps against the flexed elbow, combined with a deceleration-like impact, overloads the tendon eccentrically

[2, 5, 7, 16, 17, 20, 21, 25, 29–31]. Although the tendon can withstand three times tetanic contraction [32], various factors may alter its structural integrity and reduce its maximum load capacity [16, 21]. Distal triceps tendon ruptures may even occur spontaneously or following minimal trauma in patients with concomitant significant systemic or local pathological conditions. Pathological changes that weaken the tendon are believed to be the underlying mechanism in almost all tendon ruptures. The vast majority of reports have associated triceps tendon rupture with anabolic steroid use or steroid treatment, hyperparathyroidism, renal osteodystrophy, hypocalcemic tetany, Marfan syndrome, osteogenesis imperfecta, rheumatoid arthritis, lupus, or type I diabetes [2, 4, 7, 16, 19, 21, 29, 31, 33–35]. Connective tissue degeneration due to ciprofloxacin is also reported to increase the likelihood of tendon rupture [7]. Professional football players and body builders are believed to have a higher risk of rupture than the general population, possibly owing to their training regimen, the use of locally injected steroids in case of olecranon bursitis, and the violent nature of the sport itself [2]. Adolescent athletes with incompletely fused or recently fused physes are also susceptible to triceps tendon rupture, though this is an extremely rare event [5].

15.4 History and Physical Examination

A history of eccentric loading in flexion against the triceps contracture (e.g., fall or weightlifting) associated with acute pain and weakness provides the most reliable diagnosis. The patient presents with pain and swelling over the posterior aspect of the elbow, though the pain is frequently not dysfunctional. As a consequence, patients may underestimate the severity of the trauma after the acute event and wait several weeks before going to see the orthopedic surgeon, complaining of reduced strength and persistent pain.

In the acute setting, the physical examination reveals tenderness, swelling, muscle spasm, and ecchymosis. Although a defect proximal to the olecranon may be palpable, this is not a common finding in partial tears and obese patients [36]. The inability to actively extend against gravity is a pathognomonic sign of complete rupture. However, complete tears do not always result in the inability to actively extend against resistance owing to an intact lateral expansion or a compensating anconeus muscle [36, 37]. In such cases, assessing the reduction in strength against gravity or resistance starting from maximum elbow flexion is mandatory.

Viegas has recommended the use of a modified Thompson squeeze test as a clinical diagnostic tool [38]. During this passive extension test, the patient lies prone with the elbow at the edge of the examination table. The forearm is then allowed to hang over the edge of the table so that it is flexed at 90° in a relaxed position. When the examiner firmly squeezes the triceps muscle in a patient with complete disruption of the triceps tendon and the lateral expansion as well, he will not observe a passive extension of the elbow. No study has yet demonstrated the sensitivity and specificity of this diagnostic test.

In an unpublished study, Giannicola proposed a new diagnostic test for triceps tendon rupture called the "posterior hook test." This test is similar to the hook test described by O'Driscoll et al. for distal biceps tendon avulsion [39]. To perform the posterior hook test, the patient stands with the examiner behind him. The patient is the asked to contract and relax the triceps muscle with the forearm fully extended. The examiner's index finger is inserted into the superomedial side of the olecranon, laterally to the ulnar nerve in an attempt to hook the medial portion of triceps tendon. In contrast to O'Driscoll's test, in the posterior hook test, it is impossible to insert the finger beneath the tendon during the triceps contraction in healthy patients; indeed, the examiner will encounter a cord-like structure belonging to the triceps tendon that prevents the index finger from sliding in a medial-to-lateral direction along the humeral bone surface. By contrast, in patients with a triceps tendon tear, this cord-like structure is not encountered and the examiner's finger can reach the central and lateral bone surfaces of the distal humerus. The

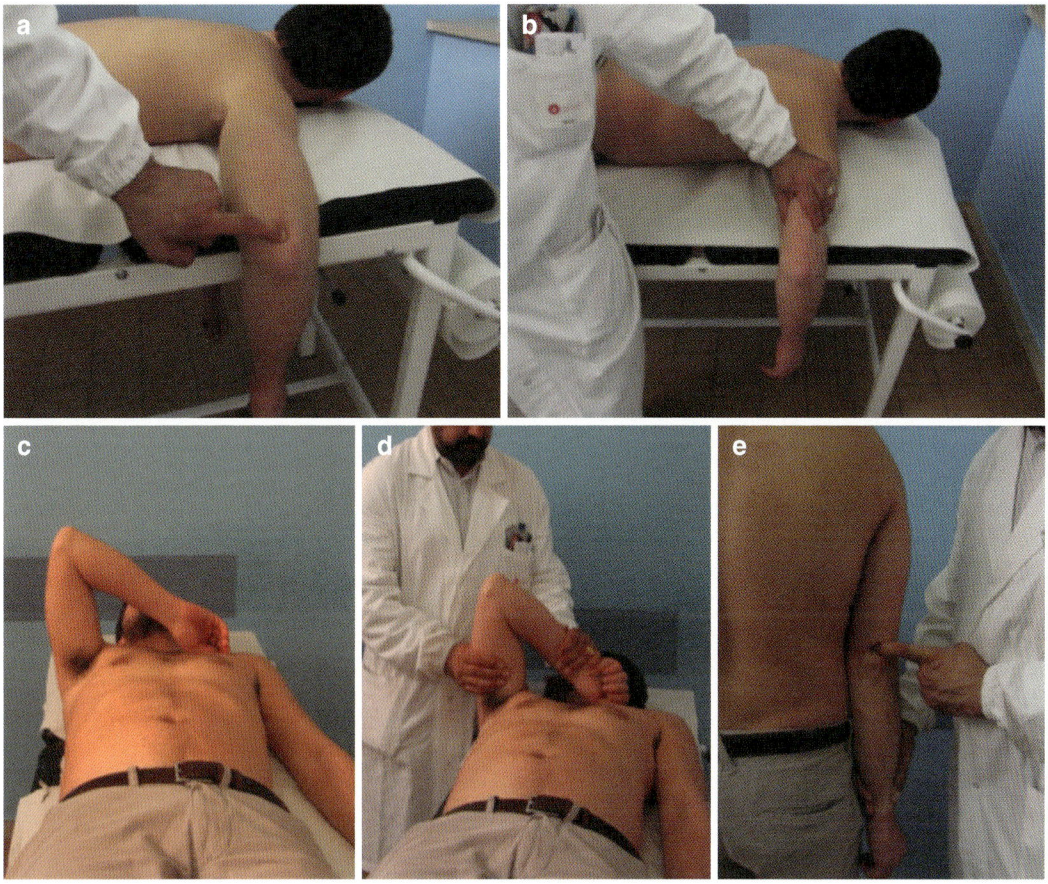

Fig. 15.3 Clinical test used for the diagnosis of triceps tendon tear. (**a**) In case of distal triceps tendon rupture, a palpable defect proximal to the olecranon may be apparent. This evidence of rupture is called "gap sign." (**b**) The "Viegas squeezing sign." (**c**) The inability to actively extend against gravity is usually a sign of complete rupture, with involvement of the lateral expansion, whereas (**d**) the ability to actively extend against gravity associated with the inability to extend against resistance may be a sign of partial rupture. (**e**) The "posterior hook sign"

clinical tests preferred by the authors are showed in Fig. 15.3.

Diagnostic difficulties, low clinical suspicion, and underestimation of injury severity may result in delayed diagnosis and surgical intervention, with consequent prolonged disability [16, 36]. Diagnosis of triceps tendon rupture requires a high degree of suspicion; indeed, in one recent study, almost 50 % of acute triceps ruptures were found to have been initially misdiagnosed [16]. Concerning chronic tears, the most common complaints are pain, mild extension lag, and weakness. In such cases the lack of swelling and acute pain enhance the reliability of the clinical examination.

15.5 Imaging

AP and lateral radiographs of the affected elbow should always be performed. The lateral radiograph may show the presence of small olecranon avulsion fragments, which is referred to as the "flake sign" and is considered almost pathognomonic of a triceps tendon rupture (Fig. 15.4a) [5, 31]. Similarly, the presence of dystrophic calcification or heterotopic ossification (an indirect sign of tendon degeneration) at the level of triceps tendon insertion should be interpreted as a sign of probable triceps rupture (Fig. 15.4b). When Giannicola et al. analyzed the tendons from ten patients with a triceps tear, they found

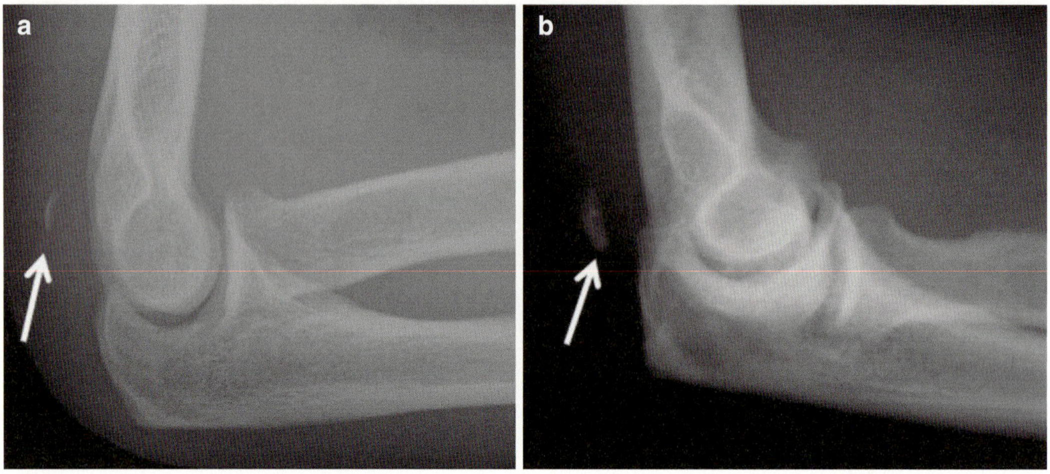

Fig. 15.4 (**a**) Standard LL radiograph showing a small avulsion fragment from the olecranon (*arrow*) named "flake sign." (**b**) Figure showing the presence of dystrophic calcification in the context of the triceps tendon, which represents a sign of tendon degeneration

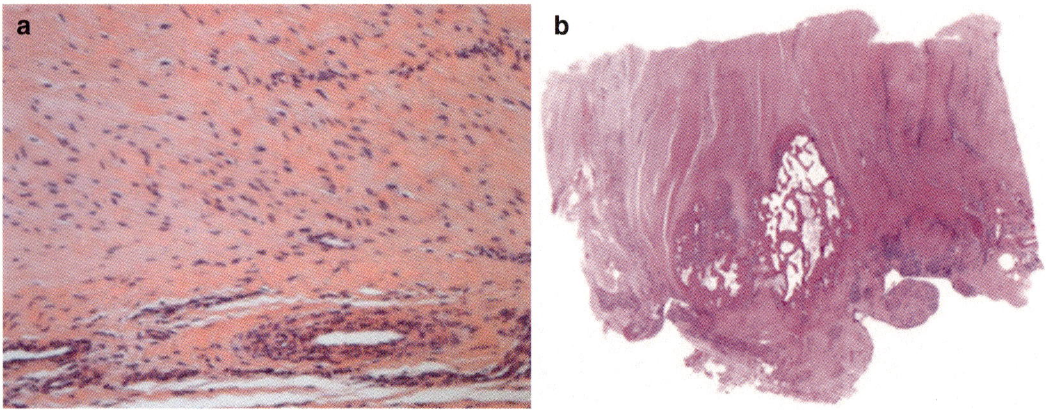

Fig. 15.5 Histological sections of a ruptured tendon showing (**a**) increased cellularity and vascularization along with chronic inflammatory infiltrates and (**b**) the presence of metaplastic osseous and cartilaginous inclusions

metaplastic bone tissue within the tendon in 20 % of cases. In particular, the histological analysis revealed a microscopic picture of enthesopathy characterized by degenerative changes, including thinning, fragmentation and tearing of collagen fibers, increased cellularity, and vascularization and focal areas of ossification along with chronic inflammatory infiltrates (Fig. 15.5).

MRI and ultrasonography may prove useful in challenging cases and in preoperative planning to determine the location and extent of the tear [40–42]. Axial and sagittal MRI is considered the gold standard because it accurately demonstrates the integrity of the triceps tendon [2, 16, 43, 44]. Furthermore, MRI can distinguish between both partial and complete rupture and superficial and deep tears of the triceps tendon and can assess retraction degree of completely torn tendon. Partial rupture is characterized by a small fluid-filled defect within the distal triceps tendon (bright area on T2-weighted images), with edema extending to the surrounding subcutaneous tissues. Complete rupture of the triceps tendon is instead characterized by a large fluid-filled gap between the distal end of the triceps tendon and the olecranon process [42]. The distal edge of the torn tendon is retracted and yields heterogeneous signal intensity. In the authors' clinical experience, T2-weighted images on the sagittal plane performed with the elbow flexed at about 90° are the sequences that provide the most reliable diagnosis.

15.6 Associated Lesions

The association between triceps tears and concomitant injuries has been described by several authors. The most frequent concomitant lesion is the radial head fracture, probably owing to the similar underlying mechanism of injury [45–47]. Levy et al. have described a series of 15 patients in whom this association was present and have found that the mechanism of trauma in the majority of patients (12/15) was a fall on an outstretched arm without direct injury to the elbow [45, 46]. Recently, Yoon et al. described a case series of four patients with particular triad injury consisting of triceps avulsion, radial head fracture, and medial collateral ligament lesion [47]. Other associated lesions include ulnar collateral ligament laxity [48], ulnar nerve compression through hematoma [18], radial nerve compression through compartment syndrome [25], wrist fracture [19], ulnar collateral ligament avulsion with flexor/pronator group injury [17], and distal humerus fracture [32].

15.7 Classification

No shared classification system for distal triceps rupture has been previously recognized. We used the Giannicola's classification (Fig. 15.6) [49], which describes these injuries

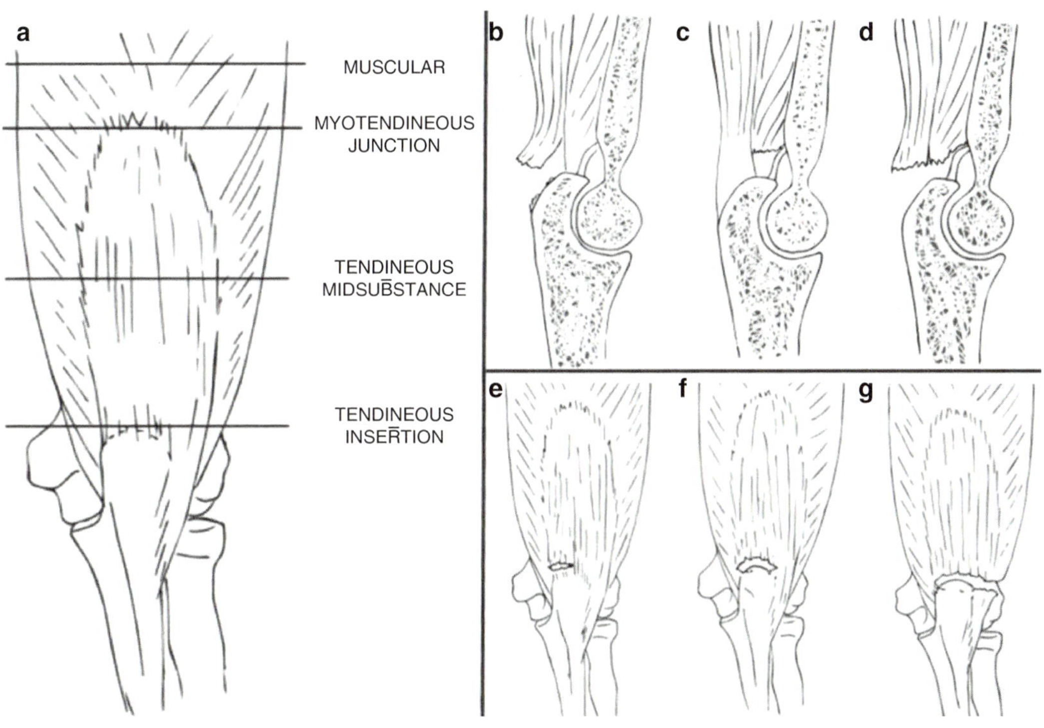

Fig. 15.6 Figure showing Giannicola's classification of triceps ruptures: (**a**) the tear may occur at the level of the muscle belly, musculotendinous junction, midsubstance of the tendon, or insertion; (**b**) the depth of the tendinous lesion may involve the superficial layer with the isolated tear of the lateral and long head tendon (superficial tear); (**c**) the deeper layer (medial head) may be involved alone (deep tear) or (**d**) in association with the superficial tendinous layer (full-thickness tear); the degree of the tendinous or/and muscular tear allows triceps lesions to be divided into either (**e**) partial or (**f**) complete tears; and (**g**) the extension of the lesion to the lateral expansion categorizes the tears with or without the involvement of lateral expansion

according to (1) the *location* of the tear (muscle belly, musculotendinous junction, tendinous body, tendon-bone insertion); (2) the *depth* of the tendinous lesion (superficial with the isolated involvement of lateral and long edges, deep with isolated involvement of medial edge and a combination of both); (3) the *degree* of the tendinous or/and muscular tear (complete or partial); and (4) the *involvement of the lateral expansion* (intact or torn).

The majority of published studies have described triceps tears only as a partial or complete rupture in the muscle belly, musculotendinous junction, or tendinous insertion, thereby preventing any reliable comparison of the outcomes. A more standard classification should be adopted in future studies to allow diagnostic and therapeutic guidelines to be drawn up.

In a particular subset of patients with triceps tear, a portion of the olecranon is avulsed together with the tendon [29, 38, 50]. This is more commonly observed in skeletally immature patients in whom the ossification center of the olecranon is not fused; by contrast, proximal olecranon fracture is the most frequently associated lesion in adults. We believe that these types of injury should be classified, respectively, as detachment of the ossification center and olecranon fracture, rather than as triceps ruptures. We thus excluded these types of lesions from this chapter. Indeed, tendon degeneration, which is the main predisposing factor to these injuries, is highly unlikely in skeletally immature patients. We believe that only triceps lesions characterized by small bony avulsion fragments of the olecranon footprint (i.e., the flake sign) should be considered true triceps tendon tears in adults, because the majority of ruptures in such cases occur at the degenerated tendon insertion.

15.8 Treatment

No guidelines on the treatment of triceps tendon injuries are available, even for athletes. This is due to several factors, which include the rarity of this type of injury and the lack of a widely accepted classification. This has resulted in few studies, most of which are retrospective and with low level of evidence, and in the lack of RCTs on this topic.

Triceps tears are generally managed according to tear location and extension. Some authors have reported that the nonsurgical treatment of an acute tear affecting less than 50 % of the triceps tendon [5], along with the belly muscle, triceps aponeurosis, and lateral expansion lesions, yields satisfactory results in non-professional sports players, in the majority of cases. Other authors believe that this type of lesion warrants surgery to ensure rapid recovery of elbow function, particularly in athletes [2, 51]. A greater agreement is shown in the literature regarding the need for surgical treatment in case of complete or near-complete tears, both in low- and high-demand patients [16, 36, 52].

15.9 Conservative Treatment

Although partial triceps tendon ruptures have historically been treated nonoperatively, this is not a consensus opinion. Some authors believe that partial tears at the muscle belly and musculotendinous junction and within the tendon can be managed nonsurgically, particularly in low-demand patients [5, 19]. Bos et al. described a patient with a partial injury treated with posterior splinting of the elbow in 30° flexion for 6 weeks, followed by active motion [53]. Full ROM and normal strength were achieved, respectively, at 3 and 6 months, with the MRI at 3 months showing fibrous tissue continuity. Farrar and Lippert also reported a successful outcome in a patient whose elbow was splinted at 30° flexion for 3 weeks; full ROM and strength were achieved at 9 months [22]. Harris et al. described a patient with a 70 % right- sided rupture and a 50 % left-sided rupture, as seen at the MRI [19]. As this patient refused immobilization, arm slings were prescribed. The patient began weightlifting 4 weeks following injury and regained normal function by 41 weeks.

Other authors believe that it is not always possible to predict the healing of partial tears at the tendon insertion [54]. Although they may show healing signs initially, with reduced pain and improved function, the patient will often become symptomatic as activity levels increase; it is thus advisable to observe recovery progression over a 6- to 12-week period before deciding if delayed surgery is needed [54]. Lempainen et al. reported failed conservative treatment of a partial musculotendinous junction tear in six athletes who subsequently underwent delayed surgical treatment [55]. Delayed surgical treatment in conservatively treated partial tears has also been reported in the general population by other authors [16, 20, 29, 34, 56, 57].

Mair et al. reported that six out of ten professional football players with partial tears who were treated nonsurgically did not experience any residual pain or weakness [2]. Three players were treated by means of bracing for the remainder of the season, followed by surgery to correct residual pain and weakness, whereas one player sustained a complete rupture upon returning to play despite the bracing. Authors concluded that surgery was required in 40 % of the patients treated conservatively. This suggests that, although treatment should be individually tailored, surgery should be preferred in professional sports players, even in partial tears. Mair et al. thus recommended nonoperative management in professional sports players only in cases of tendon "strain," in which a gradual recovery can be achieved by means of physical activity alone.

To sum up, conservative treatment may be performed in partial tears of the triceps tendon; patients may return to play after about 4–6 months, when symptoms have resolved and strength has returned to nearly normal. However, close observation of the patient is mandatory during this period to rule out any worsening of the lesion; the persistence of pain and weakness are the most negative prognostic factors.

15.10 Surgical Treatment

Primary repair is recommended in patients with acute and chronic complete or near- complete triceps tendon tears associated with a significant loss of triceps strength, as well as in complete muscle belly or musculotendinous junction with a significant gap. As above mentioned, surgical treatment may also be beneficial for acute partial tears in high-demand patients or in cases of failed nonsurgical treatment. Surgical treatment is contraindicated in patients that have serious comorbidities or are medically unstable, as well as in noncompliant patients. Although primary repair should be performed as soon as possible, it has been adopted as late as 8 months after injury [5, 16, 56]. Van Riet et al. noted good results in all eight patients who presented and underwent primary repair within 3 weeks after injury, but in less than half of the patients (6/15) who presented after 25 days [16]. These seem to suggest that an early intervention offers the best chances to perform primary repair, thereby avoiding challenging reconstruction procedures.

Several procedures have been described for primary repair, including reinsertion of triceps tendon with the trans-osseous technique and suture anchors [7, 10, 16, 18, 22, 52]. By contrast, relatively little is known about belly muscle or musculotendinous junction repair, because such lesions are extremely rare [30]. With regard to tendon insertion tears, the most investigated technique is a direct attachment with #2 or #5 nonabsorbable cross-suture (Bunnell or Krackow whipstitch technique) through cruciate drill holes through the olecranon [7, 10, 16, 18, 22, 33]. Another less common surgical procedure for primary repair is the suture anchor technique [52]. It provides the positioning of the anchors in the middle of the tendon footprint and the tying of locking stitches applied to either side of the tendon. Yeh et al. recently described the "anatomic triceps tendon footprint repair" in a biomechanical study; the authors used suture anchors to create a suture bridge (double-row) in order to restore the pre-injury anatomy and create a wider area of tendon-bone contact [10]. They concluded that this technique not only restores the pre-injury anatomy more effectively but also reduces repair-site motion compared to other types of repair.

For intra-tendinous tears, proximal to the insertion site, the same cross-suture techniques used to treat tendon insertion tears are usually adopted [16]. Fewer investigations have been conducted on the treatment of musculotendinous and intramuscular tears. Musculotendinous junction lesions tend to extend more to the medial side of the muscle, though they may also affect the belly [58–60]. Lempainen et al. achieved satisfactory results, after conservative treatment had failed, in six athletes with such lesions treated surgically with side-to-side suture [55]. However management of triceps rupture at the musculotendinous junction may be challenging owing to the poor quality of the tissue available for primary repair. Indeed, Wagner and Cooney recommended the use of the V-Y triceps tendon advancement technique with plantaris augmentation to effectively repair this type of lesion [59].

Intramuscular tears and their treatment have been poorly investigated and the best approach is still debated. Only two of the seven cases reported in the literature presented a complete rupture of all three heads of the triceps [30, 61], whereas only the long head was involved in another two of these cases [60, 62]; the medial head was involved in one of the three remaining cases [58], an unclearly defined partial lesion in another [58]. Penhallow also reported about one patient with a complete rupture of the long head and a partial tear of the medial head [63]. Four out of these seven cases were treated surgically with a side-to-side suture, while the remaining three did not undergo any surgery. The repair was not carried out in one of the four patients who underwent surgery because surgical exploration showed that the muscle was already scarred and had adhered [58]. With regard to intramuscular tears, Singh and Pooley suggest that the extent of the injury and the functional requirements of the patient must be taken into account when deciding whether conservative or surgical treatment is more appropriate [30].

15.11 Primary Repair: Surgical Technique

The patient may be placed in the supine, prone (author's preferred), or lateral position, under general or local anesthesia, according to the surgeon's preference. With the prone patient, the upper extremity is draped free and is hung over an arm rest so as to allow the elbow to be manipulated comfortably. The silicone ring tourniquet may be preferred to the pneumatic tourniquet because it allows the operating field to be extended proximally; this may prove particularly useful in chronic tears, in which an extended proximal release is needed to mobilize the tendon adequately. A posterior incision is performed slightly lateral or medial to the olecranon. The ulnar nerve is identified and protected, though not decompressed or transposed, particularly in acute cases. Dissection through skin and subcutaneous tissues leads to the identification of lesion; this is always more challenging in chronic cases, owing to the presence of the bursa and fibrous tissues that tend to cover the tendon. After this pathological tissue has been removed, the edges of the ruptured tendon are exposed and debrided back to the normal-appearing tendon; the balance of tendon tear in terms of tissue quality, size, and retraction is then performed. Small avulsed bony fragment need to be excised. A single or double #5 nonabsorbable suture is inserted through the tendon using a Krackow whipstitch technique. The mobilization and reduction of the tendon are then evaluated. Extended release of the triceps muscle from the posterior aspect of the humerus and from the intermuscular septa and subcutaneous tissue is performed when significant retraction of the tendon is present; in such cases the ulnar and radial nerves are decompressed. Following debridement of the olecranon footprint with a high-speed burr, cruciate 2 mm drill holes are made, starting at the footprint site and exiting the proximal ulna distal to the olecranon region. The nonabsorbable sutures are then passed through the cruciate holes and the tendon is reattached to the olecranon by tying the suture with the elbow in extension. Stability of the reattachment may be assessed intraoperatively by moving the elbow in extension-flexion. Primary repair in chronic cases should provide flexion to 45°. The wound is then irrigated and closed in layers. One or two subcutaneous drains are applied for 24/48 h. The arm is immobilized in 45° extension. The main steps of primary repair are illustrated in Fig. 15.7.

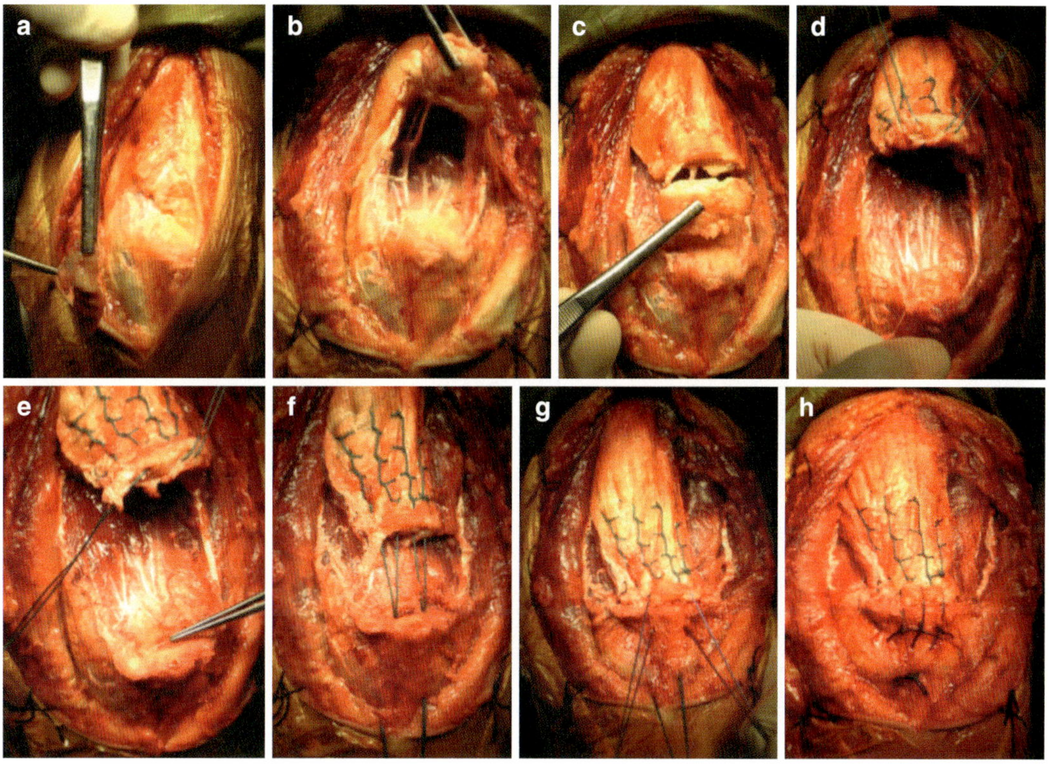

Fig. 15.7 Intraoperative photographs showing the main surgical steps of primary distal triceps tendon reinsertion. (**a**) After a posterior skin incision, an olecranon bursectomy is performed to identify the tendon tear. (**b**) The ruptured tendon is exposed and the tendon tear is classified: in this case the lesion involves the superficial layer of the triceps tendon (long and lateral head), whereas the medial (deep) head of the triceps is intact. (**c**) The stump of the avulsed tendon is debrided back to normal-appearing tendon. (**d**) A double Krackow suture is performed and (**e**) the olecranon footprint is decorticated with a high-speed burr. (**f**) Two cruciate drill holes across the olecranon footprint and exiting the proximal ulna are made, and the sutures are then passed through the drill holes. (**g**) With the elbow in extension, the sutures are tied and (**h**) additional reinforcement sutures are performed

15.12 Results and Complications in Primary Repair

The results achieved after primary repair of acute triceps ruptures in professional sports players are satisfactory in the majority of cases (Table 15.1) [2, 19, 24, 30, 55, 58, 64]. As few published reports provide detailed quantitative data, such as an isokinetic evaluation or subjective and objective outcomes based on standardized functional scores, a retrospective clinical comparison and a review of such reports are not easy. Indeed, in the majority of these studies, the only parameters assessed were the range of motion and the muscle strength. Sollender et al. surgically treated four weightlifters affected by complete rupture of the triceps tendon insertion, reporting full recovery of strength and ROM in all four patients at 7 years of follow-up [64]. The only complication was a re-rupture of the triceps tendon during early aggressive weightlifting performed 6 weeks after surgery; re-operation yielded a satisfactory final outcome. Mair et al. adopted surgery to treat 11 football players affected by complete tears of the triceps tendon; by the final follow-up examination (average 3 years), all of these patients had regained full range of motion, and none complained of residual pain or had discernible weakness [2]. In that study, a re-rupture 6 weeks after surgery in one patient required revision surgery, while another patient retired from professional activity after surgery. Singh and Pooley performed surgery

Table 15.1 Studies regarding triceps tendon injuries in athletes

Authors	Study design	No. of elbow	Sport	Treatment	Results (follow-up)	Complications
Sherman (1984)	Case report	1	Weightlifter professional	Surgery	Complete recovery (6 months)	No
Aso (1984)	Case report	1	Volleyball player	Conservative	Complete recovery (19 months)	No
Sollender (1998)	Case series	4	Weightlifters (oral steroid use)	Surgery	75 % complete recovery (6, 7 years)	1 re-rupture at 6 weeks
Singh (2002)	Case report	1 (intramuscular rupture)	Ice hockey player professional	Surgery	Playing at professional level (6 months)	No
Mair (2004)	Case series	21 (10 partial, 11 complete)	Football players professional	Partial: conservative	Partial: 60 % healed without symptoms (3 years)	Partial: 1 complete rupture after return to play; 3 required surgery for symptoms
				Complete: surgery	Complete: 72 % full active ROM, no symptoms (3 years)	Complete: 1 re-rupture at 7 weeks with return to play, 1 re-rupture at 6 week without return to play
Harris (2004)	Case report	2 partial (bilateral)	Weightlifter	Conservative	Normal function (41 weeks)	No
Lempainen (2011)	Case series	10 (6 myotendinous 3 avulsion from olecranon 1 avulsion from scapula)	Power sports with heavy weight training	Surgery	90 % good-excellent (5 year)	No
Khiami (2012)	Case report	1	Weightlifter	Surgery	Full sports activity(4 months)	No

on a professional ice hockey player with an intramuscular triceps rupture, reporting no complications; the player was able to return to sports 6 months after surgery [30]. Lempainen et al. surgically treated nine athletes, who were involved in power sports requiring heavy weight training, affected by triceps tears: six had musculotendinous tears while the remaining three had tendon avulsions [55]. The authors reported 4 excellent, 4 good, and 1 fair results at a mean follow-up of 5 years and a return to sports after 4–6 months. The patient with the fair result showed a markedly thin and weak triceps muscle.

To sum up, a review of the current literature on professional sports players shows that the majority of cases resume their normal activity and that surgical treatment of the triceps tears yields good functional results and low complication and re-rupture rates.

15.13 Salvage Procedures in Chronic Tendon Insufficiency

In current literature, no studies about the results obtained in athletes treated for chronic tendon insufficiency with salvage procedures are available.

Chronic ruptures, defined as injuries that are at least 6 weeks old, usually result from a delay either in the diagnosis or between the time of injury and the request for treatment [13]. Treatment of triceps chronic lesions usually depends on the quality of tissue and on the degree of retraction. If the tendon quality is good and retraction is minimal, delayed primary repair can be performed as described above.

Several reconstructive procedures have instead been adopted in cases with poor tendon quality, in which there may be a significant gap between the stump of the retracted tendon and the footprint, even after an extensive release [6, 21, 59, 65, 66]. In 1984, Clayton performed a triceps fascial turndown in a case report (inverted V-Y technique), obtaining a good outcome. Farrar and Lippert used a forearm fascial flap to repair the tendon [22]. It should be borne in mind, however, that these techniques are neither reliable nor reproducible in cases with marked soft tissue deficiency at the insertion site.

The anconeus slide, or anconeus rotation flap technique, described by Sanchez-Sotelo and Morrey, is used for minor defects and when the anconeus is intact (Fig. 15.8a) [21]. The muscle is mobilized from its insertions to the lateral triceps; the sleeve of the extensor musculature is attached distally and medially to fully cover the site of the triceps attachment with the elbow in 30° flexion. The authors described four patients with full regain of ROM and strength and no pain during activity, at a mean follow-up of 49 months. Comparable results were achieved when the same technique was used by Van Riet [16].

Cases with marked soft tissue deficiency or a devitalized anconeus may be treated by means of other techniques, such as tendon augmentations. In 2002 Sanchez-Sotelo and Morrey reconstructed triceps tendon with an Achilles tendon and a calcaneus fragment allograft (Fig. 15.8b) [21]. The distal calcaneus block in this operation is fastened into a V-shape osteotomy of the proximal olecranon using a cancellous screw. The proximal Achilles tendon allograft is then stitched using nonabsorbable suture to the triceps muscle and tendon with the elbow in 30° flexion. The authors reported satisfactory results at a mean follow-up of 38 months.

Other authors have adopted hamstring autograft in challenging cases (Fig 15.8c) [40, 67]. The semitendinosus tendon autograft is woven in a Bunnell fashion through the remaining proximal triceps tendon. A transosseous tunnel, centered between the articular surface and the posterior cortex, is then drilled through the proximal olecranon, 1 cm distal from its tip. The two free ends of the hamstring tendon are passed through the transosseous tunnel in a retrograde fashion, and the elbow is placed in full extension as the tendon stump is reduced to the olecranon. This technique has yielded satisfactory results [6, 67], though the strength recovery is slower than that achieved by means of the Achilles tendon allograft. Indeed, some authors believe that the Achilles tendon allograft technique may provide better long-term results than the hamstring

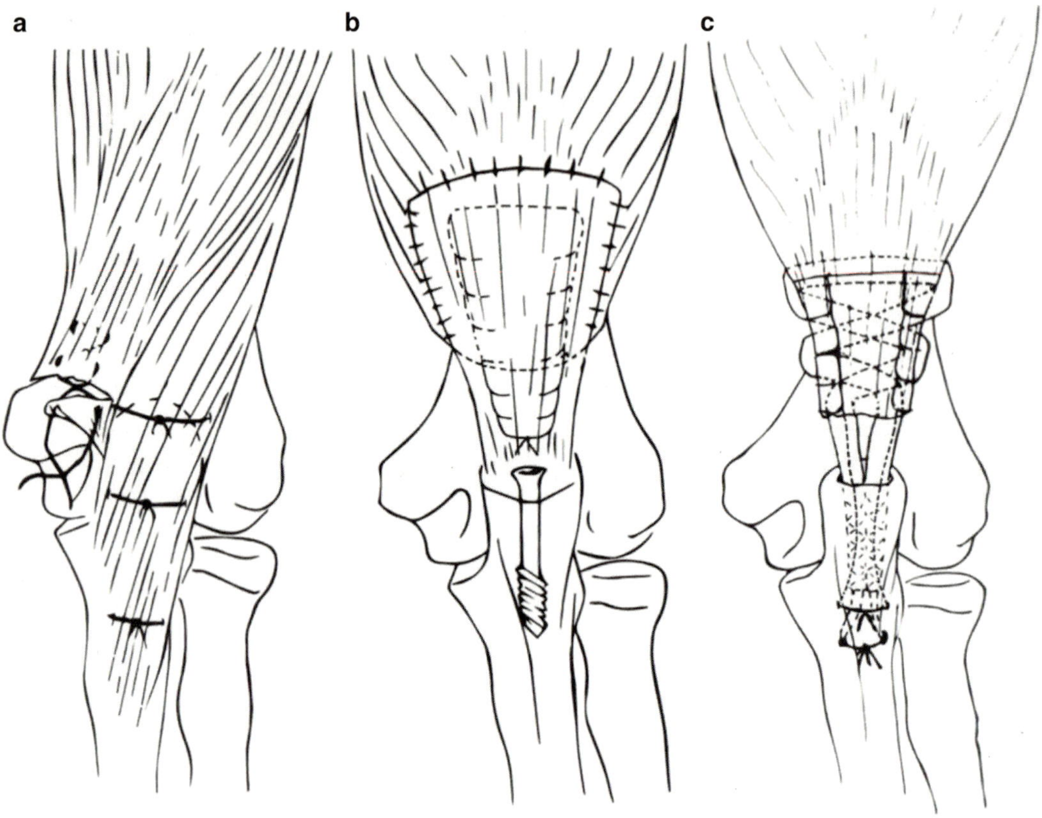

Fig. 15.8 (**a**) The "anconeus slide" technique. The anconeus muscle is elevated from the ulna and the humerus insertions to the lateral triceps, oriented over the tip of the olecranon, and reattached to the olecranon in 30° flexion. The central and medial portion of the triceps are sutured to the extensor mechanism to reinforce it. (**b**) Reconstruction with an Achilles tendon allograft. A cancellous screw is used to fix the distal calcaneus bone graft to the osteotomy of the proximal olecranon. The remainder of the reconstruction consists in reattaching the Achilles tendon to the triceps tendon and muscle using #2 or #5 high strength running sutures. Lastly, other single or cross-stitch sutures are used to attach the aponeurosis of the Achilles tendon to the triceps. (**c**) Hamstring autograft reconstruction. The autograft semitendinosus tendon is woven in a Bunnell fashion through the remaining proximal triceps tendon. A transosseous tunnel is then drilled through the proximal olecranon and the two free ends of the hamstring tendon are passed through the transosseous tunnel and fixed to the proximal ulna

autograft [6, 21, 67]. It may thus be advisable to adopt the Achilles tendon allograft technique when treating athletes.

15.14 Postoperative Care

Reports on postoperative rehabilitation in the literature vary. While some authors propose similar postoperative treatment and rehabilitation protocol in non-athletes and amateurs, few information are available regarding professional athletes. Blackmore et al. who reviewed the literature on this topic provided a detailed report of postoperative care [43]. They recommended that the elbow should be immobilized in a cast in 30° flexion for 2 weeks after surgery, followed by immobilization in a hinged elbow brace at 45°, 60°, and 90° flexion for the subsequent 3 weeks. Full active flexion and extension are allowed 6 weeks after surgery, whereas extension strengthening is started at 12 weeks. Passive full flexion, if needed, is allowed at 8 weeks. Lastly, unrestricted activity is allowed after the fifth month.

The sports clinician faces the additional question of whether and when the patient should return to sport. For athletes with a partial triceps tendon injury, several weeks of sports activity suspension may be adequate before they resume play. Nine professional football players described in one study returned to full-contact sports activity with a brace support and completed their seasons after a mean recovery period of 5 weeks [2]. Similarly, a male high-level bodybuilder with bilateral partial triceps tendon tears was able to return to his normal weightlifting regimen without a brace support after a 4 weeks healing period [19]. Athletes should be aware that some degree of pain and weakness may persist despite a recovery period [2, 19]. Moreover, an immediate return to athletic activities may raise the risk of a complete rupture or chronic extensor dysfunction [2, 18, 20, 64]. In the largest case series of professional sports players, Mair et al. reported that only one patient returned to full-contact professional football after 7 weeks without sustaining a re-rupture, while the other ten patients required a longer rehabilitation period [2].

In conclusion, a mean rehabilitation period of 4–6 months is recommended before professional sports activities are resumed because an earlier return may expose the athlete to a risk of re-rupture [16, 30, 64]. The duration of postoperative care may also vary from patient to patient according to the tension and quality of the tendon repair, other concomitant injuries, and the patient's medical history; this applies above all to patients who have undergone reconstructive procedures and in whom the healing process is consequently longer.

References

1. Anzel SH, Covey KW, Weiner AD, et al. Disruption of muscles and tendons: an analysis of 1,014 cases. Surgery. 1959;45:406–14.
2. Mair SD, Isbell WM, Gill TJ, et al. Triceps tendon ruptures in professional football players. Am J Sports Med. 2004;32:431–4.
3. Koplas MC, Schneider E, Sundaram M. Prevalence of triceps tendon tears on MRI of the elbow and clinical correlation. Skeletal Radiol. 2011;40(5):587–94.
4. Kandemir U, Fu FH, McMahon PJ. Elbow injuries. Curr Opin Rheumatol. 2002;14:160–7.
5. Vidal AF, Drakos MC, Allen AA. Biceps tendon and triceps tendon injuries. Clin Sports Med. 2004;23: 707–22, xi.
6. Weistroffer JK, Mills WJ, Shin AY. Recurrent rupture of the triceps tendon repaired with hamstring tendon autograft augmentation: a case report and repair technique. J Shoulder Elbow Surg. 2003;12:193–6.
7. McCulloch PC, Spellman J, Bach Jr BR. Familial triceps tendon ruptures. Orthopedics. 2008;31:600–2.
8. Gray H. Anatomy of the human body. In: Gross C, editor. Anatomy of the human body. Philadelphia: Lea & Febiger; 1959. p. 460–1.
9. Keener JD, Chafik D, Kim HM, et al. Insertional anatomy of the triceps brachii tendon. J Shoulder Elbow Surg. 2010;19:399–405.
10. Yeh PC, Stephens KT, Solovyova O, et al. The distal triceps tendon footprint and a biomechanical analysis of 3 repair techniques. Am J Sports Med. 2010;38: 1025–33.
11. Madsen M, Marx RG, Millett PJ, et al. Surgical anatomy of the triceps brachii tendon: anatomical study and clinical correlation. Am J Sports Med. 2006; 34:1839–43.
12. Windisch G, Tesch NP, Grechenig W, et al. The triceps brachii muscle and its insertion on the olecranon. Med Sci Monit. 2006;12:BR290–4.
13. Yeh PC, Dodds SD, Smart LR, et al. Distal triceps rupture. J Am Acad Orthop Surg. 2010;18:31–40.
14. Hughes RE, Schneeberger AG, An KN, et al. Reduction of triceps muscle force after shortening of the distal humerus: a computational model. J Shoulder Elbow Surg. 1997;6:444–8.
15. Gerbeaux M, Turpin E, Lensel-Corbeil G. Musculo-articular modelling of the triceps brachii. J Biomech. 1996;29:171–80.
16. Van Riet RP, Morrey BF, Ho E, et al. Surgical treatment of distal triceps ruptures. J Bone Joint Surg Am. 2003;85:1961–7.
17. Daglar B, Delialioglu OM, Ceyhan E, et al. Combined surgical treatment for missed rupture of triceps tendon associated with avulsion of the ulnar collateral ligament and flexor-pronator muscle mass. Strateg Trauma Limb Reconstr. 2009;4:35–9.
18. Duchow J, Kelm J, Kohn D. Acute ulnar nerve compression syndrome in a powerlifter with triceps tendon rupture: a case report. Int J Sports Med. 2000;21: 308–10.
19. Harris PC, Atkinson D, Moorehead JD. Bilateral partial rupture of triceps tendon: case report and quantitative assessment of recovery. Am J Sports Med. 2004;32:787–92.
20. Weng PW, Wang SJ, Wu SS. (2006) Misdiagnosed avulsion fracture of the triceps tendon from the olecranon insertion: case report. Clin J Sport Med. 2006;16:364–5.
21. Sanchez-Sotelo J, Morrey BF. Surgical techniques for reconstruction of chronic insufficiency of the triceps: rotation flap using anconeus andendo achillis allograft. J Bone Joint Br. 2002;84:1116–20.

22. Farrar III EL, Lippert III FG. Avulsion of the triceps tendon. Clin Orthop Relat Res. 1981;161:242–6.
23. Searfoss R, Tripi J, Bowers W. Triceps brachii rupture: case report. J Trauma. 1976;16:244–6.
24. Sherman OH, Snyder SJ, Fox JM. Triceps tendon avulsion in a professional body builder. A case report. Am J Sports Med. 1984;12:328–9.
25. Brumback RJ. Compartment syndrome complicating avulsion of the origin of the triceps muscle: a case report. J Bone Joint Surg Am. 1987;69:1445–7.
26. Gilcreest EL. Rupture of muscles and tendons. JAMA. 1925;84:1819–22.
27. Haldeman KO, Soto-Hall R. Injuries to muscles and tendons. JAMA. 1935;104:2319–24.
28. Newmark III H, Olken SM, Halls J. Ruptured triceps tendon diagnosed radiographically. Australas Radiol. 1985;29:60–3.
29. Kibuule LK, Fehringer EV. Distal triceps tendon rupture and repair in an otherwise healthy pediatric patient: a case report and review of the literature. J Shoulder Elbow Surg. 2007;16:e1–3.
30. Singh RK, Pooley J. Complete rupture of the triceps brachii muscle. Br J Sports Med. 2002;36:467–9.
31. Rettig AC. Traumatic elbow injuries in the athlete. Orthop Clin North Am. 2002;33:509–22, v.
32. Gupta RR, Murthi AM. Distal humeral fracture with associated triceps tendon avulsion in a renal transplant recipient. Orthopedics. 2010;10:204–7.
33. Tsourvakas S, Gouvalas K, Gimtsas C, et al. Bilateral and simultaneous rupture of the triceps tendons in chronic renal failure and secondary hyperparathyroidism. Arch Orthop Trauma Surg. 2004;124:278–80.
34. Clayton ML, Thirupathi RG. Rupture of the triceps tendon with olecranon bursitis: a case report with a new method of repair. Clin Orthop Relat Res. 1984;184:183–5.
35. Lambert MI, St Clair Gibson A, Noakes TD. Rupture of the triceps tendon associated with steroid injections. Am J Sports Med. 1995;23:778.
36. Sharma SC, Singh R, Goel T, et al. Missed diagnosis of triceps tendon rupture: a case report and review of literature. J Orthop Surg (Hong Kong). 2005;13:307–9.
37. Petre BM, Grutter PW, Rose DM, et al. Triceps tendons: a biomechanical comparison of intact and repaired strength. J Shoulder Elbow Surg. 2011; 20:213–8.
38. Viegas SF. Avulsion of the triceps tendon. Orthop Rev. 1990;19:533–6.
39. O'Driscoll SW, Goncalves LB, Dietz P. The hook test for distal biceps tendon avulsion. Am J Sports Med. 2007;35(11):1865–9.
40. Kaempffe FA, Lerner RM. Ultrasound diagnosis of triceps tendon rupture: a report of 2 cases. Clin Orthop Relat Res. 1996;332:138–42.
41. Zionts LE, Vachon LA. Demonstration of avulsion of the triceps tendon in an adolescent by magnetic resonance imaging. Am J Orthop. 1997;26:489–90.
42. Kijowski R, Tuite M, Sanford M. Magnetic resonance imaging of them elbow: part II. Abnormalities of the ligaments, tendons, and nerves. Skeletal Radiol. 2005;34:1–18.
43. Blackmore SM, Jander RM, Culp RW. Management of distal biceps and triceps ruptures. J Hand Ther. 2006;19:154–68.
44. Thornton R, Riley GM, Steinbach LS. Magnetic resonance imaging of sports injuries of the elbow. Top Magn Reson Imaging. 2003;14:69–86.
45. Levy M, Fishel RE, Stern GM. Triceps tendon avulsion with or without fracture of the radial head – a rare injury? J Trauma. 1978;18(9):677–9.
46. Levy M, Goldberg I, Meir I. Fracture of the head of the radius with a tear or avulsion of the triceps tendon. J Bone Joint Surg Br. 1982;64:70–2.
47. Yoon MY, Koris MJ, Ortiz JA, et al. Triceps avulsion, radial head fracture, and medial collateral ligament rupture about the elbow: a report of 4 cases. J Shoulder Elbow Surg. 2012;21(2):e12–7.
48. Tatebe M, Horii E, Nakamura R. Chronically ruptured triceps tendon with avulsion of the medial collateral ligament: a report of 2 cases. J Shoulder Elbow Surg. 2007;16:e5–7.
49. Giannicola G, Sacchetti FM, Bullitta G, et al. Distal triceps tendon ruptures. Poster. 24th congress of the European Society for surgery of the shoulder and the elbow. Dubrovnik, Croatia 19–22 September 2012. 2012
50. Tarallo L, Zambianchi F, Mugnai R, et al. Distal triceps tendon repair using Krakow whipstitches, K wires, tension band and double drilling technique: a case report. J Med Case Rep. 2015;9(1):504.
51. Strauch RJ. Biceps and triceps injuries of the elbow. Orthop Clin North Am. 1999;30:95–107.
52. Pina A, Garcia I, Sabater M. Traumatic avulsion of the triceps brachii. J Orthop Trauma. 2002;16:273–6.
53. Bos CF, Nelissen RG, Bloem JL. Incomplete rupture of the tendon of triceps brachii: a case report. Int Orthop. 1994;18:273–5.
54. Morrey BF, editor. Functional evaluation of the elbow. In: Morrey BF, editor. The elbow and its disorders. 4th ed. Philadelphia: WB Saunders; 2009; p. 536–46.
55. Lempainen L, Sarimo J, Rawlins M, et al. Triceps tears in athletes: different injury patterns and surgical treatment. Arch Orthop Trauma Surg. 2011; 131(10):1413–7.
56. Inhofe PD, Moneim MS. Late presentation of triceps rupture: a case report and review of the literature. Am J Orthop (Belle Mead NJ). 1996;25:790–2.
57. Athwal GS, McGill RJ, Rispoli DM. Isolated avulsion of the medial head of the triceps tendon: an anatomic study and arthroscopic repair in 2 cases. Arthroscopy. 2009;25:983–8.
58. Aso K, Torisu T. Muscle belly tear of the triceps. Am J Sports Med. 1984;12:485–7.
59. Wagner JR, Cooney WP. Rupture of the triceps muscle at the musculotendinous junction: a case report. J Hand Surg Am. 1997;22:341–3. 15.
60. O'Driscoll SW. Intramuscular triceps rupture. Can J Surg. 1992;35:203–7.

61. Montgomery AH. Two cases of muscle injury. Surg Clin Chic. 1920;4:871–7.
62. Sheps D, Black B, Reed M, et al. Rupture of the long head of the triceps muscle in a child: case report and review of the literature. J Trauma. 1997;42:318–20.
63. Penhallow DP. Report of a case of ruptured triceps due to direct violence. N Y Med J. 1910;91:76–7.
64. Sollender JL, Rayan GM, Barden GA. Triceps tendon rupture in weight lifters. J Shoulder Elbow Surg. 1998;7:151–3.
65. Sai S, Fujii K, Chino H, Inoue J, et al. Old rupture of the triceps tendon with unique pathology: a case report. J Orthop Sci. 2004;9:654–6.
66. Dos Remedios C, Brosset T, Chantelot C, et al. Repair of a triceps tendon rupture using autogenous semi-tendinous and gracilis tendons: a case report and retrospective chart review [French]. Chir Main. 2007;26:154–8.
67. Wolf JM, McCarty EC, Ritchie PD. Triceps reconstruction using hamstring graft for triceps insufficiency or recurrent rupture. Tech Hand Up Extrem Surg. 2008;12:174–9.

16 Posterior Impingement of the Elbow

Michel P.J. van den Bekerom
and Denise Eygendaal

16.1 Introduction and Scope of the Problem

The increase in the number of participants in overhead sports as baseball, tennis, football, and volleyball has resulted in a rise in the incidence of elbow injuries in recent decades. In baseball, the most described and studied overhead sport, the incidence of upper extremity injuries is related to the number of years of participation, as well as to the age of the athlete; elbow pain is reported in 20 % of the 8- to 12-year-old group, 45 % of the 13- to 14-year-old group, and 58 % of high school and college athletes [10, 11]. The highest rates of pediatric elbow injuries occur in little league baseball, tennis, and gymnastics. The most common site of elbow pain in the young athlete is the medial side [9]. Posteromedial elbow impingement, as a part of the valgus extension overload syndrome, was originally described by Wilson and colleagues in 1983 [12] and involves the formation of soft-tissue swelling, posteromedial chondromalacia, posteromedial osteophytes, loose bodies due to fractured osteophytes, and the risk of proximal ulna stress fractures.

M.P.J. van den Bekerom • D. Eygendaal (✉)
Shoulder and Elbow Unit, Department of Orthopedic surgery, OLVG, Amsterdam, The Netherlands

Denise Eygendaal, Upper limb unit, Department of Orthopedic surgery, Amphia Hospital, Breda, The Netherlands

Department of Orthopedic Surgery, Academic Medical Centre, Amsterdam, The Netherlands
e-mail: bekerom@gmail.com; denise@eygendaal.nl

16.2 In Which Specific Sports; Why in This Specific Sports

Posteromedial impingement of the elbow occurs in the overhead athlete. Sports such as baseball, football, volleyball, javelin throwing, water polo, badminton, and tennis are examples of overhead sports that subject the shoulder and the elbow to extreme ranges of motion, forces, and accelerations/decelerations over many repetitions. As a consequence, extraordinary demands on the elbow joint are generated. Specific injuries in these athletes can be caused by chronic stress overload or repetitive micro traumatic stress, observed during the overhead motion [21, 22].

The overhead throwing motion can be broken down into six phases: (1) windup, (2) early cocking, (3) late cocking, (4) acceleration, (5) deceleration, and (6) follow-through [7, 8] (Fig. 16.1).

As the elbow extends at over 2,300 °/s, a medial shear force of 300 N and lateral compressive force of 900 N are produced [1, 2]. In addition, the valgus stress applied to the elbow during the acceleration phase of throwing is 64 Nm [1, 2]. The posterior compartment is subject to tensile, compressive, and torsional forces during acceleration and deceleration phases. This valgus stress at the elbow is associated with biomechanical variables: late trunk rotation, reduced shoulder external rota-

L.A. Pederzini et al. (eds.), *Elbow and Sport*, DOI 10.1007/978-3-662-48742-6_16

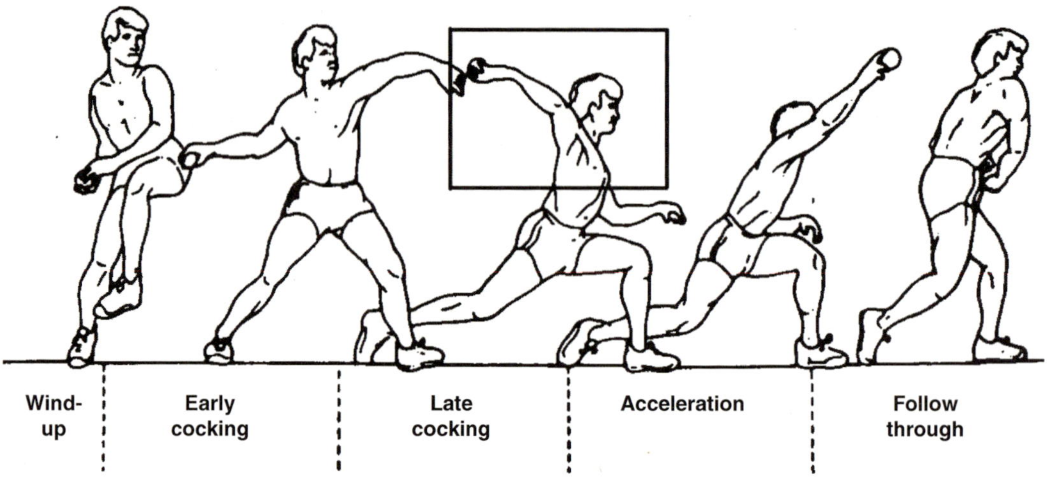

Fig. 16.1 The overhead throwing motion can be broken down into six phases: (1) windup, (2) early cocking, (3) late cocking, (4) acceleration, (5) deceleration, and (6) follow-through

tion, reduced total rotation, and increased elbow flexion appear to be overhand pitchers to reduced elbow valgus torque [3, 4]. Another research suggests that the rising incidence of shoulder and elbow injuries in pitchers may not be caused by the curveball mechanics [5]. This mechanism may result in valgus extension overload within the posterior compartment, potentially leading to chondromalacia, osteophytes and loose bodies formation, proximal ulna stress fractures, triceps pathology, or physeal injury (Fig. 16.2).

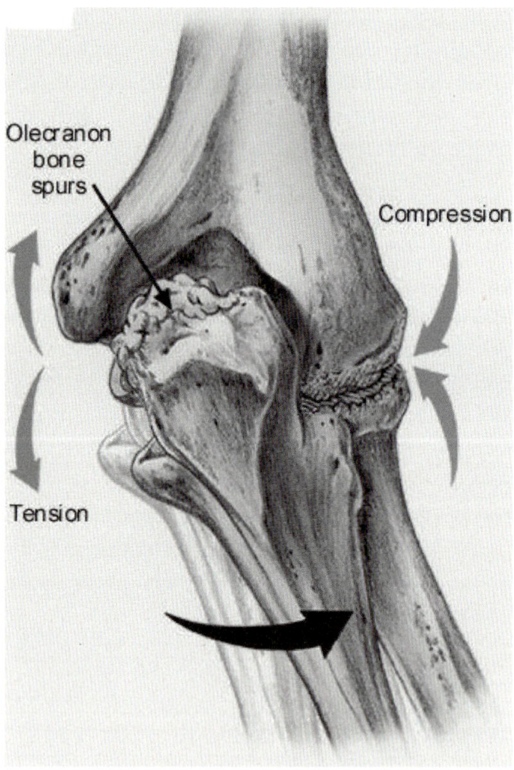

Fig. 16.2 Valgus extension overload within the posterior compartment, potentially leading to chondromalacia, osteophytes and loose bodies formation, proximal ulna stress fractures, triceps pathology, or physeal injury

16.3 History and Physical Examination

Overhead athletes complain of medial/olecranon pain during follow-through phase of throwing. Athletes who have pain during earlier phases of throwing (late cocking) more likely have other pathologies, as ulnar collateral ligament (UCL) insufficiency, posteromedial impingement complaints and loose bodies, or an inability to fully extend the arm due to pain, posterior olecranon/fossa osteophytes, or loose bodies. Checking for factors relating to (changes in) training and performance is mandatory.

Besides the routine elbow physical examination, including determination of the carrying angle of the arm, the valgus extension overload test is valuable (VEOLS). The VEOLS test or valgus extension snap maneuver was first described by Andrews: a moderate valgus stress is applied to the elbow with simultaneous palpation of the posteromedial tip of the olecranon while the elbow is moved from 30° of flexion to full extension. To be noted that valgus laxity has been described in the dominant arm of asymptomatic overhead athletes. It is important to evaluate and document the location and mobility of the ulnar nerve within the cubital tunnel during flexion in all patients undergoing elbow arthroscopy. An arthroscopy should never be performed without knowing the exact location of the ulnar nerve [19]. The examiner should keep in mind that there is a large variation in ROM and carrying angle in the overhead athletes.

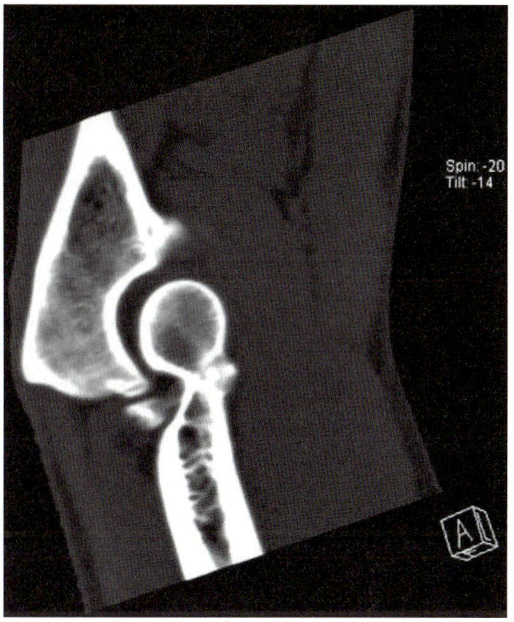

Fig. 16.3 CT scan can be useful for the assessment of osteophytes, stress fractures, avulsion fractures, or loose bodies

16.4 Radiology

Imaging of elbow in overhead athletes should include plain radiographs with anteroposterior and lateral views. An axial oblique view may be helpful to detect osteophytes on the olecranon or on the borders of the posterior fossa, where loose bodies can be identified as well. For this additional view, the elbow should be bent at 110° with the arm on the cassette. The beam should then be angled at 45° toward the ulna. CT scan can be useful for the assessment of osteophytes, stress fractures, avulsion fractures, or loose bodies (Fig. 16.3). In posteromedial impingement the osteophytes are located on the medial side of the olecranon tip and not on both sides and in other locations in the elbow as it happens commonly in osteoarthritis [16]. Magnetic resonance imaging (MRI) with or without intra-articular contrast is considered the gold standard imaging modality for the athlete's elbow. The sensitivity of the MRI scan for posterior soft tissue or loose bodies is nearly 90 % [13]. MRI findings also show high correlation with arthroscopic evaluation [14].

Dynamic ultrasound allows a real-time evaluation of the moving elbow and can help to assess the stability of the UCL and thereby guide in the diagnosis of posteromedial elbow impingement [15].

16.5 Conservative Treatment

Treatment of posteromedial impingement starts with nonoperative measures such as physiotherapy and NSAIDs, in combination with rest, ice, compression, and elevation (RICE). This treatment should also include other joints as the shoulder. Sometimes steroid injections can give some pain relief if there is only soft-tissue impingement. Nonoperative treatment of posteromedial elbow impingement was initially reported in javelin throwers in 1946 by Waris [6]. If conservative treatment fails, arthroscopy of the elbow can then a successful choice.

16.6 Operative Treatment

When performing elbow arthroscopy, we prefer general anesthesia because it allows more comfort for the patient and muscle relaxation, which prevents patient's movement during surgery (therefore decreasing the risk of nerve injuries) and avoids complications associated with a regional block [20]. We also prefer the lateral decubitus, because it offers increased stability, access to the arm, and unrestricted elbow motion, compared to the supine position [17]. This position is also favorable for the anesthesia. Standard equipment necessary for shoulder and knee arthroscopy can be utilized for elbow arthroscopy. Before starting the arthroscopy, bony landmarks, arthroscopic portals, and location of the ulnar nerve have to be marked on the skin. After inflation of the tourniquet to 250 mmHg, the joint is then injected with physiologic saline from posterior to allow full distension of the capsule [18] and shift the neurovascular structures away from the joint [5]. When the fluid is in the joint, the elbow will extend a little. In case of a posteromedial impingement without loose bodies and without contracture, a posterior arthroscopy can be sufficient to treat this pathology. In case of loose bodies, the anterior compartment should be inspected; even in the case these loose bodies are in the posterior compartment on the CT or MRI scan. Through the postero-central "trans-tricipital" portal and the proximal posterolateral portal, the posterior compartment can be reached and loose bodies can be removed, impinging osteophytes debrided back to a normal olecranon contour, and articular cartilage lesions can be addressed. Capsular contracture may also be addressed with anterior and posterior arthroscopy.

16.7 Results After Treatment

In the literature, there is often ambiguity between posterior and posteromedial impingement and these terms have often been used interchangeably. As such, it is a challenge to tease true cases of [29] posteromedial impingement out of the outcomes data. Fideler and colleagues reported on 113 professional baseball players (97 pitchers) who underwent arthroscopic treatment for posterior impingement of their dominant elbow. Given the demographic data, it is likely that most of these patients were cases of posteromedial impingement. Seventy-four percent of these athletes had good to excellent results, meaning that they were able to return to their sport for a minimum of 24 months. However, motion only objectively improved in 22 % of patients and 10 % required a subsequent UCL reconstruction. Andrews et al. [23] reported on 34 professional baseball players with posteromedial impingement who underwent arthroscopic debridement. They found a 68 % return to play rate, but a 41 % reoperation rate, often for [30] debridement of recurrent osteophytes and/or UCL reconstruction. Reddy and colleagues reported on 172 patients that underwent elbow arthroscopy, 96 of which for posterior impingement. The study population was dominated by baseball players, suggesting again that these were mostly cases of posteromedial impingement. The specific outcomes for the posterior impingement cases were not reported, but overall 56 % of patients had an excellent result and 36 % ended with a good result [31].

Pitfalls of the Treatment

1. Baseball players who underwent partial olecranon excision for posterior impingement did not have universally excellent results, 42 % of these patients requiring a second operation and several undergoing UCL reconstruction. It cannot be concluded whether removal of the osteophytes and a part of the olecranon uncovered UCL insufficiency or whether this procedure resulted in increased strain on the UCL, making it susceptible to rupture when the athlete returns to throwing [23, 24]. Resection of the olecranon osteophytes may "unmask" subtle UCL insufficiency [25]. We therefore recommend that only the osteophyte and no native olecranon

should be removed during arthroscopy [22, 23].

2. The advantage of posterior elbow arthroscopy is that the posteromedial part of the joint can be reached easily, but the ulnar nerve is located superficial to the joint capsule and the posterior bundle of the ulnar collateral ligament in the medial gutter. Therefore caution should be used when debriding this area to prevent nerve injury.
3. Unexperienced arthroscopic surgeons can mistake the secondary bone formation in the olecranon fossa, for the border of the native fossa, especially in long-standing cases.

Pearls of the Treatment/Prevention

Preventing or reducing the occurrence of (posterior) elbow complaints in the overhead athlete requires anatomical knowledge of the elbow structures involved in the stages of the overhead (throwing or hitting) motion. This knowledge increases the likelihood of developing conditioning programs that accurately target the structures involved, as well as preventing biomechanical adaptations, not only in the elbow but also in other joints as the shoulder and wrist, equally involved in the whole overhead motion and therefore in the development of injuries.

Techniques and adaptations may reduce the occurrence of injury. The risk factor with the strongest correlation to elbow injury in the overhead athlete is amount of pitching [26]. Fleisig and Andrews defined recommendation to prevent elbow injuries to youth baseball pitchers with safety rules, recommendations, education, and common sense [27].

Rehabilitation after injury or surgery of the elbow follows a progressive and sequential order to ensure that healing tissues are not overstressed [28]. Many treatment protocols have been developed and these protocols vary greatly throughout the available literature and are not really based on high-level scientific evidence. A rehabilitation program that limits the period of immobilization, early achieves full range of motion, progressively restores strength and neuromuscular control, and gradually incorporates sport specific activities is essential to a successful return to the previous level of sports and competition as quickly and safely as possible [28].

References

1. Werner SL, Fleisig GS, Dillman CJ, et al. Biomechanics of the elbow during baseball pitching. J Orthop Sports Phys Ther. 1993;17:274–8.
2. Fleisig GS, Escamilla RF. Biomechanics of the elbow in the throwing athlete. Oper Tech Sports Med. 1996;4(2):62–8.
3. Aguinaldo AL, Chambers H. Correlation of throwing mechanics with elbow valgus load in adult baseball pitchers. Am J Sports Med. 2009;37(10):2043–8.
4. Wilk KE, Macrina LC, Fleisig GS, Aune KT, Porterfield RA, Harker P, Evans TJ, Andrews JR. Deficits in glenohumeral passive range of motion increase risk of elbow injury in professional baseball pitchers: a prospective study. Am J Sports Med. 2014;42(9):2075–81.
5. Nissen CW, Westwell M, Ounpuu S, Patel M, Solomito M, Tate J. A biomechanical comparison of the fastball and curveball in adolescent baseball pitchers. Am J Sports Med. 2009;37(8):1492–8.
6. Waris W. Elbow injuries in javelin throwers. Acta Chir Scand. 1946;93:563–75.
7. Fleisig GS, Andrews JR, Dillman CJ, et al. Kinetics of baseball pitching with implications about injury mechanisms. Am J Sports Med. 1995;23:233–9.
8. Dillman CJ, Andrews JR. Biomechanics of pitching with emphasis upon shoulder kinematics. J Orthop Sports Phys Ther. 1993;18:402–8.
9. Gill TJ, Micheli LJ. The immature athlete. Common injuries and overuse syndromes of the elbow and wrist. Clin Sports Med. 1996;15:401–23.
10. Micheli LJ, Smith AD. Sports injuries in children. Curr Probl Pediatr. 1982;12:1–54.
11. Morrey BF, An KN. Articular and ligamentous contributions to the stability of the elbow joint. Am J Sports Med. 1983;11:315–9.

12. Wilson FD, Andrews JR, Blackburn TA, McCluskey G. Valgus extension overload in the pitching elbow. Am J Sports Med. 1983;11:83–8.
13. Bradley JP. Arthroscopic treatment of posterior impingement of the elbow in NFL lineman. J Should Elb Surg. 1995;2:119–20.
14. Cohen SB, Valko C, Zoga A, Dodson CC, Ciccotti MG. Posteromedial elbow impingement: magnetic resonance imaging findings in overhead throwing athletes and results of arthroscopic treatment. Arthroscopy. 2011;27(10):1364–70.
15. Nazarian LN, McShane JM, Ciccotti MG, O'Kane PL, Harwood MI. Dynamic US of the anterior band of the ulnar collateral ligament of the elbow in asymptomatic major league baseball pitchers. Radiology. 2003;227:149–54.
16. Lim YW, van Riet RP, Mittal R, Bain GI. Pattern of osteophyte distribution in primary osteoarthritis of the elbow. J Should Elb Surg. 2008;17(6):963–6.
17. O'Driscoll SW, Morrey BF. Arthroscopy of the elbow. Diagnostic and therapeutic benefits and hazards. J Bone Joint Surg Am. 1992;74:84–94.
18. O'Driscoll SW, Morrey BF, An KN. Intraarticular pressure and capacity of the elbow. Arthroscopy. 1990;6:100–3.
19. Lynch GJ, Meyers JF, Whipple TL, Caspari RB. Neurovascular anatomy and elbow arthroscopy: inherent risks. Arthroscopy. 1986;2:190–7.
20. Anderson CN, Saffran MR. Chapter 2: arthroscopic technique. In: Pederzini LA, editor. Elbow arthroscopy: Springer Berlin Heidelberg. doi:10.1007/978-3-642-38103-4_2, _ ISAKOS 2013.
21. van den Bekerom MP, Eygendaal D. Posterior elbow problems in the overhead athlete. Sports Med Arthrosc. 2014;22(3):183–7.
22. Eygendaal D, Safran MR. Postero-medial elbow problems in the adult athlete. Br J Sports Med. 2006;40(5):430–4.
23. Andrews JR, Timmerman LA. Outcome of elbow surgery in professional baseball players. Am J Sports Med. 1995;23:407–13.
24. Kamineni S, ElAttrache NS, O'Driscoll SW, et al. Medial collateral ligament strain with partial posteromedial olecranon resection. A biomechanical study. J Bone Joint Surg Am. 2004;86:2424–30.
25. Ahmad CS, Park MC, Elattrache NS. Elbow medial ulnar collateral ligament insufficiency alters posteromedial olecranon contact. Am J Sports Med. 2004;32(7):1607–12.
26. Olsen SJ, Fleisig GS, Dun S, Loftice J, Andrews JR. Risk factors for shoulder and elbow injuries in adolescent baseball pitchers. Am J Sports Med. 2006;34:905–12.
27. Fleisig GS, Andrews JR. Prevention of elbow injuries in youth baseball pitchers. Sports Health. 2012;4(5): 419–24.
28. Wilk KE, Reinold MM, Andrews JR. Rehabilitation of the thrower's elbow. Clin Sports Med. 2004;23(4): 765–801.
29. Fideler BM, Kvitne RS, Jordan S, ElAttrache N, Yocum L, Jobe FW. Posterior impingement of the elbow in professional baseball players: results of arthroscopic treatment. J Should Elb Surg. 1997;6:169–70.
30. Reddy AS, Kvitne RS, Yocum LA, ElAttrache NS, Glousman RE, Jobe FW. Arthroscopy of the elbow: a long-term clinical review. Arthroscopy. 2000;16: 588–94.
31. Moskal MJ. Review article. Arthroscopic treatment of posterior impingement of the elbow in athletes. Clin Sports Med. 2001;20:11–24.

Rehabilitation of the Elbow

17

Rob Tamminga and Val Jones

17.1 Introduction

To counteract for the physical forces placed on the structures above, an athlete's upper limb develops marked physical adaptations [1, 2].

Over recent decades, there has been a sharp rise in the number of participants in sport. Whilst the elbow may suffer an acute injury, such as dislocation and/or fracture, after participation in contact sports, the most common mechanism of elbow injury in sport is associated with repetitive overhead activities. Up to 30 % of participants engaged in activities such as throwing, bowling, tennis, swimming and volleyball complain of elbow problems [3–6]. The most common athletic injuries include lateral and medial tendinopathies, ulnar or medial collateral ligament (UCL/MCL) injury and valgus extension overload (VEO).

VEO describes a specific, unique pattern of injuries to the elbow [7]. A number of forces act on the elbow, during throwing, including tensile stress along the medial compartment, compressive forces laterally and shear stress seen posteriorly [7]. The forces produced often exceed the tensile strength of primary restraints of the elbow, such as the ulnar collateral ligament, predisposing the joint to injury [8, 9].

Other common sporting injuries to the elbow are listed below (Table 17.1), and it should be remembered that the patterns of injuries seen in adolescents, such as growth plate-related injuries, differ from those seen in adults [10, 1].

Table 17.1 Commonly encountered injuries

Ulnar collateral ligament tears
Ulnar neuritis
Flexor-pronator sprain, tear or tendinopathy
Medial epicondyle apophysitis or avulsion (little league elbow)
Lateral epicondylar tendinopathy
Olecranon osteophytes
Olecranon stress fractures
Osteochondritis dissecans
Loose bodies

17.2 Physical Adaptations to Overhead Activities

Adaptations in range of motion, ligamentous laxity and muscular compensation are seen in the throwing limb compared to the contralateral upper limb. This means comparisons with the

R. Tamminga, MD (✉)
Clinical Physiotherapist in Shoulder and Elbow Division of Departement Sport and Orthopedic Care, Medicort, Utrecht, The Netherlands
e-mail: rtamminga@medicort.nl, rtamminga57@gmail.com

V. Jones, MD
Lead physiotherapist for the Sheffield Shoulder and Elbow Unit, Sheffield Teaching Hospital, Sheffield, UK

L.A. Pederzini et al. (eds.), *Elbow and Sport*, DOI 10.1007/978-3-662-48742-6_17

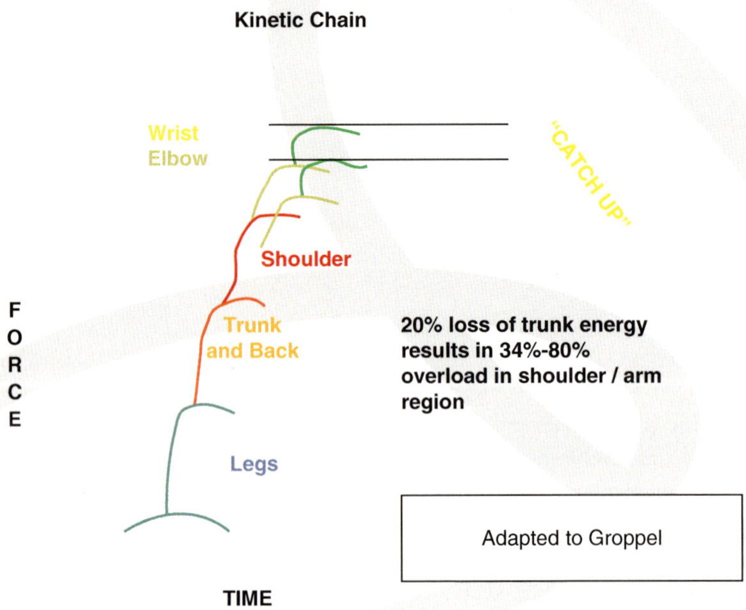

non-injured limb may not be adequate, when restoring an athlete back to their pre-injury baseline [10, 2]. Preseason/pre-injury assessments establishing baselines of range of motion, strength, kinetic chain evaluation and upper limb and scapula stability can help inform the rehabilitation team regarding the necessary function an individual needs to regain, to compete once again. Subjective functional outcome measures such as DASH, MEPI, Oxford Elbow Score and Dutch Elbow Score can also be utilised to help monitor an athlete's progress over time [11].

A body of evidence shows the presence of medial elbow laxity, significant elbow flexion contractures and a significant decrease in wrist flexibility in the dominant arm of overhead athletes [12]. There is also an increased strength profile for the dominant arm in the glenohumeral joint internal rotators, elbow, wrist and forearm muscles and grip strength, seen in tennis players, baseball pitchers and javelin throwers [13–18].

However, it should be noted that muscle group strength ratios are sport specific. In some overhead activities such as volleyball, tennis and handball, high elbow extensor to flexor ratios are seen [18], whereas in activities such as judo, there is an almost equal ratio of elbow extensors to flexors [19]. This should be borne in mind when designing individual rehabilitation programmes.

17.3 General Rehabilitation

The aim of rehabilitation is to expose healing tissues to appropriate stress and avoid the adverse changes to tissue biomechanics and morphology seen after prolonged immobilisation. According to Wilk [10], rehabilitation following elbow injury or surgery follows a sequential, well-defined approach, where phases overlap to ensure the athlete returns to their previous functional level, as quickly and safely as possible. The approach is based on best current available evidence, adapted to each individual and their respective sport. Each phase is entered when an athlete reaches physical milestones in terms of range and strength, rather than being time dependent. Timings are also influenced by whether an athlete has been conservatively or surgically managed.

17.4 Acute Phase

The first phase is the immediate motion phase, where the goals are to reduce the deleterious effects of immobilisation, re-establish motion, decrease pain, decrease inflammation and prevent muscle atrophy [10, 20]. Movement is initiated as soon as it is safely possible, as progressive mechanical loading is more likely to restore the morphological characteristics of capsuloligamentous, osteochondral and muscular structures [21, 22]. Animal models have demonstrated that loading upregulates genetic expression for key proteins associated with tissue healing [21–23]. Clinical studies have demonstrated that immediate elbow mobilisation, even after a simple posterolateral dislocation, results in less loss of motion with no apparent increase in instability [24]. The safe arc of motion is dictated by healing constraints of soft tissues as well as the specific pathology or surgery [10].

Mobilisation exercises are performed, in a protected range, as defined by the nature of surgery or injury. Exercises must be performed frequently throughout the day and involve all planes of elbow, forearm and wrist motion. There should be a bias towards active mobilisation, as studies show muscular activation stabilises the elbow, when compared to passive mobilisation alone [25].The elbow joint is especially prone to flexion contractures; therefore, the primary goal of this phase should be to establish full pre-injury range, especially extension.

The overhead position described by Wolffe and Hotchkiss [26] is the optimal mobilisation position to achieve this goal (Fig. 17.1).This position has been demonstrated to maximise elbow stability, by minimising ulnohumeral distraction [27]. Distraction is most marked with the arm hanging dependent by the side [27], especially when wearing a cast or hinged elbow brace, so this position for exercises should be avoided. The overhead position also has the added benefit of minimising biceps EMG activity seen clinically in the painful stiff elbow [28]. It also enhances triceps activity thereby maximising elbow extension range [29]. This position is suitable for the majority of individuals with conservatively managed elbow pathology. However, in post-operative patients, it is only suitable where a triceps-sparing approach has been taken.

Initially active assisted flexion/extension is performed with the contralateral upper limb providing support where needed. The forearm position during this exercise is dictated by the capsuloligamentous structures that need protecting. With lateral compartment lesions, the forearm is placed in pronation, whereby passive tension in the common extensor origin contributes to lateral stability. It follows therefore that with medial compartment lesions, exercises are performed in supination, and stability is afforded by passive tension in the common flexor origin [25]. Exercises are progressed to active movements without assistance, as soon as comfort allows. It is very important that any exercise or alternative techniques used in this stage produce minimal pain, as neuropeptides such as substance P, involved in pain transmission, can be associated with increased myofibroblastic activity [30]. This is seen in individuals with contracted elbow capsules, a common complication seen after elbow trauma or surgery. Supplemental manual therapy may also be used in the early phase, to modulate pain, by stimulating type I/II articular receptors [10]. In elbow tendinopathy, mobilisations with movements can be applied, where they have a demonstrable effect on decreasing pain on symptomatic activities [31], e.g. grip. During this phase, focus is also placed on voluntary activation of muscles and reducing muscular atrophy. Isometric exercises of the major elbow, forearm and wrist muscle groups are performed, which have been shown to place no additional strain on healing ligamentous grafts [32]. Contractions are performed at the common flexor pronator group and the common extensor group, which are secondary stabilisers of the medial and lateral compartments, respectively [33]. Also the dynamic stabilisers, producing compression at the elbow, are targeted including triceps, biceps and anconeus [33]. Anconeus appears from both EMG and anatomical studies to be a lateral elbow stabiliser,

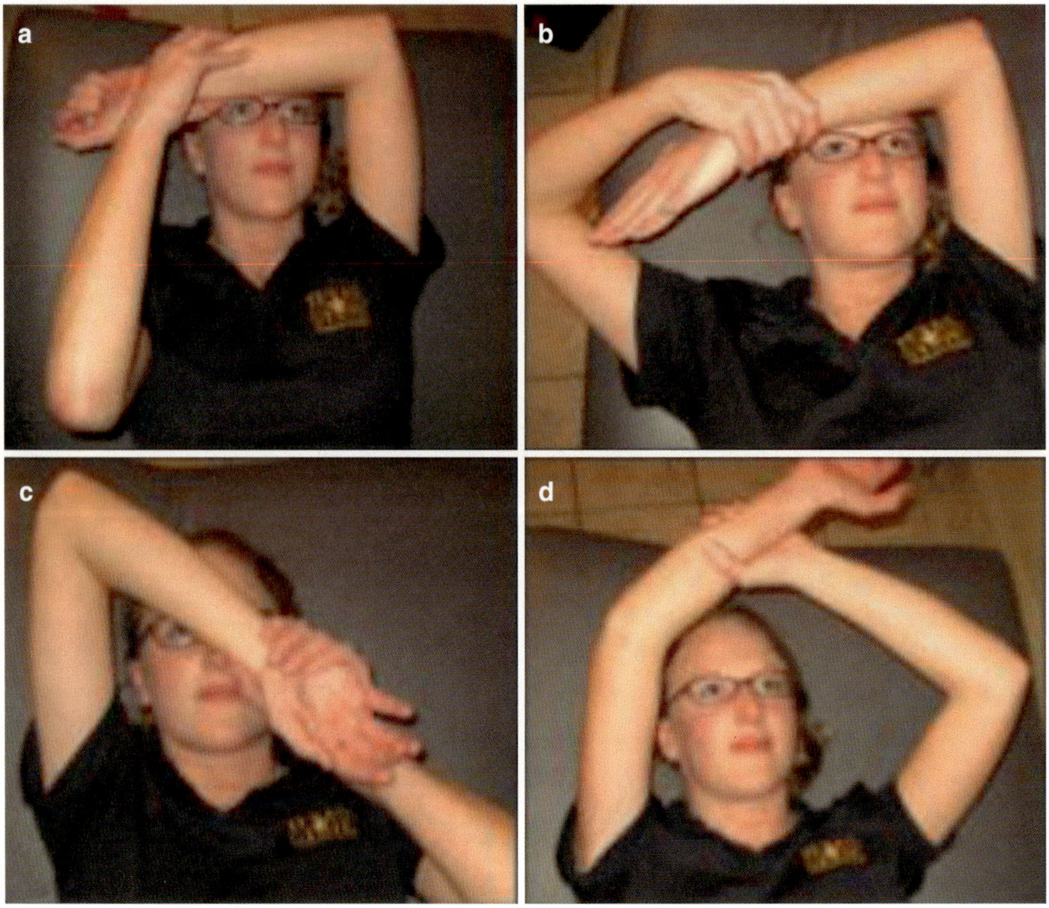

Fig. 17.1 The overhead position described by Wolffe and Hotchkiss 26 is the optimal mobilisation position to achieve this goal. This position has been demonstrated to maximize elbow stability, by minimising ulno-humeral distraction

co-apting the ulna to the humerus, reducing posterolateral rotatory displacement [34–36], and can be facilitated isometrically even when the elbow is immobilised in a plaster cast or splint.

Isometric contractions also have the additional benefit of reducing pain, via a generalised, centrally induced, pain inhibitory response. The magnitude of this effect increases with contractions of longer durations and of moderate or above intensity (40–50 % MVC) and is not constrained to the exercising limb [37–42]. Some therapists advocate the use of neuromuscular electrostimulation (NMES) to facilitate this process; however, more good quality evidence regarding its beneficial effects is limited. One consideration for post-operative patients is which surgical approach was used and the condition of the muscle origins, in order to guide early resistance work [43]. Therefore, good communication between the surgical and therapy team is essential. Shoulder isometric work may be performed with caution with resistance applied proximal to the elbow. However, care should be taken with positions of extreme glenohumeral external rotation, as they produce a valgus moment at the elbow, possibly compromising vulnerable tissues [43].

17.5 Intermediate Phase

This is started when the following is achieved, a return to pre-injury range, with minimal pain and tenderness and good strength of elbow and forearm musculature [10], usually at 4–6 weeks post-injury/surgery. Elbow extension and forearm pronation are of particular importance for effective performance in throwing sports [10, 20]. Local strengthening exercises are progressed to isotonic contractions, beginning with concentric work, then eccentric work, with emphasis placed on the secondary stabilisers [10] (Fig. 17.2). With medial compartment symptoms, emphasis should be placed on the flexor pronator mass, especially flexor carpi ulnaris, which anatomical and EMG studies have been shown to contribute to valgus stability, by reducing forces placed on ulnar collateral ligament, during throwing [44 – 47]. With tendinopathy, the key goal is improving the capacity of the tendon and muscle to manage load. Several strengthening options exist, as described previously, as well as heavy slow resistance work, all sharing a common goal of gradually increasing load, whilst carefully monitoring pain. This approach for tendinopathy has been supported by clinical trials, with long-term benefits seen compared with pharmacological and electrotherapy interventions [48–50].

Counterforce bracing is only useful in individuals where it demonstrably reduces pain or improves grip and is only worn during pain-provoking activities [51]. Emphasis is also placed on exercises improving endurance and neuromuscular control of the elbow complex [10, 20, 52]. Loss of kinaesthetic awareness of upper extremities can occur post-injury and has been shown to decrease proprioceptive accuracy in throwers [53–56]. Proprioceptive neuromuscular facilitation, rhythmic stabilisation drills and open and closed kinetic chain activities, which promote cocontraction and mimic functional positions with joint approximation, are now implemented [10]. Studies show a decrease in neuromuscular control, kinaesthetic detection strength and throwing accuracy is associated with muscular fatigue; therefore, exercises, including multiple sets [2], to promote endurance are a key component of this stage.

Shoulder flexibility is also addressed at this stage, as loss of total shoulder rotational range or

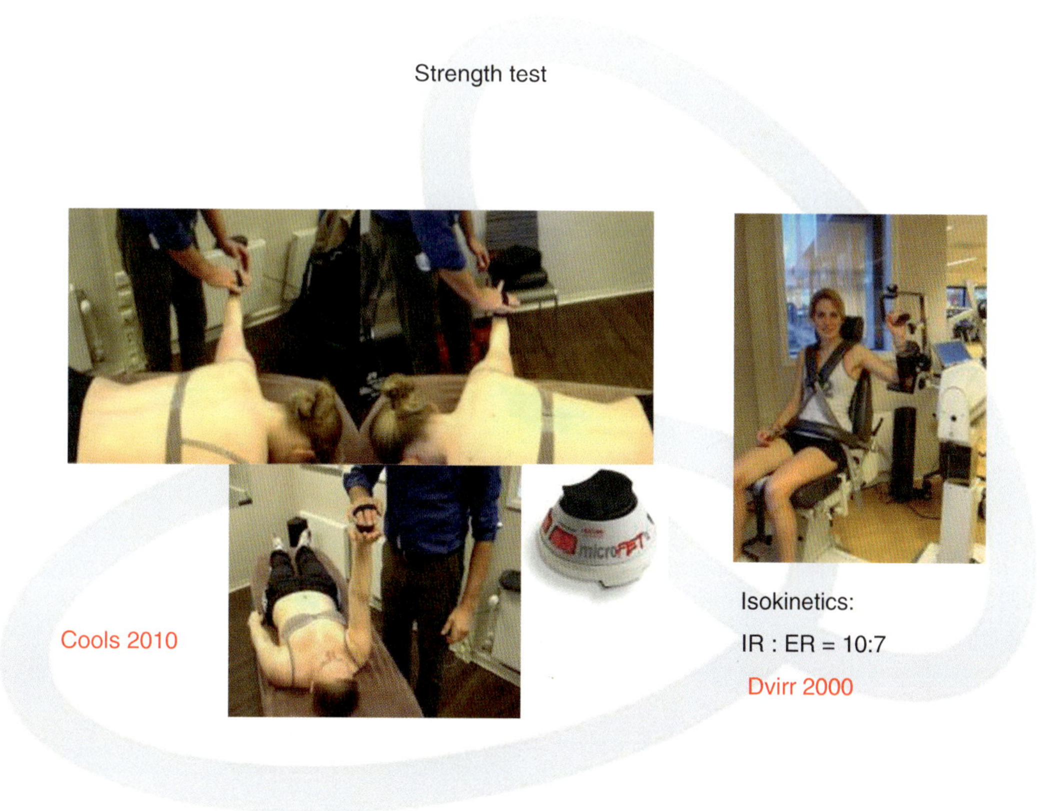

Fig. 17.2 Local strengthening exercises are progressed to isotonic contractions, beginning with concentric work, then eccentric work, with emphasis placed on the secondary stabilisers [10]

glenohumeral internal rotation deficit (GIRD) has been shown to place strain on medial elbow structures during throwing [57, 58]. It is advised that between sides, differences should be less than 18° and the difference in total range of motion should not be more than 5°. The assessment of rotational range of motion can be measured with a goniometer or an inclinometer. Posteroinferior glenohumeral capsular tightening and shrinkage, along with adaptive humeral head changes, are well-documented problems in long-term throwers [57, 58, 59]. For this group, stretches such as a sleeper stretch are thought to be effective in addressing the posterior capsular tightness [60] and significantly increase acromiohumeral distance in overhead athletes with GIRD, after a 6-week stretching programme. Care should be taken with stretches at extremes of glenohumeral external rotation, as mentioned previously.

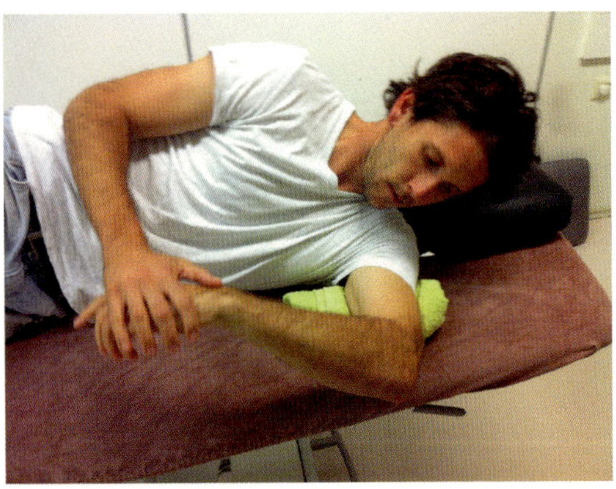

According to Ellenbecker [9] you see the modified sleepers stretch in sidelying with a towel beneath the upper arm to provide horizontal adduction to achieve more stretch on the capsule in the 90 degrees abduction position.

It is also important not to apply this to all individuals with elbow injury or pathology. It must be considered that the GIRD may be a problem, not just due to capsular pathology [57]. For this group stretching may not be as effective, and the problem should be addressed by performing eccentric and concentric rotator cuff exercises through range. It is essential that the individual is carefully assessed to ensure that any deficit is managed appropriately. Therefore, a comprehensive assessment of the shoulder and the scapula should be undertaken, as scapula dysfunction prevents optimum energy transfer in the upper limb. Glenohumeral rotational strength and scapula strength are addressed during this phase [10, 2, 20, 43] and are incorporated in the throwers TEN strengthening programme [61]. This has been designed, from EMG evidence, to illicit muscular activity most needed to provide upper limb dynamic stability [62, 63] and has been demonstrated to increase throwing velocity, following a 6-week programme [64]. Attention should be paid to global upper limb strengthening, even with elbow tendinopathy, as previous studies have shown global weakness, affecting all major shoulder groups, and the triceps, with this condition [65], probably due to pain inhibition and disuse. The use of flywheel and fly pull devices has been advocated in restoring muscle strength and neuromuscular coordination and endurance.

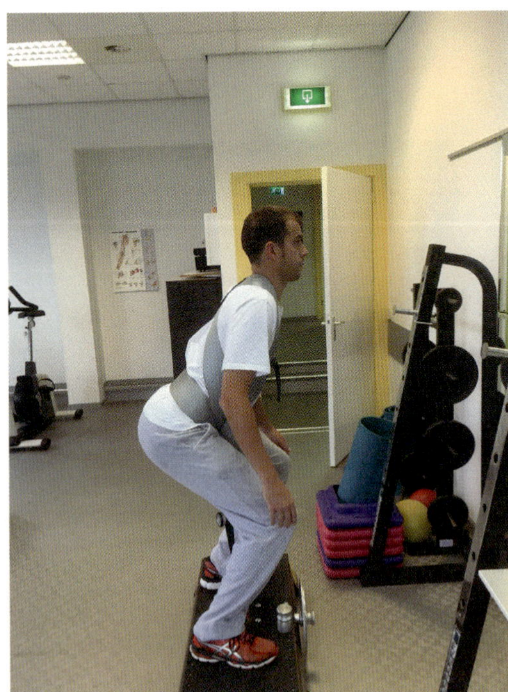

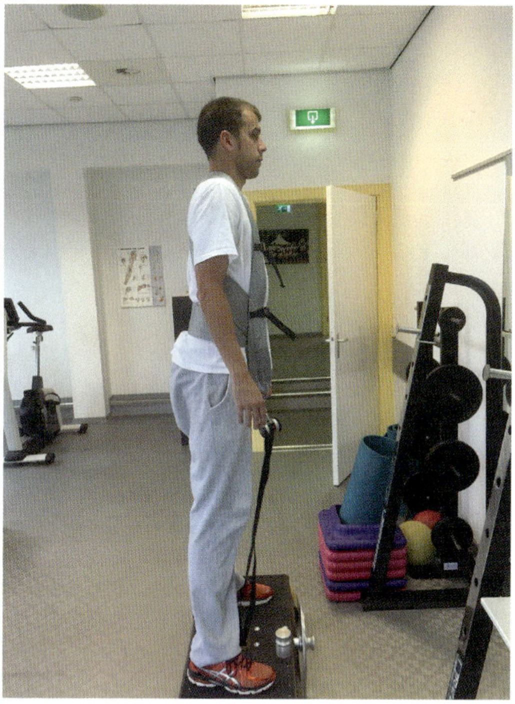

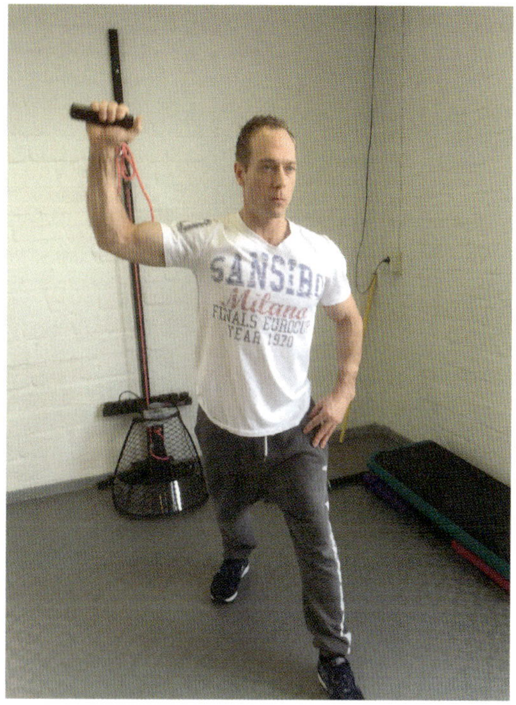

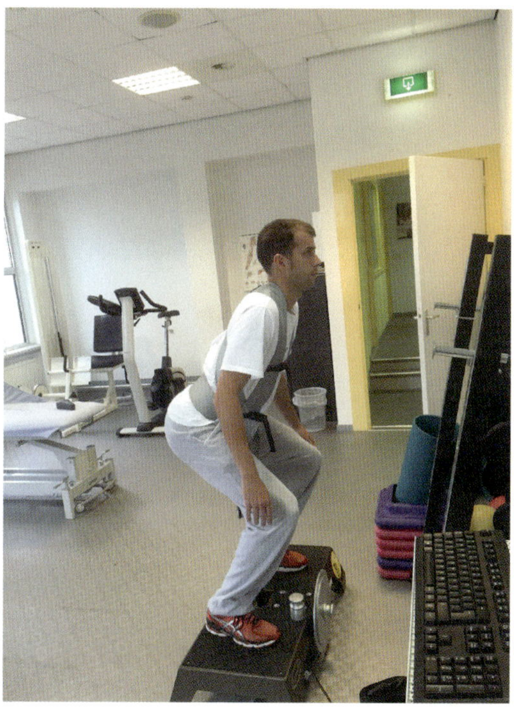

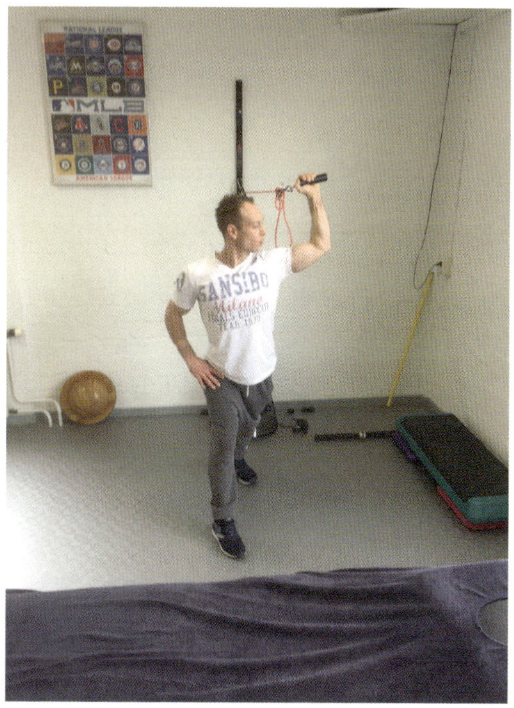

In these athletes eccentric training with maximum of coordination and kinetic chain position is provided in tennis (adolescent and ATP level) and Gymnastics (Olympic level) to restore muscle strength and coordination or maintain during the season their high level of sports in training the kinetic chain by squats or IR/ER in 90 degrees of abduction.

It is vital to concentrate not only on the upper limb but also on the whole kinetic chain at this stage in rehabilitation, the kinetic chain being a specific sequence of movement which allows efficient accomplishment of a task. Injuries or adaptations in remote areas of the chain can cause problems not only locally but also distally, as joints such as the elbow compensate for lack of force production and energy delivery through more proximal links [10, 66]. Kibler and Chandler [67] calculated a 20 % reduction in kinetic energy delivered from the hip and trunk to the upper limb and require a 34 % increase in rotational velocity of the arm, to impart the same amount of force to the hand. Hannan et al.'s study [68] has shown a link between lower limb balance deficits in throwers with medial elbow ligament injuries compared with healthy controls. These balance deficits disappear following a 3-month throwers rehab programme including the trunk and the lower limb. Therefore, in this early stage, whilst the elbow is recovering, leg and trunk exercises involving sport-specific activation patterns can be initiated, so that the base of the kinetic chain is ready for the next phase, late-stage rehabilitation.

17.6 Late-Phase Rehabilitation

This stage involves progression of activities to prepare the athlete for a return to sport. The goal of this stage is to gradually increase strength, power, endurance and neuromuscular control. Physical criteria to progress to this phase include full active range of movement, no pain or tenderness, strength that is 70 % of that of the contralateral limb and a functional score that indicates less than 15 % impairment on QuickDASH or similar subjective outcome score [10]. Usually, progression to late-stage rehabilitation will commence between 7 and 12 week and depends upon whether an athlete has been conservatively or surgically managed. Strengthening exercises emphasising higher resistance and functional sports-specific movements, including eccentric and plyometric activities, are now employed. Elbow flexion exercises are progressed to emphasise eccentric control, as biceps is an important stabiliser, during the follow-through stage of throwing. Eccentric control prevents pathological abuttal of the olecranon in the olecranon fossa. Concentric triceps activity is also emphasised during this phase, because of the triceps activity seen during the acceleration phase of throwing.

Resistance exercises should be chosen that closely stimulate the demands of an athlete's individual sport. In ground-based sports, exercises that simulate throwing or service action in tennis, with the glenohumeral joint in 90° of abduction in the scapula plane, are advocated. Regimes such as the Advanced Throwers Ten Programme incorporate exercise and movement patterns specific to the throwing motion. The programme utilises the principle of co-activation, high level neuromuscular control, dynamic stability, endurance and coordination that are vital in the overhead athlete. However, in swimmers, Swiss ball exercises, performed in the prone position with the feet off the floor, may appear to be more specific to the demands of this particular sport. Exercises to promote endurance should be emphasised during this phase, because the overhead athlete is at risk of injury, if throwing whilst fatigued. Endurance drills using lower weights and higher repetitions are advocated, which have been shown to preferentially load key muscle groups required in overhead sport. Fatigue also adversely affects proprioception; therefore, endurance activities are critical in improving coordination and joint stability. This stage should also commence plyometric exercise and controlled impact work. Plyometric drills can be a beneficial form of functional exercise for training the elbow and have been shown to increase throwing and service action speeds, increase elbow extension power and improve measures of proprioception and kinaesthesia.

Stretch of the musculotendinous unit immediately followed by shortening is key to the concept of plyometric exercise, with the stretch-shortening cycle enhancing the ability of the musculotendinous unit to produce maximum force in the shortest time. It has been suggested they should be performed in conjunction with other forms of strengthening programmes, for an athlete to gain maximum benefit. Initially plyometric exercises are performed with both upper limbs, i.e. chest pass, side pass and overhead football throw. They are then progressed to one-handed throwing in the 90/90 position, along with specific plyometric drills for the forearm musculature including wrist flips, wrist snaps and extension grips. For individuals who wish to return to contact sports, e.g. rugby, it is vital to address impact work at this stage. Previous studies have shown that increased muscle activation patterns of the elbow and wrist during forward falls increase the transition of force shock waves through the forearm [69]. With practice, individuals can select the upper extremity posture, allowing the athlete to minimise the effects of impact. Lo et al. [70] showed that practising five to ten repetitions of forward falls results in decreased impact forces in the upper limb, during subsequent falls, for the following 2 months.

17.7 Return to Sport Phase

An athlete can progress to this phase, after attaining of full range of motion, no pain or tenderness, good strength and endurance and stability of the upper extremity and scapula. Athletes should also have 0 % disability on the QuickDASH outcome score, with good compliance and knowledge of their individualised home exercise programme. Individuals should also be medically cleared, following a thorough clinical examination.

Traditional exercise programmes cannot reproduce speed or joint forces generated in sport. The only way to mimic these forces is to practice the sport concerned. Interval training programmes are progressive sport-specific regimes that gradually expose an athlete to the demands they will experience upon return to sport. Interval sports programmes (ISP) have been described for swimming, golf, tennis and throwing sports. Prior to the initiation of the ISP, throwing motion and kinetic chain stability should be assessed, wherever possible using digital imagery. A focussed warm-up programme, which can be reproduced by the athlete on returning to full participation in sport, is implemented prior to every session of the ISP. At the start of a session, an athlete's strength and flexibility are measured, with an expectation that an individual maintains 90 % of these levels, following execution of the session. The ISP should progress through 4 distinct stages: return to sport, basic programme, advanced programme and simulated competition. The amount of time spent at each stage is dictated by the type of injury/surgery athlete has sustained as well as any symptoms in response to the programme. If athletes experience pain with or after activity, a reduction in strength or range of motion, or if they have generalised upper limb soreness lasting more than 24 h, the athlete remains at that stage until symptoms resolve. The throwing interval programme gradually increases the number, intensity and type of throw, which are all progressed gradually to minimise the risk of overload at the elbow. Generally throwers begin with shorter distances at 50 % throwing intensity, increasing intensity to 100 % over a 4–6-week period. However, an athlete must be educated upon the importance of following a structured regime, as previous studies have demonstrated that athletes significantly underestimate their throwing effort, predisposing themselves to potential injury. Once an athlete can throw 40–50 times at an intensity of 80 %, without any symptoms, different styles of throw, such as breaking balls, are implemented. The final step is simulated completion/game, for a given position and level of play. Rehabilitation will continue until the individual successfully returns to sport. It should be remembered that to return an athlete to competition may take up to 9–12 months [43], dependent upon the type/site of injury and its management, with athletes throwing for short periods of time at 3 months' post-op. Athletes should be monitored frequently throughout this process with frequent communication between the athlete, coaching staff and rehabilitation team, to offer support until return to competition and to reduce the risk of injury.

17.8 Injury Prevention

The most important tenants of the prevention programme are education, identification of at-risk athletes, full rehabilitation of past or current injuries and monitoring athletes for the development of warning signs for injury. Off-season training programmes, in athletes with a previous history of tendinopathy, should include a controlled tendon loading programme, to prevent a reduction in tendon integrity and stiffness. A subsequent return to training should include appropriately spaced graduated increases in load. In the absence of such strategies, an athlete will be predisposed to an active tendinopathy upon resumption of full training.

References

1. Crotin RL, Ramsey DK. Injury prevention for throwing athletes part I: baseball bat training to enhance medial elbow dynamic stability. Strength Cond J. 2012;34(2):79–85.
2. Ellenbecker TS, Nirschl R, Renstrom P. Current concepts in examination and treatment of elbow tendon injury. Sports Health Multidisc Appro. 2012;5(2):186–94. 1941738112464761.
3. Conte S, Requa RK, Garrick JG. Disability days in major league baseball. Am J Sports Med. 2001;29(4):431–6.
4. Posner M, Cameron KL, Wolf JM, Belmont Jr PJ, Owens BD. Epidemiology of major league baseball injuries. Am J Sports Med. 2011;39(8):1676–80.
5. Priest JD, Jones HH, Nagel DA. Elbow injuries in highly skilled tennis players. Am J Sports Med. 1974;2(3):137–49.
6. Priest JD. Tennis elbow. The syndrome and a study of average players. Minn Med. 1976;59(6):367–71.
7. Wilson FD, Andrews JR, Blackburn TA, Mccluskey G. Valgus extension overload in the pitching elbow. Am J Sports Med. 1983;11(2):83–8.
8. Dillman CJ, Smutz P, Werner S. Valgus extension overload in baseball pitching. Med Sci Sports Exerc. 1991;23:S135.
9. Cain EL, Dugas JR, Wolf RS, Andrews JR. Elbow injuries in throwing athletes a current concepts review. Am J Sports Med. 2003;31(4):621–35.
10. Wilk KE, Macrina LC, Cain EL, Dugas JR, Andrews JR. Rehabilitation of the overhead athlete's elbow. Sports Health Multidisc Appro. 2012;4(5):404–14.
11. Ellenbecker TS, Mattalino AJ, Elam EA, Caplinger RA. Medial elbow joint laxity in professional baseball pitchers a bilateral comparison using stress radiography. Am J Sports Med. 1998;26(3):420–4.
12. Wright RW, Steger-May K, Wasserlauf BL, O'Neal ME, Weinberg BW, Paletta GA. Elbow range of motion in professional baseball pitchers. Am J Sports Med. 2006;34(2):190–3.
13. Ellenbecker TS. A total arm strength isokinetic profile of highly skilled tennis players. Isokinet Exerc Sci. 1991;1(1):9–21.
14. Ellenbecker TS, Roetert EP, Riewald S. Isokinetic profile of wrist and forearm strength in elite female junior tennis players. Br J Sports Med. 2006;40(5):411–4.
15. Laudner KG, Wilson JT, Meister K. Elbow isokinetic strength characteristics among collegiate baseball players. Phys Ther Sport. 2012;13(2):97–100.
16. Kovacs MS, Ellenbecker TS. A performance evaluation of the tennis serve: implications for strength, speed, power, and flexibility training. Strength Cond J. 2011;33(4):22–30.
17. Wilk KE, Arrigo C, Andrews JR. Rehabilitation of the elbow in the throwing athlete. J Orthop Sports Phys Ther. 1993;17(6):30.
18. Ellenbecker TS, Paul Roetert E. Isokinetic profile of elbow flexion and extension strength in elite junior tennis players. J Orthop Sports Phys Ther. 2003;33(2):79–84.
19. Ruivo R, Pezarat-Correia P, Carita AI. Elbow and shoulder muscles strength profile in judo athletes. Isokinet Exerc Sci. 2012;20(1):41–5.
20. Wilk KE, Reinold MM, Andrews JR. Rehabilitation of the thrower's elbow. Clin Sports Med. 2004;23(4):765–801.
21. Bring DKI, Reno C, Renstrom P, Salo P, Hart DA, Ackermann PW. Joint immobilization reduces the expression of sensory neuropeptide receptors and impairs healing after tendon rupture in a rat model. J Orthop Res. 2009;27(2):274–80.
22. Martinez DA, Vailas AC, Vanderby Jr R, Grindeland RE. Temporal extracellular matrix adaptations in ligament during wound healing and hindlimb unloading. Am J Phys Regul Integrative Comp Physiol. 2007;293(4):R1552–60.
23. Eliasson P, Andersson T, Aspenberg P. Rat Achilles tendon healing: mechanical loading and gene expression. J Appl Physiol. 2009;107(2):399–407.
24. Ross G, McDevitt ER, Chronister R, Ove PN. Treatment of simple elbow dislocation using an immediate motion protocol. Am J Sports Med. 1999;27(3):308–11.
25. Armstrong AD, Dunning CE, Faber KJ, Duck TR, Johnson JA, King GJ. Rehabilitation of the medial collateral ligament-deficient elbow: an in vitro biomechanical study. J Hand Surg. 2000;25(6):1051–7.
26. Wolff AL, Hotchkiss RN. Lateral elbow instability: nonoperative, operative, and postoperative management. J Hand Ther. 2006;19(2):238–44.
27. Lee AT, Schrumpf MA, Choi D, Meyers KN, Patel R, Wright TM, Hotchkiss RN, Daluiski A. The influence of gravity on the unstable elbow. J Shoulder Elbow Surg. 2013;22(1):81–7.
28. Page C, Backus SI, Lenhoff MW. Electromyographic activity in stiff and normal elbows during elbow flexion and extension. J Hand Ther. 2003;16(1):5–11.
29. Jones V, Stanley D.

30. Monument MJ, Hart DA, Salo PT, Befus AD, Hildebrand KA. Posttraumatic elbow contractures: targeting neuroinflammatory fibrogenic mechanisms. J Orthop Sci. 2013;18(6):869–77.
31. Bisset LM, Hing W, Vicenzino B. The efficacy of mobilisations with movement treatment on musculoskeletal pain: a systematic review and meta-analysis. In: 16th international congress of the world confederation for physical therapy. 2011. http://www.wcpt.org/wpt11.
32. Bernas GA, Thiele RAR, Kinnaman KA, Hughes RE, Miller BS, Carpenter JE. Defining safe rehabilitation for ulnar collateral ligament reconstruction of the elbow a biomechanical study. Am J Sports Med. 2009;37(12):2392–400.
33. O'Driscoll SW, Jupiter JB, King GJ, Hotchkiss RN, Morrey BF. The unstable elbow*†. J Bone Joint Surg. 2000;82(5):724.
34. Basmajian JV, GRIFFINJR W. Function of anconeus muscle an electromyographic study. J Bone Joint Surg. 1972;54(8):1712–4.
35. Bergin MJG, Vicenzino B, Hodges PW. Functional differences between anatomical regions of the anconeus muscle in humans. J Electromyogr Kinesiol. 2013;23(6):1391–7.
36. Molinier F, Laffosse JM, Bouali O, Tricoire JL, Moscovici J. The anconeus, an active lateral ligament of the elbow: new anatomical arguments. Surg Radiol Anat. 2011;33(7):617–21.
37. Misra G, Paris TA, Archer DB, Coombes SA. Dose–response effect of isometric force production on the perception of pain. PLoS One. 2014;9(2):e88105.
38. Koltyn KF, Umeda M. Contralateral attenuation of pain after short-duration submaximal isometric exercise. J Pain. 2007;8(11):887–92.
39. Kosek E, Ekholm J. Modulation of pressure pain thresholds during and following isometric contraction. Pain. 1995;61(3):481–6.
40. Kosek E, Lundberg L. Segmental and plurisegmental modulation of pressure pain thresholds during static muscle contractions in healthy individuals. Eur J Pain. 2003;7(3):251–8.
41. Lannersten L, Kosek E. Dysfunction of endogenous pain inhibition during exercise with painful muscles in patients with shoulder myalgia and fibromyalgia. Pain. 2010;151(1):77–86.
42. Staud R, Robinson ME, Price DD. Isometric exercise has opposite effects on central pain mechanisms in fibromyalgia patients compared to normal controls. Pain. 2005;118(1):176–84.
43. Ellenbecker TS, et al. Current concepts in rehabilitation following ulnar collateral ligament reconstruction. Sports Health Multidis Appro. 2009;1(4): 301–13.
44. Lin F, et al. Muscle contribution to elbow joint valgus stability. J Shoulder Elbow Surg. 2007;16(6):795–802.
45. Otoshi K, et al. The proximal origins of the flexor–pronator muscles and their role in the dynamic stabilization of the elbow joint: an anatomical study. Surg Radiol Anat. 2014;36(3):289–94.
46. Park MC, Ahmad CS. Dynamic contributions of the flexor-pronator mass to elbow valgus stability. J Bone Joint Surg. 2004;86(10):2268–74.
47. Perry J, Jobe FW. Functional anatomy of the flexor pronator muscle group in relation to the medial collateral ligament of the elbow. Am J Sports Med. 1995;23(2):245–50.
48. Pienimäki TT, Tarvainen TK, Siira PT, Vanharanta H. Progressive strengthening and stretching exercises and ultrasound for chronic lateral epicondylitis. Physiotherapy. 1996;82(9):522–30.
49. Stasinopoulos D, Stasinopoulou K, Johnson MI. An exercise programme for the management of lateral elbow tendinopathy. Br J Sports Med. 2005;39(12):944–7.
50. Svernlöv B, Adolfsson L. Non-operative treatment regime including eccentric training for lateral humeral epicondylalgia. Scand J Med Sci Sports. 2001;11(6): 328–34.
51. Ng G. The effects of forearm brace tension on neuromuscular performance in subjects with lateral humeral epicondylosis: a review: review article. Int SportMed J Elbow Injury Sport Part 2 Biomech Elbow Sport. 2005;6(2):124.
52. Fusaro I, Orsini S, Kantar SS, Sforza T, Benedetti MG, Bettelli G, Rotini R. Elbow rehabilitation in traumatic pathology. Musculoskelet Surg. 2014;98(1): 95–102.
53. Carpenter JE, Blasier RB, Pellizzon GG. The effects of muscle fatigue on shoulder joint position sense. Am J Sports Med. 1998;26(2):262–5.
54. Guskiewicz KM, Schneider RA, Prentice WE. Proprioception and neuromuscular control of the shoulder after muscle fatigue. J Athl Train. 1999;34(4):362.
55. Myers JB, Ju YY, Hwang JH, McMahon PJ, Rodosky MW, Lephart SM. Reflexive muscle activation alterations in shoulders with anterior glenohumeral instability. Am J Sports Med. 2004;32(4):1013–21.
56. Voight ML, Hardin JA, Blackburn TA, Tippett S, Canner GC. The effects of muscle fatigue on and the relationship of arm dominance to shoulder proprioception. J Orthop Sports Phys Ther. 1996;23(6): 348–52.
57. Shanley E, Rauh MJ, Michener LA, Ellenbecker TS, Garrison JC, Thigpen CA. Shoulder range of motion measures as risk factors for shoulder and elbow injuries in high school softball and baseball players. Am J Sports Med. 2011;39(9):1997–2006.
58. Wilk KE, Macrina LC, Flensing GS, Aune KT, Porterfield RA, Harker P, Evans TJ, Andrews JR. Deficits in glenohumeral passive range of motion increase risk of elbow injury in professional baseball pitchers a prospective study. Presented at the 39th annual meeting of the AOSSM, Chicago, July 2013.
59. Dines JS, et al. Glenohumeral internal rotation deficits in baseball players with ulnar collateral ligament insufficiency. Am J Sports Med. 2009;37(3):566–70.

60. Cools AM, Johansson FR, Cagnie B, Cambier DC, Witvrouw EE. Stretching the posterior shoulder structures in subjects with internal rotation deficit: comparison of two stretching techniques. Shoulder Elbow. 2012;4(1):56–63.
61. Wilk KE, Obma P, Simpson CD, Cain EL, Dugas J, Andrews JR. Shoulder injuries in the overhead athlete. J Orthop Sports Phys Ther. 2009;39(2):38–54.
62. Reinold MM, Macrina LC, Wilk KE, Fleisig GS, Dun S, Barrentine SW, Andrews JR. Electromyographic analysis of the supraspinatus and deltoid muscles during 3 common rehabilitation exercises. J Athl Train. 2007;42(4):464–9.
63. Reinold MM, Wilk KE, Fleisig GS, Zheng N, Barrentine SW, Chmielewski T, Cody RC, Jameson GG, Andrews JR. Electromyographic analysis of the rotator cuff and deltoid musculature during common shoulder external rotation exercises. J Orthop Sports Phys Ther. 2004;34(7):385–94.
64. Escamilla RF, Ionno M, ScottdeMahy M, Fleisig GS, Wilk KE, Yamashiro K, Mikla T, Paulos L, Andrews JR. Comparison of three baseball-specific 6-week training programs on throwing velocity in high school baseball players. J Strength Cond Res. 2012;26(7): 1767–81.
65. Alizadehkhaiyat O, Fisher AC, Kemp GJ, Vishwanathan K, Frostick SP. Upper limb muscle imbalance in tennis elbow: a functional and electromyographic assessment. J Orthop Res. 2007;25(12):1651–7.
66. Seroyer ST, Nho SJ, Bach BR, Bush-Joseph CA, Nicholson GP, Romeo AA. The kinetic chain in overhand pitching: its potential role for performance enhancement and injury prevention. Sports Health Multidis Appro. 2010;2(2):135–46.
67. Kibler WB, Chandler J. Baseball and tennis. In: Griffin LY, editor. Rehabilitation of the injured knee. St. Louis: Mosby; 1995. p. 219–26.
68. Hannon J, Garrison JC, Conway J. Lower extremity balance is improved at time of return to throwing in baseball players after an ulnar collateral ligament reconstruction when compared to pre-operative measurements. Int J Sports Phys Ther. 2014;9(3):356.
69. Burkhart TA, Andrews DM. Kinematics, kinetics and muscle activation patterns of the upper extremity during simulated forward falls. J Electromyogr Kinesiol. 2013;23(3):688–95.
70. Lo J, McCabe GN, DeGoede KM, Okuizumi H, Ashton-Miller JA. On reducing hand impact force in forward falls: results of a brief intervention in young males. Clin Biomech. 2003;18(8):730–6.

18 Endoscopy Around the Elbow

Gregory Bain, Hani Saeed, and Joideep Phadnis

18.1 Introduction

Endoscopic surgery around the elbow has grown to encompass a wide range of pathologies over the last few decades, owing to increased breadth, safety and reproducibility of practice. As these techniques evolve, soft tissue endoscopy about the elbow has expanded to include ulnar nerve release and transposition, olecranon bursectomy, resection of the olecranon spur and endoscopic suturing.

Ulnar nerve entrapment at the level of the elbow is the second most common entrapment neuropathy of the upper limb behind carpal tunnel syndrome [7, 17].

The sites of ulnar nerve compression are the arcade of Struthers, the cubital tunnel (most common site) and the flexor carpi ulnaris fascia [17]. Failing conservative management, treatment options include open or endoscopic [18] cubital tunnel release and open or endoscopic anterior ulnar nerve transposition if the ulnar nerve is found to be unstable or is in a hostile bed.

G. Bain, MBBS, FRACS, FA(Ortho)A, PhD (✉)
H. Saeed, MD, BPharm
Department of Orthopaedic Surgery and Trauma, Flinders University, Adelaide, SA, Australia

Department of Orthopaedic Surgery and Trauma, Flinders Medical Centre, Adelaide, SA, Australia
e-mail: greg@gregbain.com.au

J. Phadnis, MBChB, MRCS, Dip SportsMed, FRCS
Department of Orthopaedic Surgery and Trauma, Flinders Medical Centre, Adelaide, SA, Australia

Olecranon bursitis refers to inflammation of the subcutaneous synovial-lined sac of the bursa overlying the olecranon process at the proximal aspect of the ulna [5]. It is the most common form of superficial bursitis at the elbow [31]. Inflammation can result from abrasions around the elbow leading to infection, but is often caused by acute injuries during sport (i.e. direct impact to the posterior elbow), autoimmune inflammatory process (e.g. rheumatoid arthritis) or secondary to crystal deposition disease (e.g. gout or pseudogout). Patient with diabetes mellitus, uraemia, intravenous drug abuse, alcohol abuse or long-term use of steroids are at increased risk [38]. Two-thirds of cases are sterile bursitis, with one-third of cases being septic, secondary to Staphylococcus aureus and requiring bacterial cultures, drainage, irrigation and antibiotics [24].

The two conditions can be differentiated based on clinical examination [6], and surgery is indicated when conservative management has failed. Wet or dry endoscopic techniques can be performed, using incisions away from the apex of the olecranon that lead to faster healing rates and lower reoperation rates [13, 14].

Before any endoscopic procedure is performed, familiarity with the open technique is essential and provides a backup should the endoscopic procedure fail. Furthermore, a thorough understanding of surgical anatomy of the elbow is paramount due to the close proximity of neurovascular structures that can be damaged.

L.A. Pederzini et al. (eds.), *Elbow and Sport*, DOI 10.1007/978-3-662-48742-6_18

18.1.1 Surgical Anatomy

The ulnar nerve, a terminal branch of the medial cord of the brachial plexus, enters the arm with the axillary artery where it passes posterior and medial to the brachial artery, travelling between the brachial artery and vein [26].

At the level of the insertion of coracobrachialis in the middle third of the arm, the ulnar nerve pierces the medial intermuscular septum (MIMS) to enter the posterior compartment of the arm approximately 8 cm proximal to the medial epicondyle, where it lies on the anterior aspect of the medial head of triceps. The MIMS extends from the coracobrachialis proximally to the medial humeral epicondyle distally where it is a thick and distinct structure [16].

The ulnar nerve then courses anterior to the arcade of Struthers, a thin fibrous band extending from the medial head of triceps to the MIMS that is found 8 cm proximal to the medial epicondyle [16]. It then passes behind the medial epicondyle in the epicondylar groove where it continues through the cubital tunnel, a space bounded medially by the medial epicondyle and laterally by the tip of the olecranon. It is converted into a tunnel by the cubital tunnel retinaculum (arcuate ligament of Osborne), which are fibres that run perpendicular to the flexor carpi ulnaris (FCU) aponeurosis.

Next, the ulnar nerve passes between the ulnar and humeral heads of the FCU and penetrates the flexor-pronator aponeurosis about 5 cm beyond the medial epicondyle before descending into the forearm between FCU and flexor digitorum profundus as it courses down the forearm to the wrist.

18.1.2 Presentation and Investigations

A careful history is important to determine the chronicity, extent and nature of ulnar nerve compression. Symptoms can range from transient numbness, tingling or burning sensation in the ring and small fingers to clawing of these digits and intrinsic muscle atrophy in severe cases [4]. The most common symptoms are sensory disturbances along the ulnar nerve distribution, pain at the elbow and weakness of ulnar-innervated intrinsic hand muscles [12].

Pain may be present in the elbow region, and there may be a history of trauma at or near the elbow. Symptoms may worsen during the day with repeated elbow use, producing increasing weakness and sensory changes. Physical examination involves examining elbow range of motion and assessing for areas of tenderness or ulnar nerve subluxation over the epicondylar groove. In addition, the examiner should look for intrinsic muscle weakness, clawing or inability to abduct the small finger in extension. Assessing sensory changes provides additional information for localisation of ulnar nerve lesions. An elbow flexion test, where the examiner flexes the patient's elbow past 90°, supinates the forearm and extends the wrist, may be performed. This is considered positive if discomfort is reproduced, or paraesthesia along the ulnar nerve distribution occurs within 60 s [8, 33].

Examination of ulnar nerve instability, where the elbow is taken through full range of movement, is used to assess for chronic subluxation and relocation of the ulnar nerve during flexion and extension, respectively. The ulnar nerve may directly be visualised for subluxation or snapping as it lies superficially over the medial humeral epicondyle [3].

In patients presenting with bursitis, there is often a history of local repetitive or direct trauma. Patients may complain of swelling at the posterior elbow, associated with increased pain exacerbated by pressure or prolonged elbow flexion. The onset of symptoms may be acute in setting of infection or trauma or chronic if secondary to autoimmune disease or crystal deposition and chronic irritation. However, patients may also present with painless swelling in the setting of chronic disease. Examination of the posterior elbow in olecranon bursitis often reveals a fluctuant swelling felt over the olecranon process. There may be tenderness on palpation, especially in the acute setting. Skin inspection may reveal areas of abrasion or local infection, rheumatoid nodules or gouty tophi. Elbow range of movement is often normal, but may be reduced in severe cases.

Examination should also be directed at assessing if previous surgery has been performed. Significant scarring around the elbow joint may make endoscopic surgery increasingly difficult or unsafe, and an open technique may be required.

18.1.3 Imaging

Plain radiographs are required for assessment of anatomy, such as deformity secondary to trauma, bony spurs or fragments, shallow olecranon groove or destructive lesions.

Ultrasound examination may be useful in assessing specific compressive pathologies and allow for real-time visualisation of the nerve through its course. It is particularly useful in the assessment of bursitis, as it allows for the demonstration of effusions, inflammatory collections or presence of loose bodies [19].

18.2 Treatment Options

18.2.1 Endoscopic Ulnar Nerve Release

Several endoscopic techniques for ulnar nerve release have been published, including those by Hoffman (Storz), Cobb (Integra) and Tsai (glass tubes). Using the Hoffman technique, the subcutaneous plane is opened with tunnelling forceps and a hooded endoscope is introduced [11].

The hooded endoscope acts to keep the workspace open, making visualisation possible and allowing scissors and cautery to be introduced [2].

Cobb's technique makes use of the Integra Endo Release System, utilising a cannula specifically designed for cubital tunnel release, to protect the ulnar nerve whilst the roof of the cubital tunnel is released [1]. Tsai utilises glass tubes to house an endoscope and guide a meniscus knife [35].

The senior author published a technique utilising the Agee MicroAire endoscopic carpal tunnel device. This device has a trigger to activate a retractable cutting blade from a protected sheath immediately distal to the endoscopic tip, allowing for direct visualisation of both blade and

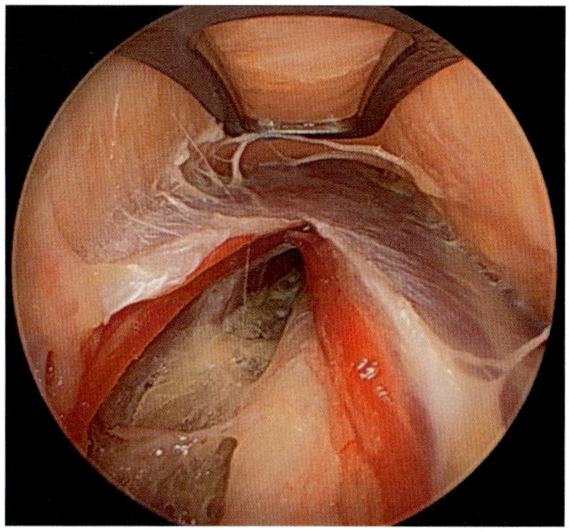

Fig. 18.1 Endoscopic ulnar nerve release utilising the hooded scope as developed by Hoffman and Storz. The ulnar nerve is seen below the flexor carpi ulnaris (Copyright Dr. Gregory Bain)

tissue at all times. Blunt dissection to the level of the cubital retinaculum is made, and the Agee device is introduced directly adjacent to the nerve, and the overlying constrictive tissue is released with the nerve and its branches in view at all times [7, 17] (Fig. 18.1).

Rehabilitation following endoscopic repair involves early active range-of-motion activities and a return to normal activities as tolerated.

18.2.2 Endoscopic Ulnar Nerve Anterior Transposition

If the ulnar nerve is found to be unstable, an endoscopic anterior transposition can be performed [29]. A standard ulnar nerve release is performed. The MIMS is excised. Care is required to ensure any adjacent vessels are identified and cauterised if required. The ulnar nerve is then mobilised and transposed anterior to the medial epicondyle (Fig. 18.2). Once the nerve is checked proximally and distally to ensure no kinking, the subcutaneous fat is sutured to the soft tissue over the medial epicondyle. Rehabilitation involves placing the elbow into a sling in flexion for 1 week to allow for soft tissue healing and stabilisation of the nerve in its new bed.

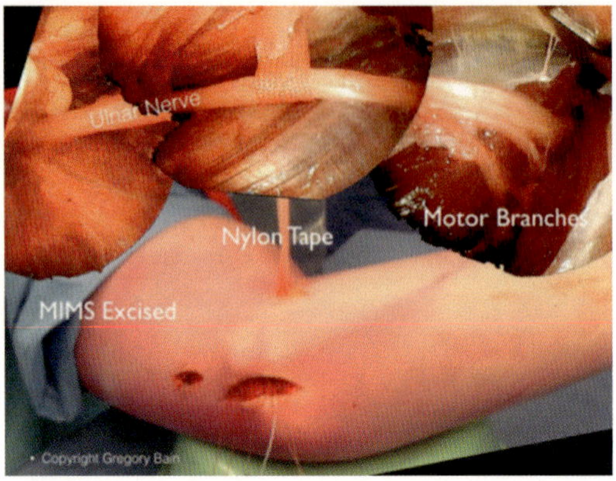

Fig. 18.2 Endoscopic ulnar nerve transposition. Below is the elbow with the main working portal over the medial epicondyle. A proximal portal was used to retract the ulnar nerve at the time of resection of the medial intermuscular septum (*MIMS*). An anterior portal has a nylon tape to retract the nerve. The composed photo shows the ulnar nerve held transposed by the nylon tape and the multiple motor branches dissected free (Copyright Dr. Gregory Bain.)

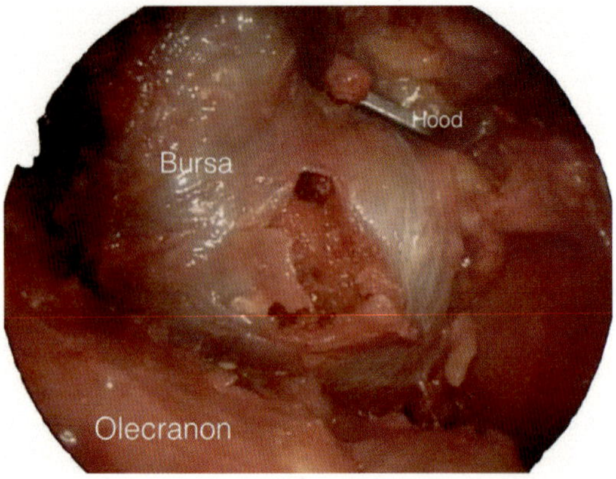

Fig. 18.3 Endoscopic olecranon bursa resection utilising dry endoscopy. Note the hood suspends the soft tissues and skin. The bursa is released and then excised whilst maintaining the skin over the olecranon, optimising healing (Copyright Dr. Gregory Bain)

18.2.3 Olecranon Bursitis

Surgery traditionally involves open bursectomy, with incision over the point of the olecranon. However, wound healing can be a problem owing to the area of bridging skin. Endoscopic techniques allow for faster healing with improved outcome.

Utilising the wet technique, two separate 1.5 cm longitudinal portals are made 2 cm proximal and distal to the margins of the bursa, in the midline. Distension is maintained via saline inflow and arthroscopic cannula to prevent fluid draining away. The scope can then be placed into the bursa, resecting the bursa from inside-out until normal tissue planes are visualised. Care should be taken to protect the overlying skin and to prevent any perforations that may develop into sinuses.

The senior author's preferred technique is the dry endoscopic procedure, specifically for treatment of sterile olecranon bursitis [36], utilising the Storz endoscopic equipment described above (Fig. 18.3). A 2 cm incision distal to the bursa is made to allow the introduction of the hooded scope, and the subcutaneous tissues are elevated off the bursa and olecranon. A separate proximal portal is made, and a pituitary rongeur is used to resect the bursa and cautery to control bleeding and fluid accumulation postoperatively (Fig. 18.4). To prevent recurrence in the dead space, the elbow should be placed in a sling at 90° of flexion.

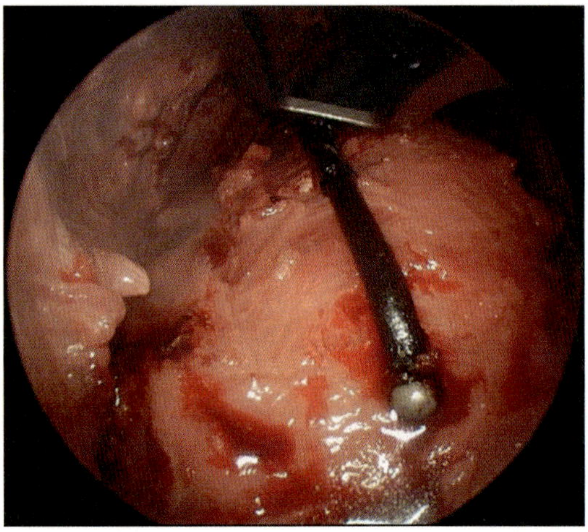

Fig. 18.4 After endoscopic resection of olecranon bursa, the tourniquet is deflated and cautery is used on any significant bleeding points identified (Copyright Dr. Gregory Bain)

18.2.4 Olecranon Spurs

Once the position of the spur is identified using fluoroscopy, dry endoscopy can be used to resect

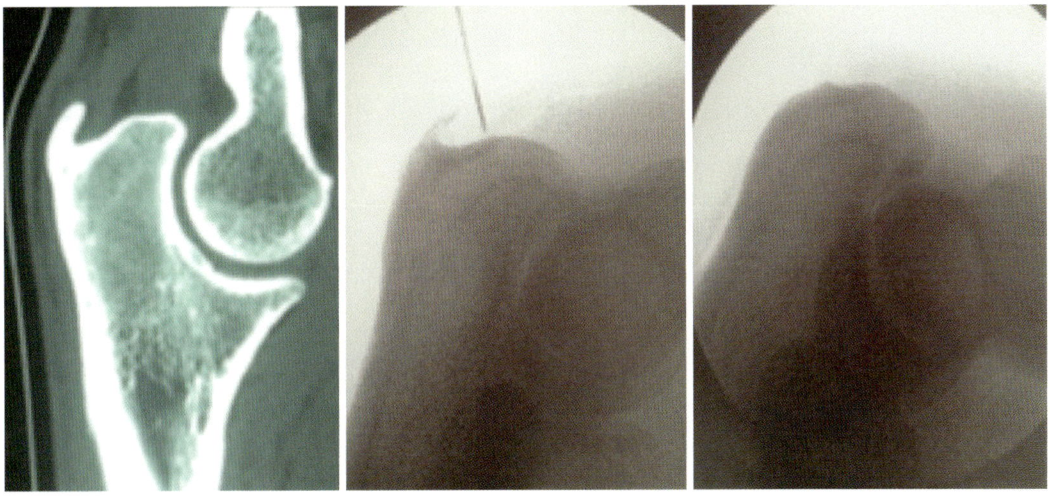

Fig. 18.5 Olecranon spur as seen on CT scan. Intra-operatively, fluoroscopy is used to identify the position of the spur and post-operatively to ensure complete resection (Copyright Dr. Gregory Bain)

the spur by introduction of high-speed burr. Fluoroscopy can then be used to ensure complete resection (Fig. 18.5).

18.2.5 Dry Elbow Arthroscopy

Dry arthroscopy has been utilised in elbow, providing greater appreciation of the anatomy of the elbow joint, reducing the risk of fluid extravasation and compartment syndrome. When the joint is distended with air, the synovial and articular surfaces are able to reflect light, allowing superior clarity and better understanding of subtle findings of the soft tissues and articular cartilage (Fig. 18.6). This technique has been shown to be particularly useful in synovitis, as fluid distension in wet arthroscopy may compress the soft tissues, change the shape of the synovium and reduce its vascularity [30, 34].

However, there are relative contraindications to using dry arthroscopic techniques. When radiofrequency ablation is required, wet arthroscopy should be used to provide cooling effect to the joint and prevent risk of chondrocyte damage. Furthermore, there is a theoretical risk of air embolus when arthroscopy is performed under air pump pressure and when a tourniquet is not inflated. Therefore, this technique should not be used with an air pump until further research is available [34].

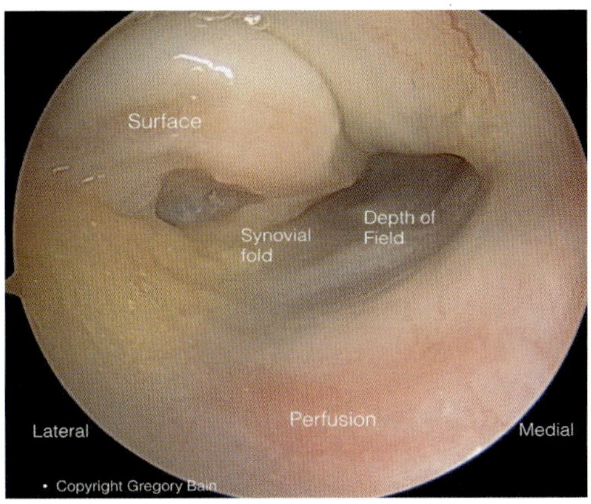

Fig. 18.6 Dry elbow arthroscopy, note the quality of the image and the depth of field. The synovial fluid on the surface of the articulation reflects the light, providing a better understanding of the surface itself. In the normal fluid arthroscopy, the synovial folds are flattened and the small vessels are compressed. However with dry arthroscopy, the synovial fold maintains its shape, and the small vessels perfuse the synovium and can be seen (Copyright Dr. Gregory Bain)

It can also be used for any of the therapeutic procedures, such as synovectomy, resection of osteophytes and capsulectomy (Fig. 18.7).

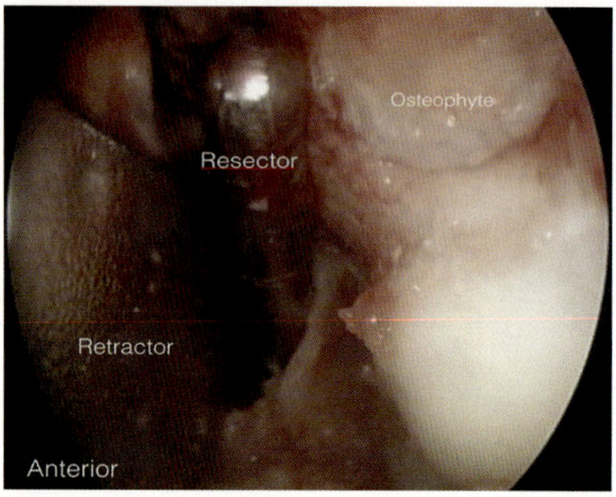

Fig. 18.7 Dry elbow arthroscopy is being used here for anterior humeral osteophyte resection. Intermittent irrigation is used to clear any debride from the resector (Copyright Dr. Gregory Bain)

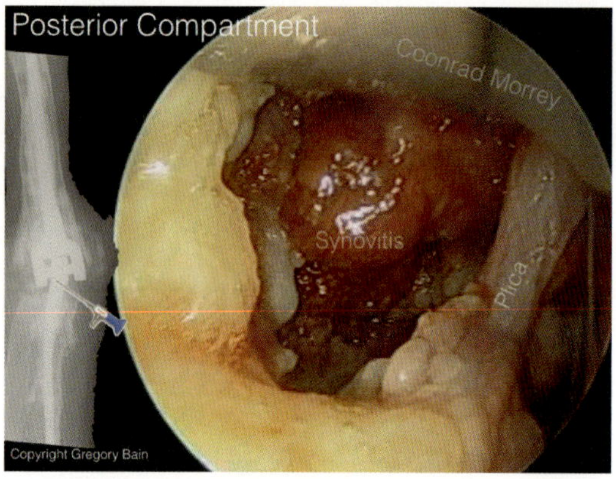

Fig. 18.8 Arthroscopic assessment of a patient with a suspected elbow arthroplasty infection shows synovitis and plica that was excised (Copyright Dr. Gregory Bain)

18.2.6 Arthroscopy and Elbow Arthroplasty

Arthroscopic management of elbow arthroplasty has been utilised as a valuable adjunct in the diagnosis of painful or swollen arthroplasty. Arthroscopy in this setting allows for targeted biopsies for microbiological diagnosis and for assessment of mechanical factors before an informed decision regarding definitive management is made [34]. Mechanical diagnosis can be made, and sometimes running repairs can be performed (Fig. 18.8).

18.2.7 Endoscopic Suturing

The senior author has performed deep suturing endoscopically using barbed sutures (Fig. 18.9). These are ideal for endoscopic repairs, as they do not require knot tying. The sutures can be inserted in the same way as we perform microsurgery. They can be used to repair deep fascia and other soft tissues [36].

18.2.8 Other Procedures

Soft tissue endoscopy has grown to encompass a range of pathologies (Table 18.1). In the elbow, endoscopy has been successfully utilised in biceps bursoscopy and distal biceps tendon repairs [9, 15, 37]. which is described in more detail in another chapter in this series. In the forearm, endoscopic techniques have been used for decompression of the anterior interosseous nerve [22, 25], pronator syndrome [27], and performing fasciotomy in cases of chronic exertional compartment syndromes [10, 32].

Furthermore, endoscopic soft tissue release of DeQuervain's tenosynovitis and intersection syndrome has been successfully performed [21]. Endoscopic harvesting of the radial artery has been utilised in patients undergoing coronary artery bypass grafting (CABG) with an overall patency at 10 years of 82 % [23].

18.3 Outcomes

A prospective study comparing the outcomes of the open versus endoscopic ulnar nerve release reported better patient satisfaction with the endoscopic technique and a lower complication rate, including elbow pain, scar tenderness and medial elbow paraesthesia [17]. Endoscopic decompression has been shown to be as effective as the open decompression, with additional advantages of being less invasive, a smaller incision, less vascular insult to the nerve and

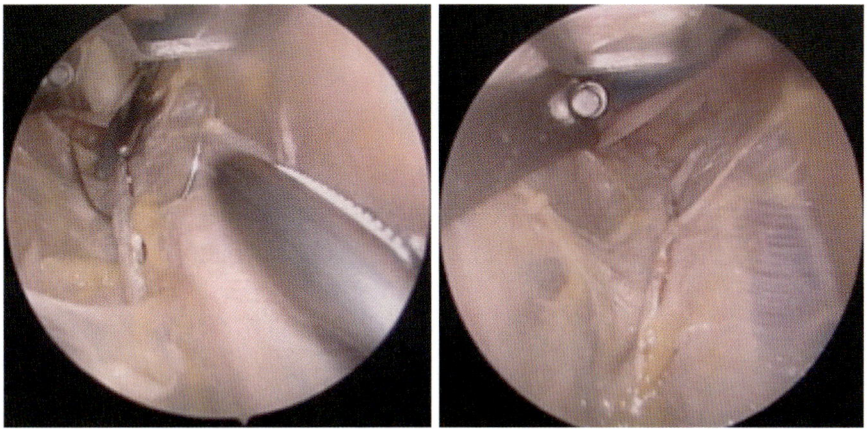

Fig. 18.9 Endoscopic suturing using barbed sutures in a cadaveric model. The suture technique is similar to the microsurgery. Once positioned, the sutures are pulled tight, and the barbs of the suture hold the suture in place (Copyright Dr. Gregory Bain)

Table 18.1 Indications for endoscopic procedures about the elbow, forearm and wrist

Procedure	Indication
Releases	Ulnar nerve release at cubital tunnel anterior interosseous nerve release
	DeQuervain's tenosynovitis, intersection syndrome
	Forearm fasciotomy in chronic exertional compartment syndrome
Excision	Bursectomy (olecranon bursitis)
	Tenosynovectomy (e.g. of the extensor tendons)
	Excision of lesions (e.g. olecranon rheumatoid nodules)
	Olecranon spur resection
Harvesting	Vessel graft (e.g. radial artery for CABG)
	Nerve graft (e.g. distal PIN, MCNFA)
	Tendon graft (e.g. FCR, palmaris longus)
	Bone graft (e.g. distal radius and olecranon)
Nerve transposition	Ulnar nerve transposition
Stabilisation	Repair of distal biceps tendon
	Fixation of ulnar fractures/ulnar osteotomies
Reconstruction	Tendon transfer (e.g. extensor indicis to EPL)

CABG coronary artery bypass graft, *PIN* posterior interosseous nerve, *MCNFA* medial cutaneous nerve of the forearm, *FCR* flexor carpi radialis, *EPL* extensor pollicis longus

faster recovery [17, 20]. Furthermore, Cobb et al. [21] have shown that patients experience less pain with quicker functional recovery and return to work. Meta-analyses have shown that in situ decompression has comparable outcomes with anterior transposition but with fewer complications [28, 39]. Additionally, endoscopic technique of olecranon bursectomy has shown faster healing and lower reoperation rates when compared to open technique, leading to shorter hospital stays [13, 14].

18.4 Complications

Potential complications, especially in the early phases of using these new techniques, are related to a lack of appreciation of the anatomy from an endoscopic perspective, familiarity with endoscopic dissection techniques or inexperience with effective use of instrumentation.

Pearls of Treatment

Before any soft tissue endoscopic procedure is performed, familiarity with the open technique is essential and should be utilised as a backup if the procedure cannot be performed endoscopically. A thorough understanding of the surgical anatomy is paramount owing to proximity of neurovascular structures and risks of damage. When using scissors to incise internal structures, for example, the fascia, care should be taken to have limited opening of the scissors and do multiple small releases to ensure safety of neurovascular bundles. Below is a summary of the senior authors' tips for training and development of these techniques:

1. Become competent with the open procedure
2. Develop familiarity with the instrumentation on mock models
3. Attend cadaveric courses and trial on cadaveric models
4. Visit colleagues who are experienced in the surgical methods
5. "Mind map" the procedure, i.e. plan out the steps of the procedure prior to operating
6. Commence with diagnostic endoscopic procedures, before therapeutic
7. Have a low threshold for use of a backup open procedure, or avoid endoscopic procedure completely, if:
   (a) There are difficulties or safety concerns with the procedure
   (b) There is previous surgeries and development of severe scar tissue
   (c) There is a revision or complex case
   (d) Procedure, staffing or logistical issues are time consuming

References

1. Cobb TK. Endoscopic cubital tunnel release. J Hand Surg Am. 2010;35(10):1690–7.
2. Hoffman R. Arthroscopy and sports medicine. 2015. https://www.karlstorz.com/cps/rde/xbcr/karlstorz_assets/ASSETS/3309865.pdf.
3. Lazaro 3rd L. Ulnar nerve instability: ulnar nerve injury due to elbow flexion. South Med J. 1977;70(1):36–40.
4. Miller RG. The cubital tunnel syndrome: diagnosis and precise localization. Ann Neurol. 1979;6(1):56–9.
5. Snider RK. Olecranon bursitis. In: Snider RK, editor. Essentials of musculoskeletal care. 2nd ed. Rosemont: American Academy of Orthopaedic Surgeons; 1997. p. 156–9.
6. Stell IM. Septic and non-septic olecranon bursitis in the accident and emergency department—an approach to management. J Accid Emerg Med. 1996;13(5):351–3.
7. Bain GI, Bajhau A. Endoscopic release of the ulnar nerve at the elbow using the Agee device: a cadaveric study. Arthroscopy. 2005;21(6):691–5.
8. Buehler MJ, Thayer DT. The elbow flexion test. A clinical test for the cubital tunnel syndrome. Clin Orthop Relat Res. 1988;233:213–6.
9. Earnes MH, Bain GI. Distal biceps tendon endoscopy and anterior elbow arthroscopy portal. Tech Should Elbow Surg. 2006;7:139–42.
10. Hijjawi J, Nagle DJ. Endoscopic-assisted fascial decompression for forearm exertional compartment syndrome: a case report and review of the literature. Hand. 2010;5(4):427–9.
11. Hoffmann R, Siemionow M. The endoscopic management of cubital tunnel syndrome. J Hand Surg Br. 2006;31(1):23–9.
12. Iyer V, Thirkannad S. Focal hand dystonia in a patient with ulnar nerve neuropathy at the elbow. Hand (NY). 2010;5(4):453–7.
13. Kerr DR, Carpenter CW. Arthroscopic resection of olecranon and prepatellar bursae. Arthroscopy. 1990;6(2):86–8.
14. Ogilvie-Harris DJ, Gilbart M. Endoscopic olecranon bursal resection: the olecranon bursa and prepatellar bursa. Arthroscopy. 2000;16(3):249–53.
15. Phadnis J, Bain GI. Endoscopic assisted distal biceps footprint repair. Techniques in hand upper extremity surgery. 2015;19(2):55–9.
16. Spinner M, Kaplan EB. The relationship of the ulnar nerve to the medial intermuscular septum in the arm and its clinical significance. Hand. 1976;8:239–42.
17. Watts AC, Bain GI. Patient-rated outcomes of ulnar nerve decompression: a comparison of endoscopic and open in situ decompression. J Hand Surg Am. 2009;34(8):1492–8.
18. Zajonc H, Momeni A. Endoscopic release of the cubital tunnel. Hand Clin. 2014;30(1):55–62.
19. Blankstein A, Ganel A, Givon U, Mirovski Y, Chechick A. Ultrasonographic findings in patients

with olecranon bursitis. Ultraschall Med. 2006; 27(6):568–71.

20. Cobb TK, Tyler J, Sterbank P, Lemke J. Efficiency of endoscopic cubital tunnel release. Hand. 2008;3:191.
21. Cobb TK, Walden AL, Merrell PT, Lemke JH. Setting expectations following endoscopic cubital tunnel release. Hand. 2014;9(3):356–63.
22. Damer t HG, Hoffmann R, Kraus A, Stowell RL, Lubahn J. Minimally invasive endoscopic decompression for anterior interosseous nerve syndrome: technical notes. J Hand Surg. 2013;38(10):2016–24.
23. Dimitrova KR, Dincheva GR, Hoffman DM, DeCastro H, Geller CM, Tranbaugh RF. Results of endoscopic radial artery harvesting in 1577 patients. Innovations. 2013;8(6):398–402.
24. Ho Jr G, Tice AD, Kaplan SR. Septic bursitis in the prepatellar and olecranon bursae: an analysis of 25 cases. Ann Intern Med. 1978;89(1):21–7.
25. Keiner D, Tschabitscher M, Welschehold S, Oertel J. Anterior interosseous nerve compression syndrome: is there a role for endoscopy? Acta Neurochir. 2011;153(11):2225.
26. Khoo D, Carmichael SW, Spinner RJ. Ulnar nerve anatomy and compression. Orthop Clin North Am. 1996;27(2):317–38.
27. Lee AK, Khorsandi M, Nurbhai N, Dang J, Fitzmaurice M, Herron KA. Endoscopically assisted decompression for pronator syndrome. J Hand Surg. 2012;37(6):1173–9.
28. Macadam SA, Gandhi R, Bezuhly M, Lefaivre KA. Simple decompression versus anterior subcutaneous and submuscular transposition of the ulnar nerve for cubital tunnel syndrome: a meta-analysis. J Hand Surg Am. 2008;33(8):1314 e1–e12.
29. Morse LP, McGuire DT, Bain GI. Endoscopic ulnar nerve release and transposition. Tech Hand Up Extrem Surg. 2014;18(1):10–4.
30. Phadnis J, Sabharwal A, Bain GI. Dry arthroscopy of the elbow. Techniques in shoulder and elbow. In Press.
31. Pien FD, Ching D, Kim E. Septic bursitis: experience in a community practice. Orthopedics. 1991;14(9):981–4.
32. Pozzi A, Pivato G, Kask K, Susini F, Pegoli L. Single portal endoscopic treatment for chronic exertional compartment syndrome of the forearm. Tech Hand Up Extrem Surg. 2014;18(3):153–6.
33. Rayan GM, Jensen C, Duke J. Elbow flexion test in the normal population. J Hand Surg Am. 1992;17(1): 86–9.
34. Saharwal A, Phadnis J, Bain GI. New techniques: the future of elbow arthroscopy. In: Savoie FH III, Field LD, Steinmann SP, editors. The elbow and wrist: AANA advanced arthroscopic surgical techniques. SLACK; In press.
35. Tsai TM, Bonczar M, Tsuruta T, Syed SA. A new operative technique: cubital tunnel decompression with endoscopic assistance. Hand Clin. 1995;11(1): 71–80.
36. TU CG, McGuire DT, Morse LP, Bain GI. Olecranon extrabursal endoscopic bursectomy. Tech Hand Up Extrem Surg. 2013;17(3):173–5.
37. Walschot LBH, Phadnis J, Bain GI. Endoscopic distal biceps repair. In: Savoie FH III, Field LD, Steinmann SP, editors. The elbow and wrist: AANA advanced arthroscopic surgical techniques. SLACK; In press.
38. Wasserman AR, Melville LD, Birkhahn RH. Septic bursitis: a case report and primer for the emergency clinician. J Emerg Med. 2009;37(3):269–72.
39. Zlowodzki M, Chan S, Bhandari M, Kalliainen L, Schubert W. Anterior transposition compared with simple decompression for treatment of cubital tunnel syndrome. A meta- analysis of randomized, controlled trials. J Bone Joint Surg Am. 2007;89(12): 2591–8.

19 Ulnar Nerve Problems in Sportsmen

M. Dervis Güner and A. Mehmet Demirtaş

19.1 Introduction

The ulnar nerve is highly susceptible to injury during overhead athletic activity. The combination of valgus forces and rapid extension results in tensile forces along the medial side and compression on the lateral portion of the elbow as well as shear forces in the posterior compartment. This combination is referred to as valgus extension overload syndrome and is the basic pathological model for most sports-related elbow injuries [1].

The ulnar nerve can be injured acutely via a direct blow to the back of the elbow during contact sports. Nevertheless, ulnar nerve injury more commonly results from traction or compressive forces at the elbow due to repetitive overuse during overhead athletic activity. Ulnar nerve dysfunction can be caused by excessive elbow valgus forces (especially in baseball pitchers), compression at the cubital tunnel associated with repetitive stress, or spur formation in the ulnar groove with subsequent nerve compression [2, 3]. Athletes can present with a tingling sensation along the ulnar side of the forearm, hand, and the fourth and fifth digits during activity and with numbness/discomfort in the fifth digit and half of the fourth digit (especially provoked by forced elbow flexion), sometimes accompanied by pain with the same distribution and loss of grip strength [4, 5].

Peripheral nerve injuries account for <0.5 % of all sports-related injuries. Sports-related peripheral neuropathies account for 6 % of all peripheral neuropathies and most commonly involve the upper extremities [6, 7]. Acute sports-related injuries usually result from a collision or fall and may require emergency treatment. Overuse injuries can often occur due to a combination of repetitive microtrauma, inadequate recovery poor conditioning and training, and faulty equipment [4]. Ulnar neuropathy at the elbow is the second most common focal neuropathy of the upper limb in athletes and nonathletes [8, 9]. Ulnar nerve injury can develop during sports training and competition via numerous mechanisms [4].

Nerve injuries are classically categorized as neurapraxia, axonotmesis, and neurotmesis [10]. Neurapraxia is the mildest form of nerve injury and is characterized by temporary motor paralysis, with or without sensory loss; focal demyelination is present, excluding the axon. As structural integrity is preserved, full nerve recovery is the rule as myelin is restored.

Axonotmesis is a nerve injury of moderate severity characterized by complete motor, sensory, and autonomic dysfunction. The axon is damaged, but the structural integrity of the endoneurium, perineurium, and epineurium, which

M.D. Güner (✉)
Department of Orthopaedics and Traumatology, Medicana International Ankara Hospital, Ankara, Turkey
e-mail: dervisguner@hotmail.com

A.M. Demirtaş
Department of Hand Surgery, Memorial Ankara Hospital, Ankara, Turkey
e-mail: demirmeh@yahoo.com

L.A. Pederzini et al. (eds.), *Elbow and Sport*, DOI 10.1007/978-3-662-48742-6_19

form the support structure surrounding the nerve, remains intact. Recovery is slow and may be incomplete. Axonal regeneration occurs at a rate of 1–7 mm d^{-1}, and such regeneration may ultimately reach its target because regeneration is directed along the nerve support structure. Neurotmesis is the most severe type of nerve injury, which is characterized by complete destruction of the nerve distal to the site of injury. Motor, sensory, and autonomic dysfunction are complete, with no hope of spontaneous recovery due to complete loss of the structural integrity of both the nerve and its surrounding support structure; recovery can only occur via direct surgical intervention.

In addition to classifying nerve injuries, it is important to define peripheral nerve injuries related to sports as acute versus subacute or chronic. Acute injuries are the result of immediate compressive, stretching, or laceration forces applied to the nerve. Although acute lesions may result from incorrect athletic technique or biomechanics, more commonly they result from a sudden trauma (e.g., a fall) or a sudden extrinsic force when an athlete is not prepared (e.g., a blindsided tackle). Subacute and chronic injuries, on the other hand, are best categorized as overuse injuries. Overuse injuries develop when the cumulative repetitive overcomes the withstanding capacity of a specific tissue [11]. Most researchers refer to repetitive microtrauma as the defining characteristic of overuse injuries.

19.2 Functional Anatomy of the Elbow Joint

The elbow is a complex modified hinge joint, consisting of three individual articulations: the ulnohumeral, radiocapitellar, and proximal radioulnar joints. In the normal elbow joint, stability is maintained by a combination of joint congruity, capsuloligamentous integrity, and balanced intact musculature [1]. The joint capsule circumferentially encloses all three elbow articulations and offers additional stability, primarily in extension [12]. The osseous anatomy of the elbow facilitates flexion-extension and pronation-supination via ulnohumeral and radiocapitellar articulation, respectively. In full extension the elbow has a normal valgus carrying angle of 11–16°. The osseous configuration provides approximately 50 % of the elbow's overall stability, primarily against varus stress when the elbow is in extension. The remaining stability of the elbow is provided by the anterior joint capsule, the medial collateral ligament (MCL) complex, and the lateral collateral ligament complex [13–15]. The MCL complex consists of the anterior oblique ligament (AOL), posterior oblique ligament (POL), and a transverse band (known as Cooper's ligament) that originates and inserts in the ulna). The AOL is known to be the most important soft tissue constraint to valgus instability of the elbow and is the strongest of the elbow's collateral ligaments, with an average failure load of 260 Nm [16, 17].

The musculotendinous structures originating from the medial epicondyle include the flexor-pronator musculature and provide additional dynamic functional resistance to valgus stress [18]. From proximal to distal, this muscle mass includes pronator teres, flexor carpi radialis (FCR), palmaris longus, flexor digitorum superficialis, and flexor carpi ulnaris (FCU). The pronator teres and FCR arise from the medial supracondylar ridge, the palmaris longus originates from the anterior midpoint of the medial epicondyle, and the FCU arises with two heads from the anterior base of the epicondyle and from the ulna [19].

The ulnar nerve is composed from the C8 and T1 nerve roots. These two roots combine to form the lower trunk of the brachial plexus and the transition into the medial cord, of which the ulnar nerve is the terminal branch. The course of the ulnar nerve continues between the medial head of the triceps brachii and the brachialis muscles. The nerve is posteromedial to the brachial artery and just posterior to the intermuscular septum. The arcade of Struthers is a band of fascia that connects the medial head of the triceps to the intermuscular septum of the arm. This fascial band crosses the ulnar nerve approximately 8 cm proximal to the medial epicondyle. The ulnar nerve then becomes more superficial and enters the ulnar sulcus approximately 3.5 cm proximal to the medial epicondyle. The nerve travels posterior to the medial epicondyle and medial to the olecranon. Then, the nerve enters the cubital tunnel. The medial head of the triceps constitutes the posterior border of the cubital tunnel, and the anterior and lateral borders are formed by the medial epicondyle and the olecranon. The roof of the cubital tunnel is defined by the arcuate (Osborne's) ligament. Osborne's ligament is a thickened transverse band between the humeral and ulnar head of the FCU. The floor of the cubital tunnel consists of the medial collateral ligament of the elbow, the elbow joint capsule, and the olecranon.

After passing through the cubital tunnel, the ulnar nerve continues deep into the forearm, between the ulnar and humeral heads of the FCU.

Potential ulnar nerve entrapment can occur at five sites in the elbow region: the arcade of Struthers, the medial intermuscular septum, the medial epicondyle, the cubital tunnel, and the deep flexor-pronator aponeurosis, although the most common site of entrapment is the cubital tunnel [20]. Recent anatomic studies have reported variability in the level of previously unidentified fibrous bands, which suggests that recurrence of symptoms following decompression could be due to inadequate release of these structures. Researchers have suggested that the proximal and distal ends of the cubital tunnel should be carefully explored to prevent incomplete release [21].

19.3 Biomechanics

The overhead throwing motion, such as the characteristic throwing of a baseball, provides a prototype for evaluating the effects of overhead athletic activity on the upper extremities. As the ball is thrown, energy is transferred from the lower extremity via a kinetic chain toward the trunk to the upper extremity, ultimately resulting in ball release from the fingers. This familiar motion is classically divided into six stages: windup, early cocking, late cocking, acceleration, deceleration, and follow-through. The most significant forces act on the shoulder and the elbow during the late cocking and acceleration phases [22]. Throwing a baseball imposes extremely high valgus stresses across the elbow during these two phases, approaching 60–65 Nm [23–25]. During the throwing motion—in baseball, for example—the elbow moves, during the late cocking and acceleration phases, from 110 to 20° of flexion, with speeds up to 3,000°s-1^{-1} [24]. Additionally, the throwing motion causes longitudinal strain to the ulnar nerve in the cubital tunnel. Maximum strain on the ulnar nerve during the acceleration phase of throwing can approach the elastic and circulatory limits of the nerve [26].

19.4 History and Physical Examination

Cubital tunnel syndrome is the most common entrapment condition of the ulnar nerve. Following carpal tunnel syndrome, cubital tunnel syndrome is the second most common compressive neuropathy of the upper extremities [9, 27]. Symptoms involving the ulnar nerve are very common in athletes that perform the throwing motion, and because of its superficial location, the nerve is susceptible to injuries. Ulnar neuropathy around the elbow can present as an isolated injury and also in combination with MCL insufficiency or chronic flexor-pronator mass tendinosis [1]. More than 40 % of athletes with valgus instability develop ulnar neuritis secondary to irritation associated with inflammation of the MCL, and as many as 60 % of athletes that perform the throwing motion and have medial epicondylitis also have concomitant ulnar nerve symptoms [9, 28–30].

Ulnar nerve entrapment results from both pathological and physiological responses to repetitive trauma [31, 32]. Mechanical factors include compression, traction, and irritation of the nerve. Compression of the ulnar nerve proximal to the cubital tunnel may be due to a tight structure (arcade of Struthers or intermuscular septum) or to hypertrophy of an adjacent muscle (anconeus epitrochlearis or medial head of the triceps). Compression at the level of the cubital tunnel may result from osteophytes, loose bodies, synovitis, or a thickened retinaculum (Osborne lesion).

Compression can also occur distal to the cubital tunnel at the FCU aponeurosis or at the deep flexor-pronator aponeurosis after the ulnar nerve passes between the two heads of the FCU [19].

The pressure within the ulnar nerve when the elbow is flexed and the wrist is extended is known to increase to three times the resting level [33], which is due to compression and physiological stretching of the nerve (the ulnar nerve normally moves 7 mm medially and stretches 4–7 mm during elbow flexion) [31, 32]. As the elbow flexes, an increase in tension on the arcuate ligament and the MCL also increases tunnel pressure. Elbow flexion, wrist extension, and shoulder abduction during the throwing motion can result in intraneural pressure increasing up to six times the resting level [33]. Any tethering of the nerve secondary to chronic changes associated with valgus overload (e.g., scar tissue, calcification of the MCL, traction spurs, and degenerative changes in the ulnar groove) further increases intraneural pressure [28, 31, 32, 34]. Traction on the nerve can also occur due to restriction of its normal mobility [31, 32]. Additional friction on the nerve can be caused by ulnar nerve subluxation or dislocation, which is present in 6 % of the general population [35]. The cumulative effects of prolonged and repeated elevated pressure result in nerve fibrosis and ischemia. During contact sports, medial collateral ligament injury may occur. Acute injuries are treated with primary repair. Decision making about associated transposition of the ulnar nerve depends on type of sports. Scar tissue of the repair and sutures may cause nerve entrapment, while on the other side, transposition of the nerve may lead to a very vulnerable medial elbow (Figs. 19.1 and 19.2).

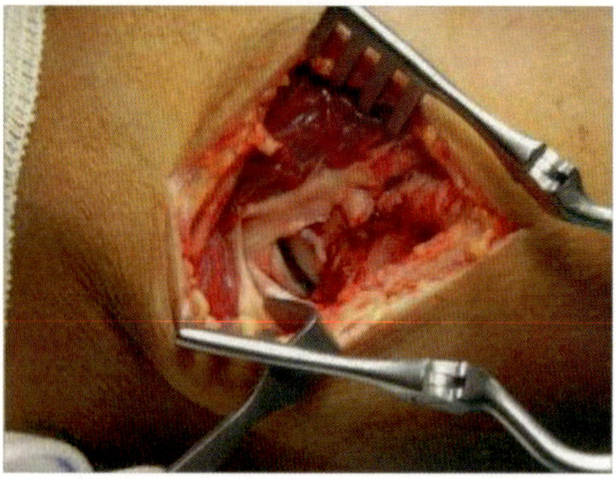

Fig. 19.1 Rupture of the medial collateral ligament in a basketball player

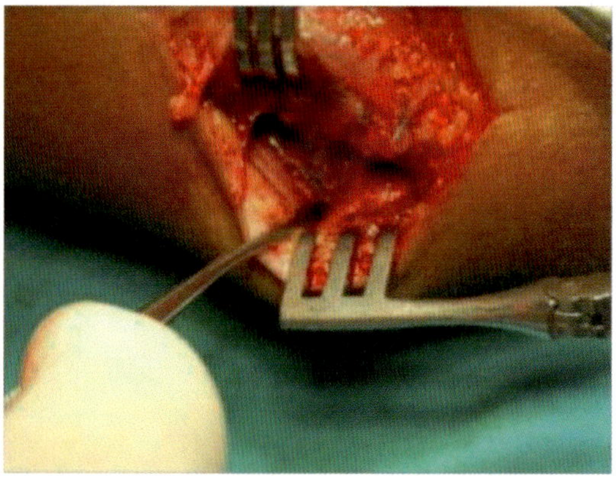

Fig. 19.2 Primary repair of the medial collateral ligament. Ulnar nerve behind the retractor left at the groove

Ulnar nerve dislocation was first described by Blattmann in 1851 [36]. This condition is referred to in the medical literature by various terms, including luxation, instability, hypermobility, and recurrent luxation/subluxation of the ulnar nerve [27, 36–38]. Each term has a unique origin and explanation and emphasizes a different clinical aspect of cubital tunnel syndrome. This rare nerve entrapment syndrome is caused by absence, rupture, or laxity of the epicondylo-olecranic ligament. Dysplasia of the retrocondylar ulnar groove also increases the likelihood of this condition [37].

Subluxation or dislocation of the ulnar nerve is uncommon in the general population, whereas it is reported with greater frequency in athletes that use their upper limbs for forceful and resisted flexion of the elbow joint [37, 39–41]. When the elbow is flexed, the nerve leaves its sulcus and is compressed by the medial humeral epicondyle. In athletes with well-developed upper limb muscles, the prominent medial head of the triceps pushes the nerve further out from the sulcus when flexing the elbow, which might cause rapid development of this pathology [42]. Subluxation/dislocation of the ulnar nerve from the ulnar groove can be palpated via elbow flexion and is often associated with a palpable click [43] (Figs. 19.3 and 19.4). Subluxation or dislocation of the nerve

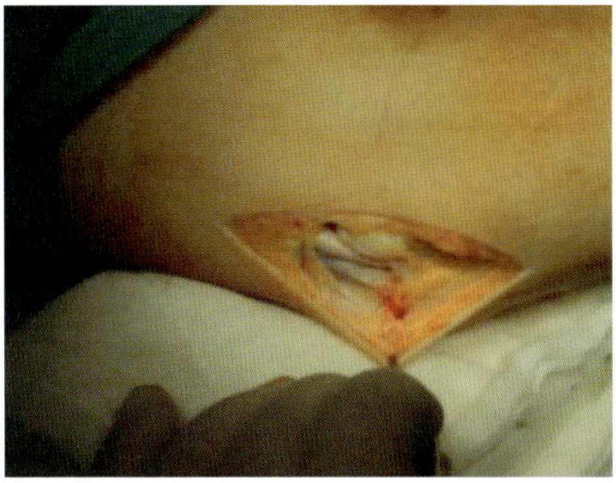

Fig. 19.3 Ulnar nerve within the groove with the elbow in extension

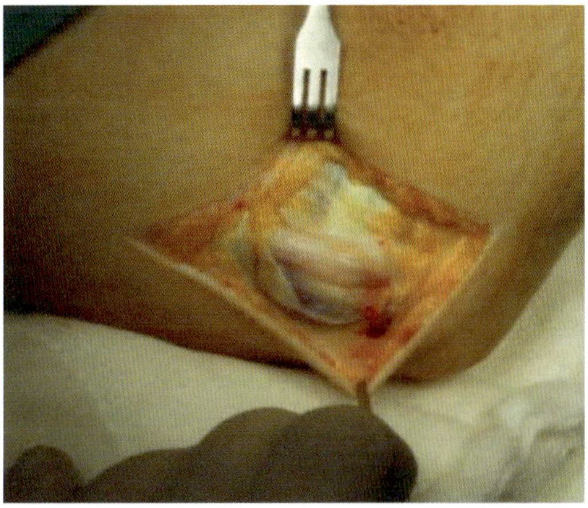

Fig. 19.4 During flexion ulnar nerve dislocates medially. Note hypertrophy of the medial triceps

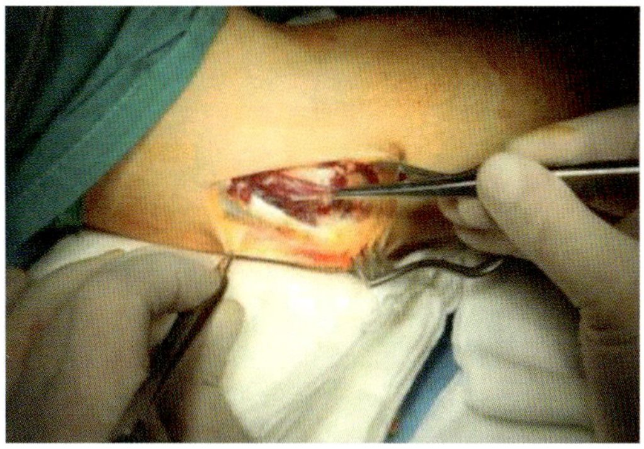

Fig. 19.5 Excision of redundant medial triceps muscle

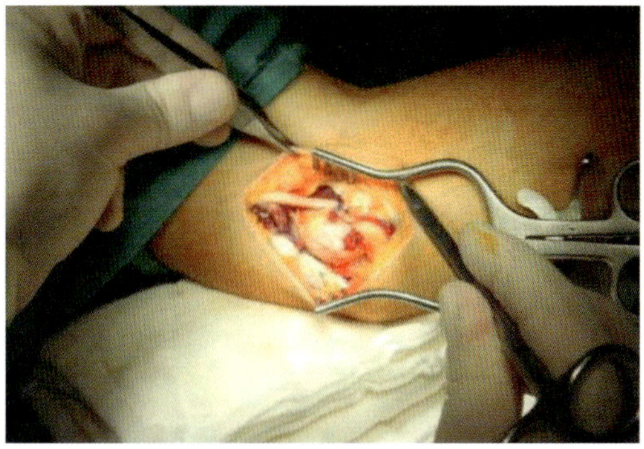

Fig. 19.6 Subfascial transfer of the ulnar nerve

may predispose to neuropathy [35]. Subluxation of the ulnar nerve should be differentiated from a hypertrophic part of the medial head of the triceps snapping over the medial epicondyle during flexion [44] (Figs. 19.5 and 19.6).

In athletes that perform the throwing motion, initial presentation of ulnar neuropathy may be pain along the medial joint line [1]. As inflammation progresses, they may also report clumsiness or heaviness of the fingers on the involved side as well as numbness and paresthesia in the fourth and fifth digits of the hand. Typically, these symptoms resolve with rest and are exacerbated by throwing or overhead activity. Athletes generally do not complain of weakness in the affected extremity—a late finding in ulnar neuropathy, as their performance is usually affected in the early stages before the development of motor changes. Painful popping or snapping sensations may also be experienced in those with recurrent nerve subluxation or dislocation [19].

Careful neurologic evaluation of the neck and upper extremity is mandatory to rule out more proximal causes of neuropathy [28, 31, 32]. Percussion along the ulnar nerve may elicit Tinel's sign. A positive elbow flexion-compression test may elicit tingling that radiates toward the fifth digit, pain at the elbow, or medial forearm pain when manual pressure is directly applied over the ulnar nerve between the posteromedial olecranon and the medial humeral epicondyle as the elbow is maximally flexed [45]. The earliest sensory changes are noted via vibrometry or monofilament threshold testing. Nerve ending density test (e.g., two-point discrimination) becomes positive later, as the condition progresses. Motor weakness, if observed, starts earlier in the intrinsic hand muscles, such as the abductor digiti minimi and adductor pollicis. Intrinsic muscle motor fibers are situated more superficially within the ulnar nerve in the cubital tunnel and are thus more susceptible to injury [19].

Froment's sign (hyperflexion of the thumb interphalangeal joint when attempting key pinch as the flexor pollicis longus is used in place of a paralyzed adductor pollicis) or Wartenberg's sign (the inability to adduct the fifth digit due to unopposed ulnar insertion of the extensor digiti quinti) are positive only in more advanced ulnar neuropathy. Atrophy of the interossei muscles or hypothenar eminence can be difficult to observe in well-developed athletes. Extrinsic muscle weakness, involving the flexor digitorum profundus and FCU, is usually associated with more severe and advanced compression, as the extrinsic motor fibers lie deep within the ulnar nerve and thus are less exposed to damage [19]; clumsiness or loss of fine dexterity may occur in such cases. Inspection and palpation of the ulnar nerve should be performed along its course through the cubital tunnel to determine its location and stability. Palpation of the ulnar nerve in its groove throughout a full range of motion should be performed to identify subluxation or dislocation; the nerve may feel "doughy" or thickened [19]. Ulnar nerve hypermobility has been identified in 37 % of elbows and can be identified by asking the patient to actively flex the elbow with the forearm in supination, followed by placing a finger at the posteromedial aspect of the medial humeral epicondyle and asking the patient to actively extend the elbow. The ulnar nerve is observed to dislocate if trapped anterior to the examiner's finger, to be perched if trapped beneath the finger, and to be stable if not palpable in the groove [38].

Diagnosis of cubital tunnel syndrome is based on a combination of clinical findings and electrodiagnostic test findings; however, in patients with clinical evidence of cubital tunnel syndrome, electromyography and nerve conduction velocities may have a false-negative rate of 10 %. False-negative electrodiagnostic test results may occur as few functional axons are required for a study to be interpreted as normal [46]. Negative tests, however, do not rule out the diagnosis of ulnar neuritis [31, 34]. Plain radiographs of the elbow, especially the cubital tunnel view, should be obtained in all patients to determine if there is elbow arthritis, which can lead to osteophytes and impingement on the cubital tunnel. In addition, radiographs may show signs of instability or previous trauma. Ultrasonography and MRI can be used to identify the presence of soft tissue masses that may compress the ulnar nerve as well as to evaluate the status of the surrounding soft tissue structures [19, 43, 47]. Dynamic sonography of the elbow may be useful for diagnosing ulnar nerve dislocation [37, 38, 48].

19.5 Treatment

Mild cubital tunnel syndrome can often be treated without surgery. There is a tendency for spontaneous recovery in patients with mild and/or intermittent symptoms if provocative causes can be avoided [46]. Nonsurgical management of ulnar neuropathy usually begins with rest, activity modification, ice, and nonsteroidal anti-inflammatory drugs (NSAIDs). Immobilization of the elbow for a brief period (2–3 weeks) may be necessary, especially in cases of ulnar nerve subluxation or dislocation. Local corticosteroid injection is not recommended. Although nonsurgical treatment has a high success rate in the general population, many athletes—especially those with associated valgus instability—experience recurrence of symptoms upon resumption of throwing and ultimately require surgical intervention. Indications for surgery include unsuccessful nonsurgical treatment, persistent ulnar nerve subluxation, symptomatic tension neurapraxia, and concomitant medial elbow problems that require surgery (e.g., valgus instability) [19].

Numerous surgical techniques have been described for the treatment of cubital tunnel syndrome, including simple in situ decompression of the cubital tunnel, anterior transposition of the ulnar nerve (subcutaneous, submuscular, or intramuscular), and medial humeral epicondylectomy with decompression of the ulnar nerve; however, there is a lack of consensus concerning which technique is superior [49]. Simple decompression and medial epicondylectomy are reported to yield poor results in athletes that perform the throwing motion and are not recommended. Simple decompression does not eliminate traction forces on the ulnar nerve, does not address pathological changes within the cubital tunnel, and cannot be performed in the presence of nerve instability. Medial epicondylectomy is associated with a high recurrence rate and destabilizes the nerve, which may predispose to subluxation or dislocation. In addition, injury to the MCL and the flexor-pronator musculature—important secondary dynamic stabilizers of the elbow—may occur and can lead to valgus instability of the elbow, with associated decreased forearm and wrist strength. Anterior subcutaneous transposition provides satisfactory results in athletes and has the advantage of minimizing disruption of the flexor-pronator musculature [50]. The subcutaneously transposed nerve, however, is vulnerable to direct trauma and may potentially develop instability [28, 31, 32]. In addition, the nerve may become secondarily compressed within the surgically created subcutaneous fasciodermal sling, leading to recurrence of symptoms.

Anterior submuscular transposition of the ulnar nerve decompresses all potential sites of entrapment and protects the transposed nerve from both direct and indirect trauma that may be encountered during athletic activity. The transposed nerve lies superficial to the pronator muscle mass and follows a direct course deep to the flexor muscle mass, where it lies adjacent to the median nerve in a fatty plane. This surgical approach also facilitates direct examination of the MCL and the underlying elbow joint for the presence of osteophytes, loose bodies, and other osseous abnormalities. In patients with concomitant valgus instability, repair or reconstruction of the MCL can be performed concurrently using the same approach [28, 31, 32, 34].

A potential disadvantage of submuscular ulnar nerve transposition is the long postoperative rehabilitation period necessary following detachment and reapproximation of the flexor-pronator origin, which must be healed before the resumption of throwing. After 1–2 weeks of immobilization, passive elbow range-of-motion exercises can begin. Active range-of-motion exercises are initiated 3–4 weeks postsurgery, followed by a strengthening program at 6 weeks. At 8 weeks' postsurgery, a supervised throwing program, beginning with light tossing, is initiated. Full, unrestricted activity is usually achieved 4–6 months' postsurgery [19].

19.6 Results

The outcome of anterior submuscular transposition of the ulnar nerve in athletes depends on the degree of preoperative ulnar nerve involvement and on the presence of associated medial elbow problems [34]. Patients with minimal sensory complaints and no motor weakness routinely recover completely and have an excellent prognosis with return to their previous level of function; however, poorer results have been observed in patients with advanced motor weakness and muscle atrophy.

Patients with concomitant medial elbow pathologies such as instability and degenerative changes are also associated with poorer results. Patients with associated valgus instability should undergo repair or reconstruction of the MCL at the time of ulnar nerve transposition, in order to optimize postoperative results. Overall, ulnar nerve transposition results in good functional outcomes in athletes performing overhead motions [28, 31, 32, 34, 50].

Pitfalls of Treatment

Injury to all branches of the medial antebrachial cutaneous nerve must be avoided.

Kinking of the ulnar nerve may occur distally, as it changes its position within the flexor carpi ulnaris and from posterior to anterior to the medial epicondyle.

The arm must be immobilized for more than 2–3 days postoperatively. Weightlifting 1-month postsurgery must be limited to 2 lbs.

Pearls of Treatment

Preoperative distribution of pain can be documented, and the entire upper extremity and cervical spine must be examined.

References

1. Eygendaal D, Safran MR. Posteromedial elbow problems in the adult athlete. Br J Sports Med. 2006; 40(5):430–4.
2. Feinberg JH, Nadler SF, Krivickas LS. Peripheral nerve injuries in the athlete. Sports Med. 1997;24(6):385–408.
3. Lorei MP, Hershman EB. Peripheral nerve injuries in athletes: treatment and prevention. Sports Med. 1993;16(2):130–47.
4. Hainline BW. Peripheral nerve injury in sports. Continuum (Minneap Minn). 2014;20(6 Sports Neurology):1605–28.
5. Hsu SH, Moen TC, Levine WN, Ahmad CS. Physical examination of the Athlete's elbow. Am J Sports Med. 2012;40:699–708.
6. Hirasawa Y, Sakakida K. Sports and peripheral nerve injury. Am J Sports Med. 1983;11(6):420–6.
7. Krivickas LS, Wilbourn AJ. Peripheral nerve injuries in athletes: a case series of over 200 injuries. Semin Neurol. 2000;20:225–32.
8. Filippou G, Mondelli M, Greco G, et al. Ulnar neuropathy at the elbow: how frequent is the idiopathic form? An ultrasonographic study in a cohort of patients. Clin Exp Rheumatol. 2010;28:63–7.
9. Norkus SA, Meyers MC. Ulnar neuropathy of the elbow. Sports Med. 1994;17:189–99.
10. Seddon HJ. Three types of nerve injury. Brain. 1943;66:238–83.
11. Krivickas LS. Anatomical factors associated with overuse sports injuries. Sports Med. 1997;24(2): 132–46.
12. Morrey BF, An KN. Articular and ligamentous contributions to the stability of the elbow joint. Am J Sports Med. 1983;11(5):315–9.
13. Morrey BF. Applied anatomy and bio- mechanics of the elbow joint. Instr Course Lect. 1986;35:59–68.
14. Schwab GH, Bennett JB, Woods GW, Tullos HS. Biomechanics of elbow insta- bility: the role of the medial collateral ligament. Clin Orthop. 1980;146: 42–52.
15. Jobe FW, Kvitne RS. Elbow instability in the athlete. Instr Course Lect. 1991;40:17–23.
16. Regan WD, Korinek S, Morrey BF, et al. Biomechanical study of ligaments around the elbow joint. Clin Orthop Relat Res. 1991;271:170–9.
17. Söjbjerg JO, Ovesen J, Nielsen S. Experimental elbow instability after transection of the medial collateral ligament. Clin Orthop Relat Res. 1987;287:186–90.
18. Davidson PA, Pink M, Perry J, Jobe FW. Functional anatomy of the flexor pronator muscle group in relation to the medial collateral ligament of the elbow. Am J Sports Med. 1995;23:245–50.
19. Chen FS M.D., Rokito AS M.D., Jobe FW M.D. Medial elbow problems in the overhead-throwing athlete. J Am Acad Orthop Surg. 2001;9:99–113.
20. Ochiai N, Honmo J, Tsunjino A, Nisiura Y. Electrodiagnosis in entrapment neuropathy by the arcade of struthers. Clin Orthop Relat Res. 2001;378: 129–35.
21. Karatsa A, Apaydin N, Uz A, Tubbs SR, Loukas M, Gezen F. Regional anatomic structures of the elbow that may potentially compress the ulnar nerve. J Shoulder Elbow Surg. 2009;18:627–31.
22. Anderson MW M.D., Alford BA M.D. Overhead throwing injuries of the shoulder and elbow. Radiol Clin N Am. 2010;48:1137–54.
23. Elliott B, Fleisig G, Nicholls R, Escamilia R. Technique effects on upper limb loading in the tennis serve. J Sci Med Sport. 2003;6(1):76–87.
24. Fleisig GS, Andrews JR, Dillman CJ, Escamilla RF. Kinetics of baseball pitching with implications about injury mechanisms. Am J Sports Med. 1995; 23(2):233–9.
25. Werner SL, Fleisig GS, Dillman CJ, Andrews JR. Biomechanics of the elbow during baseball pitching. J Orthop Sports Phys Ther. 1993;17(6):274–8.
26. Aoki M, Takasaki H, Muraki T, Uchiyama E, Murakami G, Yamashita T. Strain on the ulnar nerve at the elbow and wrist during throwing motion. J Bone Joint Surg Am. 2005;87(11):2508–14.
27. Bednar MS, Blair SJ, Light TR. Complications of the treatment of cubital tunnel syndrome. Hand Clin. 1994;10:83–92.
28. Boatright JR, DíAlessandro DF. Nerve entrapment syndromes at the elbow. In: Jobe FW, Pink MM, Glousman RE, Kvitne RE, Zemel NP, editors. Operative techniques in upper extremity sports injuries. St Louis: Mosby-Year Book; 1996. p. 518–37.
29. Conway JE, Jobe FW, Glousman RE, Pink M. Medial instability of the elbow in throwing athletes: treatment by repair or reconstruction of the ulnar collateral ligament. J Bone Joint Surg Am. 1992;74:67–83.
30. Gabel GT, Morrey BF. Operative treatment of medial epicondylitis: influence of concomitant ulnar neuropathy at the elbow. J Bone Joint Surg Am. 1995;77: 1065–9.
31. Rokito AS, McMahon PJ, Jobe FW. Cubital tunnel syndrome. Oper Tech Sports Med. 1996;4:15–20.
32. Glousman RE. Ulnar nerve problems in the athleteís elbow. Clin Sports Med. 1990;9:365–77.
33. Pechan J, Julis I. The pressure measurement in the ulnar nerve: a contribution to the pathophysiology of the cubital tunnel syndrome. J Biomech. 1975;8: 75–9.
34. Del Pizzo W, Jobe FW, Norwood L. Ulnar nerve entrapment syndrome in baseball players. Am J Sports Med. 1977;5:182.
35. Childress HM. Recurrent ulnar-nerve dislocation at the elbow. Clin Orthop. 1975;108:168–73.
36. Blattmann A. Beobachtung einer Dislokation des N. ulnaris. Dtsch Klin. 1851;435–7.
37. Xarchas KC, Psillakis I, Koukou O, et al. Ulnar nerve dislocation at the elbow: review of the literature and report of three cases. Open Orthop J. 2007; 1:1–3.
38. Calfee RP, Manske PR, Gelberman RH, et al. Clinical assessment of the ulnar nerve at the elbow: reliability of instability testing and the association of hypermo-

bility with clinical symptoms. J Bone Joint Surg Am. 2010;92:2801–8.

39. Capasso G, Testa V, Cappabianca S, et al. Recurrent dislocation of the ulnar nerve in athletes: a report of two cases. Clin J Sport Med. 1998;8:56–8.
40. Kamano M, Koshimune M, Kazuki K. Bilateral recurrent dislocation of the ulnar nerve in semiprofessional swimmer: a case report. Clin J Sport Med. 2005;15:191.
41. Apfelberg DB, Larson SJ. Dynamic anatomy of the ulnar nerve at the elbow. Plast Reconstr Surg. 1973; 51:79–81.
42. Molnar SL, Lang P, Skapinyecz J, Shadgan B. Dislocation of the ulnar nerve at the elbow in an elite wrestler. BMJ Case Rep. 2011;2011:1–3.
43. Peck E, Strakowski JA. Ultrasound evaluation of focal neuropathies in athletes: a clinically-focused review. Br J Sports Med. 2015;49:166–75.
44. Spinner RJ, Goldner RD. Snapping of the medial head of the triceps and recurrent dislocation of the ulnar nerve. Anatomical and dynamic factors. J Bone Joint Surg Am. 1998;80:239–47.
45. Novak CB, Lee GW, Mackinnon SE, Lay L. Provocative testing for cubital tunnel syndrome. J Hand Surg Am. 1994;19(5):817–20.
46. Palmer BA, Hughes TB. Cubital tunnel syndrome. J Hand Surg Am. 2010;35(1):153–63.
47. Mitchell CH, Brushart TM, Ahlawat S, Belzberg AJ, Carrino JA, Fayad LM. MRI of sports-related peripheral nerve injuries. AJR Am J Roentgenol. 2014;203(5):1075–84.
48. Jacobson JA, Jebson PJ, Jeffers AW, et al. Ulnar nerve dislocation and snapping triceps syndrome: diagnosis with dynamic sonography–report of three cases. Radiology. 2001;220:601–5.
49. Soo Bong Hahn, Yun Rak Choi, Ho Jung Kang, Eung Shick Kang. Decompression of the ulnar nerve and minimal medial epicondylectomy with a small incision for cubital tunnel syndrome: Comparison with anterior subcutaneous transposition of the nerve. J Plast Reconstr Aesthet Surg. 2010;63:1150–55.
50. Rettig AC, Ebben JR. Anterior subcuta- neous transfer of the ulnar nerve in the athlete. Am J Sports Med. 1993;21:836–40.

20 Complex Elbow Dislocations

Nuno Sevivas, Nuno Ferreira, Hélder Pereira, Manuel Vieira da Silva, Alberto Monteiro, and João Espregueira-Mendes

20.1 Introduction

Sports practice has become common and important in the daily life, in the general population. Both children and the elderly more often practice sports on a regular basis. In addition to the increasing frequency, the type of sport practiced has also been altered. Extreme sports involving greater speed, height, and a high level of physical exertion are gaining more and more fans. The

N. Sevivas (✉)
Life and Health Sciences Research Institute (ICVS), School of Health Sciences, University of Minho, Campus de Gualtar, Braga 4710-057, Portugal

ICVS/3B's – PT Government Associate Laboratory, Braga/Guimarães, Portugal

Orthopaedics department, Hospital de Braga, Braga, Portugal

Clínica Espregueira-Mendes, FIFA Medical Centre of Excellence, Estádio do Dragão, Porto, Portugal
e-mail: nuonosevias@gmil.com

N. Ferreira • M.V. da Silva
Orthopaedics department, Hospital de Braga, Braga, Portugal

Clínica Espregueira-Mendes, FIFA Medical Centre of Excellence, Estádio do Dragão, Porto, Portugal

H. Pereira
Life and Health Sciences Research Institute (ICVS), School of Health Sciences, University of Minho, Campus de Gualtar, Braga 4710-057, Portugal

ICVS/3B's – PT Government Associate Laboratory, Braga/Guimarães, Portugal

Clínica Espregueira-Mendes, FIFA Medical Centre of Excellence, Estádio do Dragão, Porto, Portugal

3B's Research Group, Biomaterials, Biodegradables and Biomimetics, Department of Polymer Engineering, University of Minho, Headquarters of the European Institute of Excellence on Tissue Engineering and Regenerative Medicine, AvePark, Zona Industrial da Gandra, S. Cláudio do Barco Caldas das Taipas, Guimarães 4806-909, Portugal

Orthopaedics department, Centro Hospitalar Póvoa de Varzim – Vila do Conde, Póvoa de Varzim, Portugal

A. Monteiro
Clínica Espregueira-Mendes, FIFA Medical Centre of Excellence, Estádio do Dragão, Porto, Portugal

J. Espregueira-Mendes
Life and Health Sciences Research Institute (ICVS), School of Health Sciences, University of Minho, Campus de Gualtar, Braga 4710-057, Portugal

ICVS/3B's – PT Government Associate Laboratory, Braga/Guimarães, Portugal
Clínica Espregueira-Mendes, FIFA Medical Centre of Excellence, Estádio do Dragão, Porto, Portugal

3B's Research Group, Biomaterials, Biodegradables and Biomimetics, Department of Polymer Engineering, University of Minho, Headquarters of the European Institute of Excellence on Tissue Engineering and Regenerative Medicine, AvePark, Zona Industrial da Gandra, S. Cláudio do Barco Caldas das Taipas, Guimarães 4806-909, Portugal

L.A. Pederzini et al. (eds.), *Elbow and Sport*, DOI 10.1007/978-3-662-48742-6_20

practice of these high-risk activities increases the number and severity of musculoskeletal traumatic lesions, namely, fractures and dislocations, that can cause severe disability. Therefore, the treatment of these extreme injuries has become more difficult despite the improvement of implants and technical options in recent years.

The elbow joint is a trocho-ginglymus joint, between the humerus, radius, and ulna, with two degrees of freedom [26]. It is composed by three distinct articulations: the ulnotrochlear, radiocapitellar, and proximal radioulnar joints which together enable flexion/extension and supination/pronation.

A stable and painless elbow motion is an important condition for the activities of daily living and the practice of sports relying on the upper limb function. The price to pay for the high mobility of the elbow is the high predisposition to instability, which makes the elbow the second most commonly dislocated major joint in adults and the first most frequent dislocation in children [19].

This epidemiological information is very useful to understand the circumstances associated with injuries and may allow delineating strategies to prevent and treat the lesions. The incidence is approximately 5–6 per 100,000 individuals during their lifetime [17, 53]. The nondominant side is involved slightly more frequently, which can only be explained by our supposed protective instinct over the dominant side.

Complex elbow dislocation is a dislocation of the elbow joint in the presence of a fracture, which usually results in greater loss of function, due to damage to the articular surfaces and the ligamentous structures that stabilize the elbow [24].

The typical patient is a young male that falls onto the outstretched hand during sport activities. A sex ratio of 1.02 to 1.7 times higher frequency in male has been described mainly at the extremes of age, with a bimodal distribution pattern [34, 53]. Approximately 44.5–75 % of elbow dislocations are secondary to sports like football > roller skating > ice skating > skateboarding in descending order. Analyzing the involved sport by patient sex, males sustained elbow dislocations more often in association with football, wrestling, and basketball, and females were more affected in gymnastics and skating activities [17, 53].

There are many possible associated injuries that may occur. We will address the management of the more prevalent categories, as follows:

- Transolecranon fracture-dislocations
- Elbow dislocation with coronoid fracture
- Elbow dislocation with radial head fracture
- Elbow dislocation with both coronoid and radial head fracture ("terrible triad")

20.2 Associated Injuries

Associated injuries complicating elbow dislocation are common and may result in significant morbidity [22]. Radial head and neck fractures occur in 5–10 % of elbow dislocations. Avulsion fractures of the medial or the lateral epicondyles occur in approximately 12 % of the cases, and coronoid fractures occur in 10 % of dislocations. The incidence of associated fractures in children is very high, approaching 50 % [19]. During childhood, while presenting open physes, a medial epicondyle avulsion is the most common associated injury. Incarceration of the fragment into the elbow joint can often occur.

Although pre- and postreduction radiographs reveal periarticular fractures in 12–60 % of dislocations, operative findings have revealed unrecognized osteochondral injuries in nearly 100 % of acute elbow dislocations [15]. Fortunately the vast majority of these injuries are small fractures, which do not require operative intervention.

Associated neurovascular injuries can be devastating but fortunately are rare. Brachial artery injury appears particularly associated with posterior dislocation and should usually be treated with ligation and vein grafting [19]. Median nerve entrapment has been reported with relocation of a dislocated elbow [22]; it may be displaced posteriorly through a space created by avulsion of the medial epicondyle or the common flexor origin, which can cause tension of the median nerve across epicondylar margin and may "notch" the bone, producing a late radiographic sign known as Matev sign [20].

Compartment syndrome can develop after an elbow dislocation due to extensive soft tissue swelling that can result in excessive increased compartment pressures. This situation should be differentiated from neurologic stretch injuries [19]. It is prudent to always have a high degree of suspicion in such cases, especially when the time elapsed between the injury and the reduction maneuver has been long. When clinically suspected and/or confirmed by intra-compartmental pressure measures, an early release of the forearm fascia and the *lacertus fibrosus*, which may exert a constricting effect, should be promptly performed.

20.3 Relevant Anatomy

Stability is provided by a complex and interrelated bony and ligamentous structures, and the constraints are often classified as either primary or secondary. The primary stabilizers are the anterior bundle of the medial collateral ligament (MCL), the ulnohumeral joint congruency, and the lateral collateral ligament (LCL) complex, while the secondary stabilizers are the anterior joint capsule, the forearm musculature, and the radial head [21, 29, 54].

20.3.1 Soft Tissues and Ligament Contributions

The LCL is a complex of ligaments, composed of four distinct structures: the annular ligament, the radial collateral ligament (RCL), the accessory lateral collateral ligament, and the lateral ulnar collateral ligament (LUCL) [42]. The LUCL in particular has been credited with a great clinical significance as a constraint against posterolateral rotatory instability, and its reconstruction after lesion is advised [35, 38].

The MCL has anterior, posterior, and transverse bundles [10, 28]. The anterior bundle runs from inferior medial epicondyle to the sublime tubercle on the medial coronoid process, and it is the primary restraint to valgus and internal rotation stress [31, 41]. This important bundle is itself composed of an anterior band, which is taut from 0 to 60°, and a posterior band, which is taut from 90 to 120°[41]; this configuration provides resistance to valgus loads throughout the whole range of motion [31]. The anterior articular capsule provides significant resistance to varus and valgus stress with the elbow in extension [27]. The muscles around the elbow joint are dynamic constraints, which help to provide stability [1, 49, 54].

20.3.2 Bone Structures Contributions

The important osseous constraints of the elbow are the olecranon, the coronoid process, and the radial head [29].

There is a strict relationship between the amount of resection of the olecranon and the resultant instability: it has been demonstrated that up to 75 % of the olecranon can be removed without compromising stability, providing that other constraints of the elbow are preserved [2, 6].

The coronoid process is clearly the most important articular stabilizer of the joint, given its role as a buttress to posterior displacement of the elbow [29, 54]. The radial head is an important secondary stabilizer to resist valgus force, especially when a deficient medial ligament complex is present [29].

Additionally, the engagement of the olecranon in the olecranon fossa, in full extension, and the engagement of the radial head and the coronoid process in the respective fossae, in flexion, give additional stability in the coronal plane [54].

20.4 Etiology

Most commonly a complex dislocation occurs from a fall on the outstretched hand or on the elbow, but in some circumstances it can result from a high-energy injury. The injury pattern and the associated lesions will be defined by the position of the elbow at the moment of trauma, the direction of the force vector, and the resistance of the different constraints.

Dislocation is considered to be the last of three sequential stages of elbow instability resulting from posterolateral rotation, with soft tissue disruption progressing from lateral to medial. The dislocating mechanism during a fall on the outstretched hand involves the body rotating internally on the elbow, which experiences an external rotation/valgus moment as it flexes [38].

Despite the disruptive forces to the ligaments of the elbow, compressive and shear forces occurring on the articular surfaces are also present and can cause significant cartilaginous injuries as well as associated fractures. Understanding the mechanism of injury is mandatory for an accurate classification and analysis of radiographs, for a correct treatment and aftercare planning.

20.5 Clinical Evaluation and Reductive Maneuvers

A global assessment, including neurovascular status, is mandatory before any reduction maneuvers and should follow advanced life support for multiple-injured patients in the setting of a high-energy injury. Patients usually present with pain, swelling, and deformity of the elbow joint with the inability to carry out active movement. Neurovascular compromise can be resolved with a prompt reduction, but when it persists or it appears after a therapeutic intervention, it may require emergent surgical exploration. Ideally, two perpendicular plane radiographs (anteroposterior and lateral) should be obtained before any attempt to reduction, but sometimes when the dislocation occurs on the field or far away from a Hospital, immediate reduction maneuvers can be performed in the presence of a trained physician, without radiographic evaluation. Expeditious atraumatic reduction maneuvers are very important because they will reduce pressure on the surrounding soft tissues and thus decrease the chance of subsequent secondary neurovascular compromise or compartment syndrome.

Reduction can usually be successfully achieved with a prone traction and countertraction maneuver, by extending the elbow while manipulating the olecranon and the coronoid and clearing the trochlea. Muscle relaxation is the key to obtain an easy and gentle reduction. Care should be taken to avoid multiple reduction attempts that increase the risk for osteochondral injuries. When a reduction is not successful due to muscle contraction, reduction should then be attempted under sedation or general anesthesia and adequate muscle relaxation.

Sometimes complex elbow dislocations can be irreducible by closed methods, and the radial head, the coronoid process, and/or the epitrochlea can be trapped in the soft tissues of the forearm or may be interposed in the joint space. These irreducible dislocations require urgent surgical intervention and should be studied and adequately planned preoperatively with a computer tomography (CT) scan.

After reduction instability should be assessed, preferably under anesthesia, for valgus, varus, and posterolateral rotatory instability. Varus and valgus instability is evaluated with the elbow in full extension and at 30° of flexion. Posterolateral rotatory instability is assessed with the lateral pivot-shift test. A positive test is manifested by a clunk that is heard and felt when the ulna and radius reduce on the humerus [1, 2].

20.6 Radiological Aspects

Radiographs should always be obtained to confirm a concentric reduction and to exclude associated injuries. Abnormal widening of the joint space may indicate entrapped osteochondral fragments, which must be removed surgically. CT scan and magnetic resonance imaging (MRI) are valuable tools, since they can give more adequate information about the associated injuries and thus for surgical planning. CT scan provides optimal definition of bones, and allows 3D reconstruction to assist in surgical planning. MRI provides further information regarding the soft tissues but is limited by posttraumatic edema in the acute setting [54].

Concomitant injuries to the wrist and the shoulder should be ruled out since they are present in 10–15 % of cases. The distal radioulnar joint and interosseous membrane should be clinically evaluated for tenderness and instability to exclude an Essex-Lopresti lesion. When these lesions are clinically suspected, the diagnosis should be complemented with the same imaging exams used for the elbow.

20.6.1 Nonoperative Treatment

In complex elbow dislocations, surgical management is often advised to restore normal anatomy and stability and thus allowing a fast mobilization and maximizing function recovery. However, nonoperative treatment may still be beneficial for some patients, especially in the presence of severe comorbidities or in the case of small fractures without recurrent instability. In such cases a conservative program, with early gentle rehabilitation and a strict follow-up to check the maintenance of a concentric reduction, is started after reduction. Our strategy is to manage these patients in a splint or more frequently a hinged elbow brace, for a short period of time, based on the extent of bony involvement and stability, followed by a pain-free mobilization program.

Before any surgical indication, the decision process must take into account the general health status of the patient, all the vital information provided by imaging examinations, the availability of adequate material (e.g., specific implants like plates, screws, and anchors), and surgical expertise to perform the surgery. Local conditions (e.g., swelling) are not absolute contraindications to surgery.

In the setting of an irreducible dislocation, an associated fracture must be suspected and ruled out. Irreducible dislocations require planned surgery after a correct evaluation with imaging exams.

The tendency for recurrence after reduction (particularly in extension) suggests an unstable joint. Anteroposterior and lateral postreduction radiographs should be obtained to confirm a concentric reduction. Large associated fractures and abnormal widening of the joint space, indicating a possible entrapped osteochondral fragment, usually require surgery.

20.6.2 Surgical Treatment

Indications for surgery, in the setting of a complex elbow dislocation, are unstable associated fractures, postreduction instability requiring 50–60° of flexion to maintain reduction, open elbow dislocation, and an acute compartment syndrome.

An unstable elbow will re-dislocate even with a well-fitting cast or splint (Fig. 20.1 a–f). If this occurs, dynamic external fixation with pins in the humerus and ulna can maintain a concentric reduction while allowing a stable range of motion.

Surgery can consist in open reduction and internal fixation of the fractures, external fixation, exploration, and repair of the medial collateral ligament and/or lateral ulnar collateral ligament. Procedures may be performed alone or combined with each other [12, 37, 51]. Dynamic external fixation is an option that can be considered when the elbow remains unstable even after surgical treatment, allowing an early mobilization while maintaining a concentric reduction (Fig. 20.2).

We will review the specific surgical procedure, according to the injury pattern, and the reported results.

20.7 Patterns of Injury and Specific Treatment

20.7.1 Transolecranon Fracture-Dislocations

In this pattern of injury, we have type III (Mayo classification) olecranon fractures, associated with elbow instability (Fig. 20.3). These uncommon lesions often result from high-energy injuries, which forces an anterior translation of the forearm in relation to the humerus; they are often misidentified with Monteggia fracture-dislocation [32, 33, 45].

Ligaments are typically not involved, so that reduction of the ulnohumeral joint is sufficient to

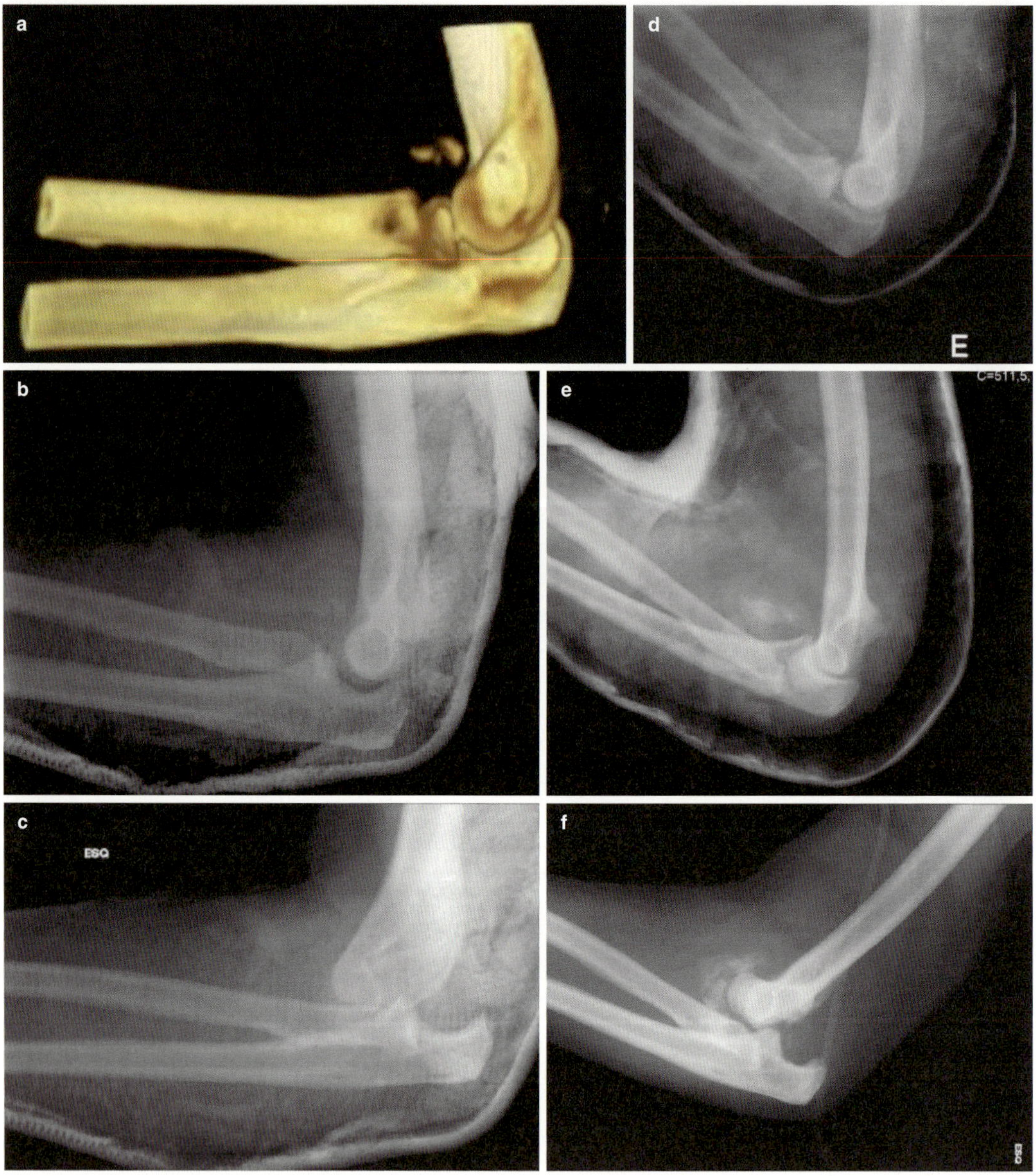

Fig. 20.1 (**a–f**) Complex elbow instability (terrible triad). Conservative treatment was attempted (due to the patient's general status). Instability recurred after hyperflexed and well-fitted cast

restore stability. The important pearls in treatment are as follows:

- Stable anatomic fixation with restoration of the trochlear notch width, preferably with contoured anatomical olecranon plates
- Fixation of concomitant coronoid process fracture
- Preservation of the olecranon tip, even if significantly comminuted, due to the attachment of triceps
- Early postoperative mobilization

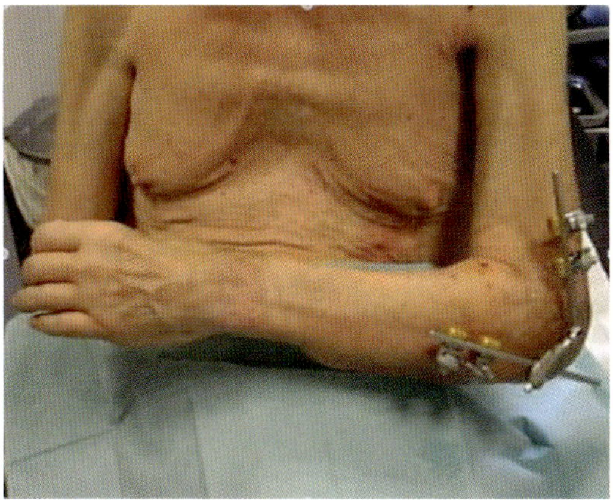

Fig. 20.2 Dynamic external fixation allowing motion while maintaining a concentric reduction

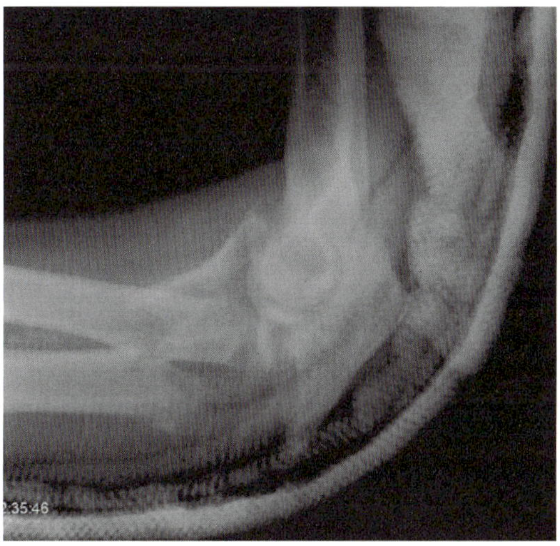

Fig. 20.3 Transolecranon fracture-dislocation

20.7.2 Elbow Dislocation with Coronoid Fracture

Fractures of the coronoid process are relatively uncommon injuries occurring in approximately 2–15 % of patients with elbow dislocation [25, 52]. The coronoid process plays a key role in elbow stability. Coronoid fractures are often associated with other lesions, but their management is usually the fundamental step, defining the postoperative stability and subsequent range of motion.

The first classification system was proposed by Regan and Morrey: coronoid fractures were classified based on the amount of coronoid involved. They observed a directly proportional correlation between poorer prognosis and larger fractures [40]. However, this system does not take into account the whole injury pattern and therefore has limited value in planning operative treatment [54]. More recently, O'Driscoll described a new classification system (Fig. 20.4) that emphasizes the importance of the anteromedial facet [36, 50]. The relevance of this anatomical reference is the relationship with sublime tubercle to which the anterior band of MCL is attached [50].

Coronoid tip fractures are often associated with terrible triad injuries and rarely occur in isolation [43]. However, in isolated tip fractures, some authors have suggested suture fixation [8], while others argue with biomechanical evidence suggesting that small (<10 % of coronoid height) fractures contribute very little to stability and any valgus instability should be addressed by repair of the MCL instead [5].

Doornberg and Ring reported the results of 18 patients with fracture of the anteromedial facet of the coronoid process and they observed concerns with elbow stability in the group with limited treatment of the fragment. On the other hand, the group with secure fixation had significantly better function, according to the system of Broberg and Morrey, and no signs of elbow instability were present [9].

The important pearls in treatment are as follows:

- Fixation of the anteromedial facet of the coronoid (Fig. 20.5) should always be performed, even when the fracture is very small, through a medial approach.
- Small tip fractures (<10 %) usually does not need fixation, but when valgus instability is present, the repair of the MCL should be done.
- Dynamic external fixation is an option that can be added when the elbow remains unstable.
- The fixation methods should be stable enough to allow an early postoperative mobilization.

O'Driscoll Coronoid Fracture Classification		
Fracture	Subtype	Description
Tip	1 2	≤2 mm of coronoid height >2 mm of coronoid height
Anteromedial	1 2 3	Anteromedial rim Anteromedial rim and tip Anteromedial rim and sublime tubercle (± tip)
Basal	1 2	Coronoid body and base Transolecranon basal coronoid fracture

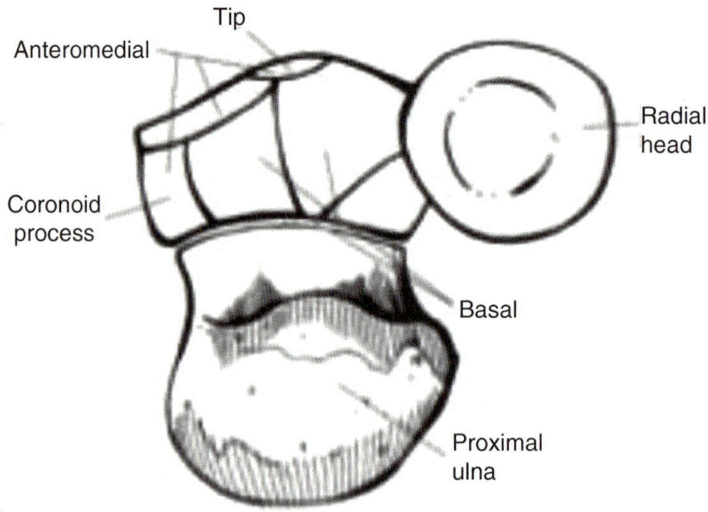

Fig. 20.4 O'Driscoll coronoid fracture classification (Printed with permission)

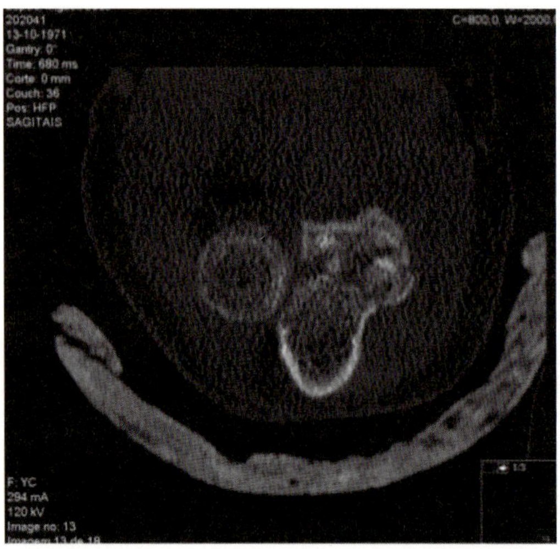

Fig. 20.5 Anteromedial facet fracture of the coronoid

20.7.3 Elbow Dislocation with Radial Head Fracture

Isolated radial head fractures following a dislocation are relatively rare injuries [55]. Josefsson et al. [16] underlined the importance of preserving the radial head to avoid recurrent instability and posttraumatic osteoarthritis. Currently, a more aggressive approach in the treatment of the radial head fractures has been adopted, trying to stabilize them with internal fixation whenever possible. When the resection is unavoidable, because reconstruction is not possible, replacement is better achieved with the use of metallic head prosthesis [18, 23, 54]. Ring et al. suggest that open reduction and internal fixation has to be reserved for minimally comminuted fractures with three or fewer articular fragments [47].

Prostheses have certain drawbacks, such as the possibility of incorrect sizing which may result in "overstuffing" of the joint, inadvertent damage to the capitellum, and loosening. However, when the radial head is not amenable to fixation due to severe comminution, prosthetic replacement in the acute setting is recommended in order to address the underlying resultant instability [44, 54].

Some authors advocate surgical repair of the MCL when radial head is excised because the increased stability allows for early mobilization avoiding valgus instability [3, 16]. However, the ligamentous complexes, particularly the MCL, can heal in the presence of sufficient stability. If the radial head is not reconstructable and prosthesis is not readily available, then the MCL should be acutely repaired in order to restore the coronal plane stability of the elbow and to allow early mobilization [54].

The important pearls in treatment are as follows:

- Internal fixation whenever possible.
- Arthroscopy can help in obtaining an anatomic reduction using minimal invasive procedures.
- Radial head resection without replacement is not recommended due to the associated instability risk.
- If replacement is required, preference is given to metallic head implants.
- In radial head replacement, correct sizing is the key point to avoid overstuffing that can subsequently wear the capitellum and to obtain a successful outcomes.
- If instability is present after radial head fracture treatment, exploration and repair of the medial collateral ligament and/or lateral ulnar collateral ligament should be the next step.

20.7.4 Terrible Triad Injuries

When a dislocation of the elbow is accompanied by fractures of both the radial head and the coronoid, also associated with disruption of the MCL complex, this is known as a "terrible triad of the elbow" [46] (Fig. 20.6). The reason for this eponym are the poor outcomes usually associated with this injury, resulting from an underappreciation of the importance of preserving the radial head or from a neglected coronoid fragment [7, 39].

The coronoid fracture's height in this pattern of injury is on average 35 % of the total height and rarely above 50 % [8]. The coronoid plays a vital role as an anterior buttress and is the key point in the treatment of these lesions. Repairing even smaller coronoid fragments has shown benefit in the final result [8, 14, 39, 46].

LCL complex disruption is prevalent in terrible triad injury and its important role as a primary posterolateral stabilizer of the elbow justifies its repair [21, 39]. On the other hand, although injuries to the MCL are also very commonly associated, being present in 50–60 % of cases, they are not universally repaired [14, 15]. Some authors assert that MCL injuries tend to heal by scarring in simple elbow dislocations and the repair of articular and LCL complex injuries will effectively transform complex elbow dislocations into a simple dislocation, thereby making MCL repair unnecessary [11]. However, other authors stated that the repair of the MCL, as shown in biomechanical studies, is fundamental and that the medial approach may be beneficial to repair fractures involving the medial facet of the coronoid [13, 14, 48] (Fig. 20.7).

In our opinion, the MCL repair must be performed only when posteromedial or valgus instability is still present intraoperatively after fractures fixation and LUCL repair [54].

The radial head fracture is treated following the same principles stated before. The important pearls in treatment are as follows:

- Repair or reconstruct the coronoid process, even when the fragment is small.
- Use an additional medial approach to the repair medial facet coronoid fractures.
- When disrupted, the LUCL should be repaired with transosseous sutures or with anchors.
- Repair the MCL when posteromedial or valgus instability persists after fracture fixation and LUCL repair or when a medial approach is used to fix a coronoid anteromedial facet fracture.
- Dynamic external fixation is an option that can be added when the elbow remains unstable.

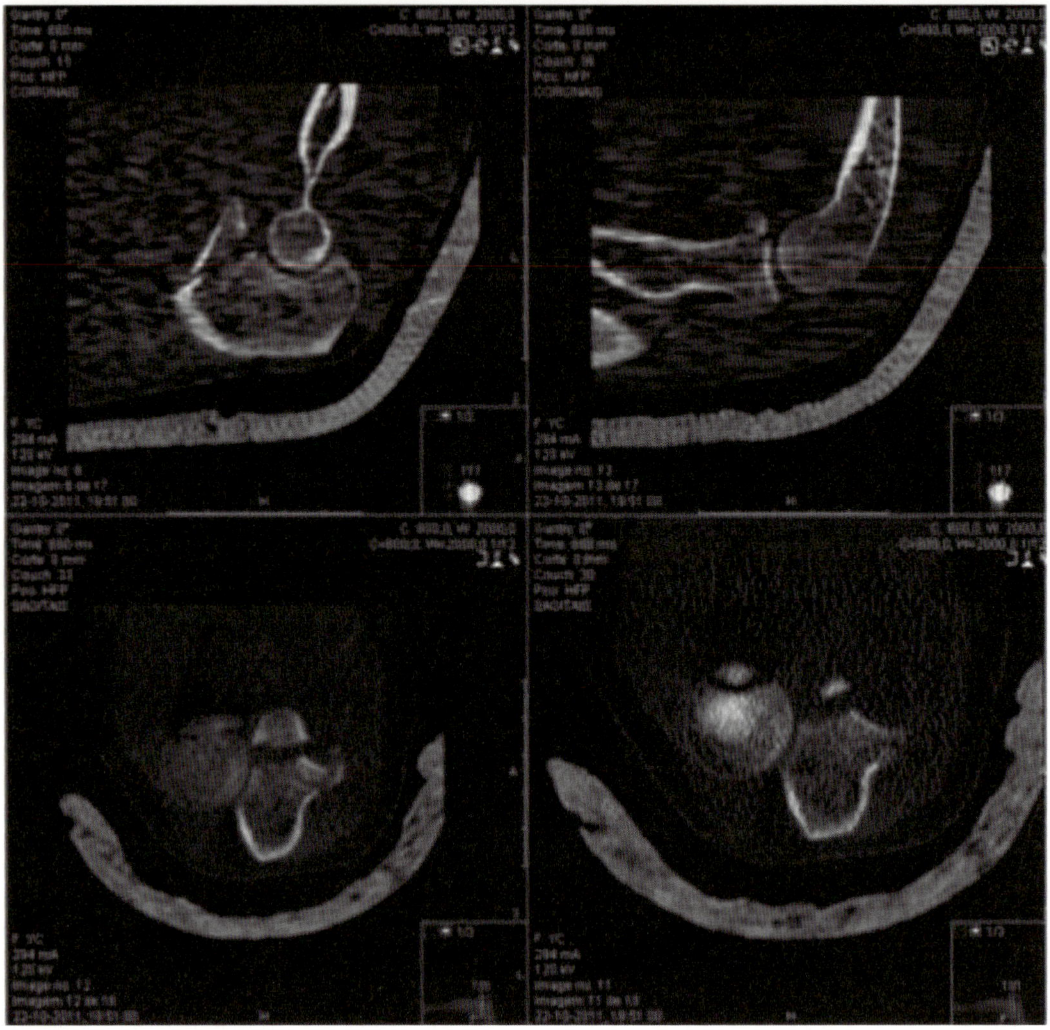

Fig. 20.6 "Elbow terrible triad"

20.8 Rehabilitation

The results of treatment after a complex elbow dislocation are not universally successful. Early mobilization is the key point, but it relies on the quality of stability achieved with the initial treatment.

Hinged elbow braces in the postoperative period can be used to give confidence to patients and to usually start an immediate and safe range of motion as defined by the surgeon; this can be increased every week while soft tissues progressively heal. However, if stability is not a concern, an early and supervised motion program, without any immobilization can give the greatest likelihood to obtain an excellent functional outcome.

Rehabilitation should be closely supervised, with an easy contact between the surgical and rehabilitation teams, and often requires a long period with multiple therapy sessions per week.

20.9 Complications

Posttraumatic stiffness is much more common than instability after a complex elbow dislocation. The likelihood of instability decreases

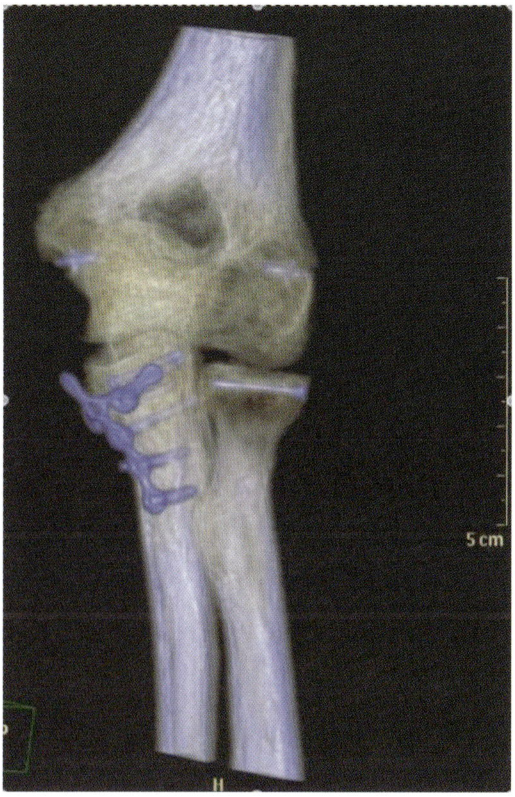

Fig. 20.7 Terrible triad with anteromedial facet fracture of the coronoid that was treated with a buttress plate by a medial approach

significantly when the correct surgical treatment has been established.

Bracing and therapy are not generally useful after 1 year. So, when the functional elbow range of motion defined by Morrey [30] is compromised and does not improve with a well-designed and supervised rehabilitation program, an open or arthroscopic arthrolysis should be considered.

Heterotopic bone formation (Fig. 20.8) occurs most frequently in the neighborhood of the lateral and medial collateral ligaments but also in the anterior capsule above the coronoid process, where it can be very disabling due to the flexion compromise. Excision is performed when there is a functional compromise but is usually delayed until reactive bone has matured, generally at 1 year.

Neurologic complications occur in up to one fifth of the cases. Symptoms range from transient paresthesia to a rare permanent palsy, and the ulnar nerve is the structure most frequently involved. Iatrogenic neurologic lesions can result from the surgical treatment, like following application of a hinged elbow external fixator, where the radial nerve is at risk [4]. Care should be taken during the surgical procedure to identify and protect all the noble structures at risk, in order to avoid extremely disabling complications for the patient and legal concerns for the surgeon.

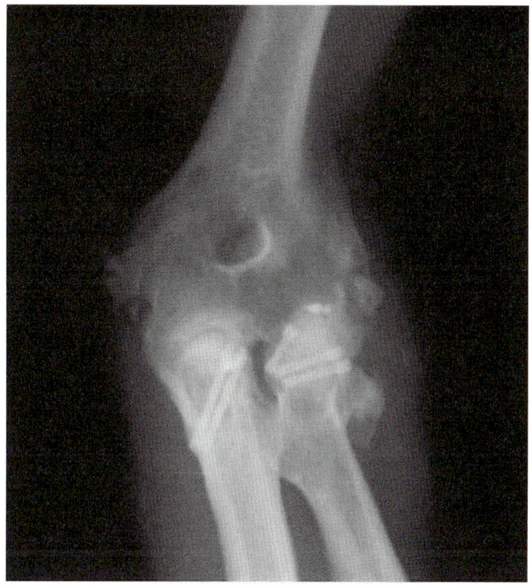

Fig. 20.8 Heterotopic bone formation

Compartment syndrome can result from intramuscular bleeding and edema formation within the flexor compartment of the forearm. Pain with passive finger and wrist extension out of proportion to the injury raises clinical suspicion. Compartment pressures can be obtained to objectively diagnose the condition and is particularly helpful in the unconscious patient, but when clinical suspicion is strong, a fasciotomy must be immediately performed.

An Essex-Lopresti injury with distal radioulnar instability may be present. This injury makes radial head reconstruction mandatory for elbow stability and axial stability of the forearm. If the radial head cannot be reconstructed, a metal prosthesis can provide axial support to the radius and improve valgus stability of the elbow. Temporary pin fixation of the distal radioulnar joint in a neutral position may be added to resist the tendency of proximal radial migration.

Conclusions

High-energy traumatic injuries affecting the elbow joint have been increasing, due to the more frequent practice of extreme sports. Complex elbow dislocation might cause severe impairments, affecting both sports practice performance and activities of daily living. An accurate diagnosis is the key step to a correct strategy and a clear algorithm aiming at the best therapeutic approach. Several technical options have been developed in recent years, which must be considered and thus require continuous study and update. Surgical treatment is hardly the end of the story and the functional recovery of the elbow joint after such injuries often dictates the need for a demanding rehabilitation protocol. These challenging injuries are better treated by a highly experienced team on elbow pathology and surgery. This team should be involved in the treatment as soon as possible in order to achieve the best possible outcome.

References

1. An KN, Hui FC, Morrey BF, Linscheid RL, Chao EY. Muscles across the elbow joint: a biomechanical analysis. J Biomech. 1981;14(10):659–69.
2. An KN, Morrey BF, Chao EY. The effect of partial removal of proximal ulna on elbow constraint. Clin Orthop Relat Res. 1986;209:270–9.
3. Ashwood N, Bain GI, Unni R. Management of Mason type-III radial head fractures with a titanium prosthesis, ligament repair, and early mobilization. J Bone Joint Surg Am. 2004;86-A(2):274–80.
4. Baumann G, Nagy L, Jost B. Radial nerve disruption following application of a hinged elbow external fixator: a report of three cases. J Bone Joint Surg Am. 2011;93(10), e51. doi:10.2106/JBJS.J.00436.
5. Beingessner DM, Stacpoole RA, Dunning CE, Johnson JA, King GJ. The effect of suture fixation of type I coronoid fractures on the kinematics and stability of the elbow with and without medial collateral ligament repair. J Should Elb Surg/Am Should Elb Surg [et al]. 2007;16(2):213–7. doi:10.1016/j.jse.2006.06.015.
6. Bell TH, Ferreira LM, McDonald CP, Johnson JA, King GJ. Contribution of the olecranon to elbow stability: an in vitro biomechanical study. J Bone Joint Surg Am. 2010;92(4):949–57. doi:10.2106/JBJS.H.01873.
7. Broberg MA, Morrey BF. Results of treatment of fracture-dislocations of the elbow. Clin Orthop Relat Res. 1987;216:109–19.
8. Doornberg JN, Ring D. Coronoid fracture patterns. J Hand Surg. 2006;31(1):45–52. doi:10.1016/j.jhsa.2005.08.014.
9. Doornberg JN, Ring DC. Fracture of the anteromedial facet of the coronoid process. J Bone Joint Surg Am. 2006;88(10):2216–24. doi:10.2106/JBJS.E.01127.
10. Floris S, Olsen BS, Dalstra M, Sojbjerg JO, Sneppen O. The medial collateral ligament of the elbow joint: anatomy and kinematics. J Should Elb Surg/Am Should Elb Surg [et al]. 1998;7(4):345–51.
11. Forthman C, Henket M, Ring DC. Elbow dislocation with intra-articular fracture: the results of operative treatment without repair of the medial collateral ligament. J Hand Surg. 2007;32(8):1200–9. doi:10.1016/j.jhsa.2007.06.019.
12. Heck S, Gick S, Dargel J, Pennig D. External fixation with motion capacity in acute dislocations and fracture dislocations of the elbow. Fixation with motion capacity. Unfallchirurg. 2011;114(2):114–22. doi:10.1007/s00113-010- 1929-y.
13. Jensen SL, Olsen BS, Tyrdal S, Sojbjerg JO, Sneppen O. Elbow joint laxity after experimental radial head excision and lateral collateral ligament rupture: efficacy of prosthetic replacement and ligament repair. J Shoul Elb Surg/Am Should Elb Surg [et al]. 2005;14(1):78–84. doi:10.1016/j.jse.2004.05.009.
14. Jeong WK, Oh JK, Hwang JH, Hwang SM, Lee WS. Results of terrible triads in the elbow: the advantage of primary restoration of medial structure. J Orthop Sci Off J Japan Orthop Assoc. 2010;15(5):612–9. doi:10.1007/s00776-010-1515-8.
15. Josefsson PO, Gentz CF, Johnell O, Wendeberg B. Surgical versus non-surgical treatment of ligamentous injuries following dislocation of the elbow joint. A prospective randomized study. J Bone Joint Surg Am. 1987;69(4):605–8.
16. Josefsson PO, Gentz CF, Johnell O, Wendeberg B. Dislocations of the elbow and intraarticular fractures. Clin Orthop Relat Res. 1989;246:126–30.
17. Josefsson PO, Nilsson BE. Incidence of elbow dislocation. Acta Orthop Scand. 1986;57(6):537–8.
18. King GJ, Zarzour ZD, Rath DA, Dunning CE, Patterson SD, Johnson JA. Metallic radial head arthroplasty improves valgus stability of the elbow. Clin Orthop Relat Res. 1999;368:114–25.
19. Kuhn MA, Ross G. Acute elbow dislocations. Orthop Clin North Am. 2008;39(2):155–61. doi:10.1016/j.ocl.2007.12.004, v.
20. Matev I. A radiological sign of entrapment of the median nerve in the elbow joint after posterior dislocation. A report of two cases. J Bone Joint Surg Br. 1976;58(3):353–5.
21. McKee MD, Schemitsch EH, Sala MJ, O'Driscoll SW. The pathoanatomy of lateral ligamentous disruption in complex elbow instability. J Should Elb Surg/Am Should Elb Surg [et al]. 2003;12(4):391–6. doi:10.1016/mse.2003.S1058274603000272.
22. Mehlhoff TL, Noble PC, Bennett JB, Tullos HS. Simple dislocation of the elbow in the adult. Results after closed treatment. J Bone Joint Surg Am. 1988;70(2):244–9.

23. Moro JK, Werier J, MacDermid JC, Patterson SD, King GJ. Arthroplasty with a metal radial head for unreconstructible fractures of the radial head. J Bone Joint Surg Am. 2001;83-A(8):1201–11.
24. Morrey BF. Complex instability of the elbow. Instr Course Lect. 1998;47:157–64.
25. Morrey BF. The elbow and its disorders. 3rd ed. Philadelphia: W.B. Saunders Company; 2000.
26. Morrey BF, Sanchez-Sotelo J. The elbow and its disorders. Philadelphia: WB Saunders Company; 2009.
27. Morrey BF, An KN. Articular and ligamentous contributions to the stability of the elbow joint. Am J Sports Med. 1983;11(5):315–9.
28. Morrey BF, An KN. Functional anatomy of the ligaments of the elbow. Clin Orthop Relat Res. 1985; 201:84–90.
29. Morrey BF, An KN. Stability of the elbow: osseous constraints. J Should Elb Surg/Am Should Elb Surg [et al]. 2005;14(1 Suppl S):174S–8. doi:10.1016/j.jse.2004.09.031.
30. Morrey BF, Askew LJ, Chao EY. A biomechanical study of normal functional elbow motion. J Bone Joint Surg Am. 1981;63(6):872–7.
31. Morrey BF, Tanaka S, An KN. Valgus stability of the elbow. A definition of primary and secondary constraints. Clin Orthop Relat Res. 1991;265:187–95.
32. Mortazavi SM, Asadollahi S, Tahririan MA. Functional outcome following treatment of transolecranon fracture- dislocation of the elbow. Injury. 2006;37(3):284–8. doi:10.1016/j.injury.2005.10.028.
33. Mouhsine E, Akiki A, Castagna A, Cikes A, Wettstein M, Borens O, Garofalo R. Transolecranon anterior fracture dislocation. J Should Elb Surg/Am Should Elb Surg [et al]. 2007;16(3):352–7. doi:10.1016/j.jse.2006.07.005.
34. Neviaser JS, Wickstrom JK. Dislocation of the elbow: a retrospective study of 115 patients. South Med J. 1977;70(2):172–3.
35. O'Driscoll SW, Bell DF, Morrey BF. Posterolateral rotatory instability of the elbow. J Bone Joint Surg Am. 1991;73(3):440–6.
36. O'Driscoll SW, Jupiter JB, Cohen MS, Ring D, McKee MD. Difficult elbow fractures: pearls and pitfalls. Instr Course Lect. 2003;52:113–34.
37. O'Driscoll SW, Jupiter JB, King GJ, Hotchkiss RN, Morrey BF. The unstable elbow. Instr Course Lect. 2001;50:89–102.
38. O'Driscoll SW, Morrey BF, Korinek S, An KN. Elbow subluxation and dislocation. A spectrum of instability. Clin Orthop Relat Res. 1992;280:186–97.
39. Pugh DM, Wild LM, Schemitsch EH, King GJ, McKee MD. Standard surgical protocol to treat elbow dislocations with radial head and coronoid fractures. J Bone Joint Surg Am. 2004;86-A(6):1122–30.
40. Regan W, Morrey BF. Classification and treatment of coronoid process fractures. Orthopedics. 1992;15(7): 845–8.
41. Regan WD, Korinek SL, Morrey BF, An KN. Biomechanical study of ligaments around the elbow joint. Clin Orthop Relat Res. 1991;271:170–9.
42. Reichel LM, Milam GS, Sitton SE, Curry MC, Mehlhoff TL. Elbow lateral collateral ligament injuries. J Hand Surg. 2013;38(1):184–201. doi:10.1016/j.jhsa.2012.10.030; quiz 201.
43. Ring D. Fractures of the coronoid process of the ulna. J Hand Surg. 2006;31(10):1679–89. doi:10.1016/j.jhsa.2006.08.020.
44. Ring D. Displaced, unstable fractures of the radial head: fixation vs. replacement – what is the evidence? Injury. 2008;39(12):1329–37. doi:10.1016/j.injury.2008.04.011.
45. Ring D, Jupiter JB, Sanders RW, Mast J, Simpson NS. Transolecranon fracture-dislocation of the elbow. J Orthop Trauma. 1997;11(8):545–50.
46. Ring D, Jupiter JB, Zilberfarb J. Posterior dislocation of the elbow with fractures of the radial head and coronoid. J Bone Joint Surg Am. 2002;84-A(4):547–51.
47. Ring D, Quintero J, Jupiter JB. Open reduction and internal fixation of fractures of the radial head. J Bone Joint Surg Am. 2002;84-A(10):1811–5.
48. Rosell P, Clasper J. Roles of the medial collateral ligament and the coronoid in elbow stability. J Bone Joint Surg Am. 2003;85-A(3):568; author reply 568–569.
49. Safran MR, Baillargeon D. Soft-tissue stabilizers of the elbow. J Should Elb Surg/Am Should Elb Surg [et al]. 2005;14(1 Suppl S):179S–85. doi:10.1016/j.jse.2004.09.032.
50. Sanchez-Sotelo J, O'Driscoll SW, Morrey BF. Medial oblique compression fracture of the coronoid process of the ulna. J Should Elb Surg/Am Should Elb Surg [et al]. 2005;14(1):60–4. doi:10.1016/j.jse.2004.04.012.
51. Schep NW, De Haan J, Iordens GI, Tuinebreijer WE, Bronkhorst MW, De Vries MR, Goslings JC, Ham SJ, Rhemrev S, Roukema GR, Schipper IB, Sintenie JB, Van der Meulen HG, Van Thiel TP, Van Vugt AB, Verleisdonk EJ, Vroemen JP, Wittich P, Patka P, Van Lieshout EM, Den Hartog D. A hinged external fixator for complex elbow dislocations: a multicenter prospective cohort study. BMC Musculoskelet Disord. 2011;12:130. doi:10.1186/1471-2474-12- 130.
52. Selesnick FH, Dolitsky B, Haskell SS. Fracture of the coronoid process requiring open reduction with internal fixation. A case report. J Bone Joint Surg Am. 1984;66(8):1304–6.
53. Stoneback JW, Owens BD, Sykes J, Athwal GS, Pointer L, Wolf JM. Incidence of elbow dislocations in the United States population. J Bone Joint Surg Am. 2012;94(3):240–5. doi:10.2106/JBJS.J.01663.
54. Tarassoli P, McCann P, Amirfeyz R. Complex instability of the elbow. Injury. 2013. doi:10.1016/j.injury.2013.09.032.
55. Van Riet RP, Morrey BF, O'Driscoll SW, Van Glabbeek F. Associated injuries complicating radial head fractures: a demographic study. Clin Orthop Relat Res. 2005;441:351–5.

Posterolateral Instability in Sportsmen

21

Tyler Clark, Mike O'Brien, and Felix H. Savoie III

21.1 Introduction

O'Driscoll [1] first described how a damaged lateral collateral ligament (LCL) complex could lead to posterolateral rotatory instability (PLRI) of the elbow. O'Driscoll defined diagnostic signs that could lead a physician to diagnose recurrent elbow instability, and more importantly, he described multiple procedures on how to repair this pathology [1]. Although O'Driscoll is credited with defining PLRI, it was a topic that multiple physicians have described before including patients with recurrent signs and symptoms, as well as reports and outcomes of repairs of the lateral ligament complex [2]. It has become an interest to many treating sports medicine specialists as the lateral complex provides varus and posterolateral rotatory stability important to athletes and everyday patients [3]. Since O'Driscoll's paper, our understanding of this condition has greatly increased, allowing improved care and outcomes for our patients and athletes who suffer from this condition.

T. Clark, MD • M. O'Brien, MD
F.H. Savoie III, MD (✉)
Department of Orthopaedics, Tulane University,
New Orleans, LA, USA
e-mail: fsavoie@tulane.edu

21.2 Anatomy

The elbow is a hinged joint that relays on various bones, muscles, and ligaments that provide static and dynamic stability to the joint. The elbow greatly relies on the ulnohumeral joint, medial collateral ligament (MCL) complex, and the lateral collateral ligament complex.

The LCL complex consists of the radial collateral ligament, the lateral ulnar collateral ligament, the annular ligament, and the accessory lateral collateral ligament which form a Y-shaped structure [4–6]. The LCL complex originates from the lateral epicondyle. Macroscopically, the radial collateral ligament and ulnar lateral collateral ligament are indistinguishable [7–9]. The ligament has an average width of 8 mm and lengths of 20 mm. The crista supinatoris, just distal to the radial notch, is where the lateral ulnar collateral ligament (LUCL) attaches [5, 7]. The LUCL is part of the capsuloligamentous complex and is the most posterior structure [10, 11]. The LUCL on average has an insertional footprint of 142 mm^2, an origin footprint of 136 mm^2, and a surface area of 532 mm^2 [12]. The radial collateral ligament inserts and blends into the annular ligament, which encircles the radial head. This ligament is blended with the extensor and supinator muscle origins [10, 13].

The LCL complex is the primary ligamentous stabilizer to PLRI and varus stress [7, 14]. This ligament prevents ulnohumeral rotation in the long axis of the ulna [1]. The ligament is also in

L.A. Pederzini et al. (eds.), *Elbow and Sport*, DOI 10.1007/978-3-662-48742-6_21

line with the flexion axis of the elbow, placing it under uniform tension throughout the flexion arc of the elbow [8].

21.3 Pathology

To produce instability, studies show that it is required for both the LUCL and radial collateral ligament to be disabled [4, 5, 7, 14, 15]. The complex most commonly avulses off of the lateral condyle, which usually occurs from an elbow dislocation. Elbow dislocations most often happen in the sporting population as compared to the general population [16]. The mechanism usually involves an axial compression and valgus force to a slightly flexed, supinated, externally rotated extremity [4, 17]. Although most LCL injuries are proximal soft tissue avulsions, other injury patterns encountered include mid-substance rupture, distal soft tissue avulsion, humeral condylar avulsion fracture, and proximal ulnar bony avulsions [18].

Other injury patterns other than elbow dislocation that causes LCL disruption include patients affected by tennis elbow whom have received multiple steroid injections and patients who have had arthroscopic or open elbow surgery for lateral epicondylitis whom are at risk for iatrogenic injury [4, 15, 19]. Other methods of LCL disruption include those suffering from cubitus varus and those who have undergone radial head excision [5].

Once the ligament has avulsed off of the condyle, it is unable to reattach and heal to its anatomic position secondary to the persistent subluxation of the joint. The proximal free portion of the LCL will move distally upon avulsion and will lie on the joint surface of the capitellum [16].

O'Driscoll has created a classification system for elbow instability due to lateral ligamentous pathology. He reports that his findings begin laterally and, as the disease progresses, circles to medially based structure involvement [20] (Table 21.1).

Table 21.1 Classification of elbow instability

Stage	Definition
1	The elbow subluxates in a posterolateral rotatory direction and will have a positive lateral pivot shit test due to lateral ulnar collateral ligament disruption
2	The elbow incompletely dislocates and the coronoid becomes perched under the trochlea due to all lateral based structures being disrupted including some anterior and posterior capsule involvement
3	Elbow completely dislocates so that coronoid is behind humerus and is due to lateral and medial sided disruption
3a	Anterior band of the medial collateral ligament (MCL) remains intact after dislocation and reduction and elbow is stable to valgus stress
3b	Anterior band of the MCL is disrupted and after reduction the elbow is unstable to valgus stress
3c	Completely stripped ligaments and soft tissue of the elbow remain unstable after reduction and splinting

21.4 Patient History and Symptoms

Most commonly, the patient will present with nonspecific pain and clicking about the elbow. While the traumatic dislocation may produce obvious instability, it is much more common for the athlete to present with a more subtle form of instability, due to multiple small injuries. The injured athlete with these more subtle patterns will not give a clear history of a precipitating event, but rather will, more commonly, describe a gradual onset with slow worsening of lateral elbow pain. When O'Driscoll first described this condition, his patients presented with symptoms consistent with recurrent dislocation of the elbow or of the proximal radioulnar joint [1]. Many patients report a history of an elbow dislocation. Almost half of elbow dislocations occurred in sport, including basketball, football, and wrestling in males and gymnastics and skating in females [19].

Patients who partake in racquet sports such as tennis, squash, and racquetball tend to present with signs and symptoms of lateral epicondylitis (tennis elbow); however, a small cohort of patients will injure their LCL complex displaying symptoms of PLRI [19]. Patients with a history of traumatic elbow injury treated with radial head excision will also display symptoms of PLRI [21].

Patients tend to report instability symptoms when the elbow is extended and the forearm is supinated [1]. Other common complaints include pain, giving way, locking, clicking, or snapping of the elbow [1, 2, 4]. These symptoms usually present with the elbow in terminal extension and with the forearm in supination [21]. A common activity patients will describe that exacerbates their symptoms will be carrying a grocery bag and that the elbow feels unstable [5]. Patients will seldom present with recurrent or complete elbow dislocations [22].

21.5 Physical Exam

Inspection of the injured elbow will often not show any abnormalities, but close visualization may reveal slight swelling along the posterolateral gutter and plica. Palpation is critical in this evaluation to discern the difference between lateral epicondylitis, radial tunnel syndrome, instability, and radiocapitellar arthritis. Sportsmen with instability will not be tender over the radial tunnel and lateral epicondyle but more posteriorly along the back of the radiocapitellar joint. Limited pronation and supination with lateral compression will not be painful, but when valgus force and increased supination in about 100° of flexion is added, the patient will often be tender along the proximal end of the radial ulnohumeral ligament (RUHL) complex and also have increased feelings of instability (Fig. 21.1).

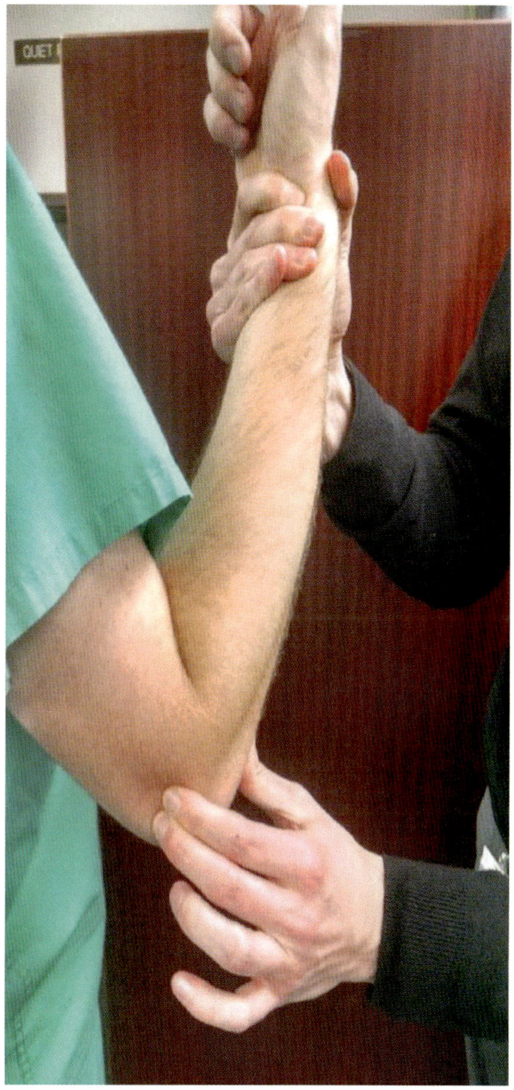

Fig. 21.1 Diagnostic maneuver for PLRI, demonstrating a valgus force applied to a fully supinated forearm at 100° of flexion

O'Driscoll [1] first described the lateral pivot shift test for PLRI. He describes testing with the extremity above the head of the patient, with the shoulder externally rotated. The test begins with the patient's forearm fully supinated; the physician then grasps the wrist and flexes the elbow from extension while applying valgus, supinating, and axial forces to the extremity. If PLRI exists, at approximately 40° of flexion, the dislocated radiohumeral joint will be most visible as a posterior prominence and a skin dimple proximal to the radial head. Continued flexion will result in reduction of the joint, and the dimple should disappear. This test is most accurate under anesthesia (Figs. 21.2 and 21.3); however, patients will present with apprehension when awake from the procedure [1].

In most patients, the O'Driscoll test cannot be performed while awake, so our institution uses a modified test where we palpate the posterior radiocapitellar joint while more gently supinating the

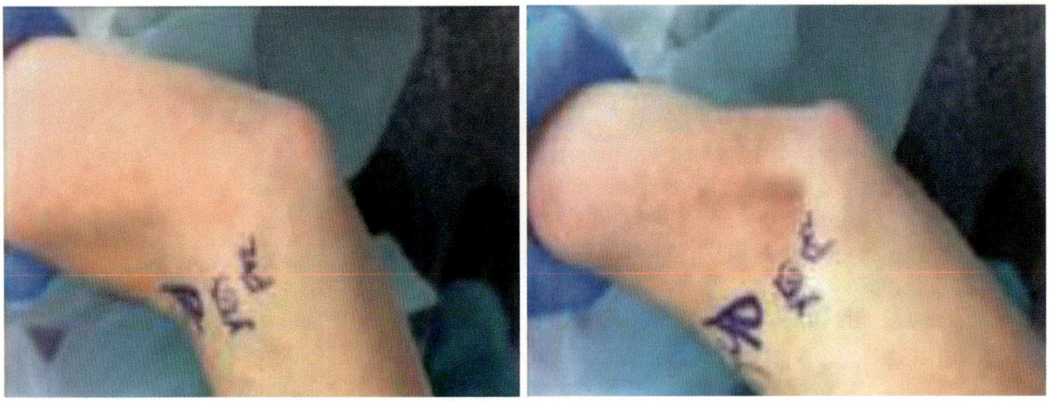

Figs. 21.2 and 21.3 Before and after pictures of the elbow prior to the lateral pivot shift test, demonstrating the dimpling of the skin at the radiohumeral joint

Table 21.2 Diagnostic physical exam maneuvers for PLRI

Test	Physical exam procedure
Posterolateral rotatory drawer	Pull posteriorly on the lateral side of the proximal forearm. Positive result signified by presence of dimple or apprehension
Table top relocation rest	Patient begins with one arm, forearm in supination and presses up on table. Test positive if apprehension at 40° of flexion, and patient relieved if physician presses on radial head
Prone push-up	Patient begins with elbows flexed at 90°, arms abducted, and forearms supinated lying prone on floor. Positive result with dimple or apprehension upon push-up
Chair push-up	Patient begins with elbows flexed at 90°, arms abducted, and forearms supinated seated in chair. While patient pushes down on chair, test is positive if dimple or apprehension

forearm and providing a slight valgus stress. In extension, there is no shifting or pain, but as the elbow is flexed to 90–110°, the radial head can be felt to shift posteriorly and away from the humerus.

Other tests have been determined from further research into this topic that provides physicians a wide array of exam maneuvers to help provide diagnosis for their patients [4, 15] (Table 21.2).

21.6 Imaging

The initial work-up for LCL injury imaging should begin with anteroposterior and lateral radiographs of the elbow. Radiographs of patients' elbows consistent with LCL disruption may show some posterior displacement of the radial head relative to the capitellum or a drop sign (slight widening of the ulnohumeral joint, >3 mm) [4, 19]. Other times a small avulsion fragment off of the lateral epicondyle may be present; however, most patients with PLRI present with negative plain radiographs [23] (Fig. 21.4). Stress films may also be obtained, including anteroposterior films with varus loading. A positive finding would show gapping at the lateral joint of the elbow [23]. A stress lateral can be performed with the forearm maximally supinated and a lateral pivot shift being performed. A positive finding would show a widened ulnohumeral joint and an inferiorly subluxated radial head [23].

Magnetic resonance imaging (MRI) may be used to further evaluate the joint in question. Coronal imaging, slices that are <2 mm slices, provides the best visualization of the collateral ligament complexes [11] (Fig. 21.5). In younger patient populations, the LUCL will appear striated on imaging [24]. MRI tends to show LCL tears at the proximal origin of the humeral condyle. If the patient has PLRI, there can be posterior displacement of the ulna and radial head in

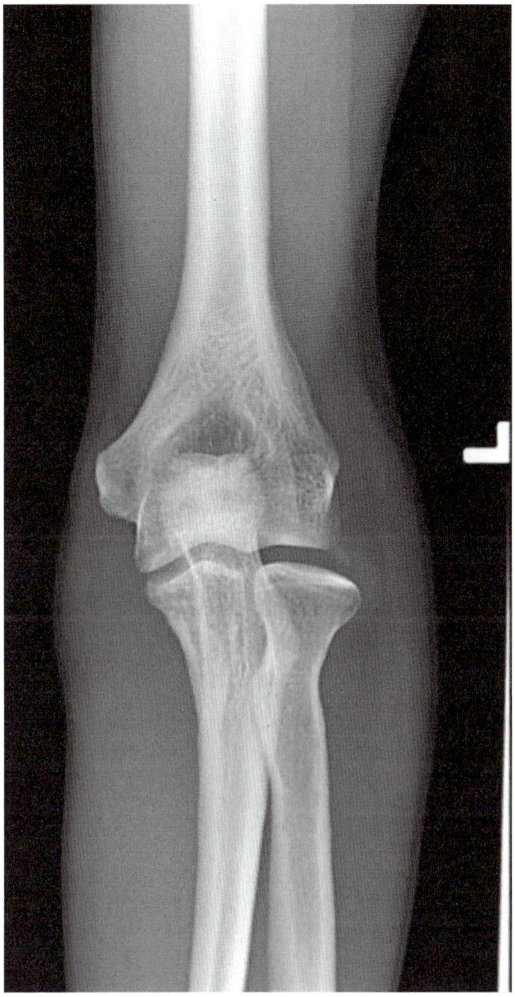

Fig. 21.4 Anterior posterior (AP) radiograph of the elbow, showing an avulsion fracture of the lateral epicondyle consistent with an LCL complex injury

regard to the humerus, and this has been coined as "perched elbow" [19]. It is recommended to detect ulnar lateral collateral ligament abnormalities that MRI is obtained with three-dimensional gradient-echo and fast-spin-echo sequences [11]. The addition of contrast can aid in the diagnosis [25, 26]. LCL injuries will present as ligament redundancy, attenuation, or discontinuity on imaging [11]. An avulsion fracture may also be seen at the proximal ligamentous attachment or underlying marrow edema in the humerus [27].

In most cases, the magnetic resonance arthrogram represents the most definitive test.

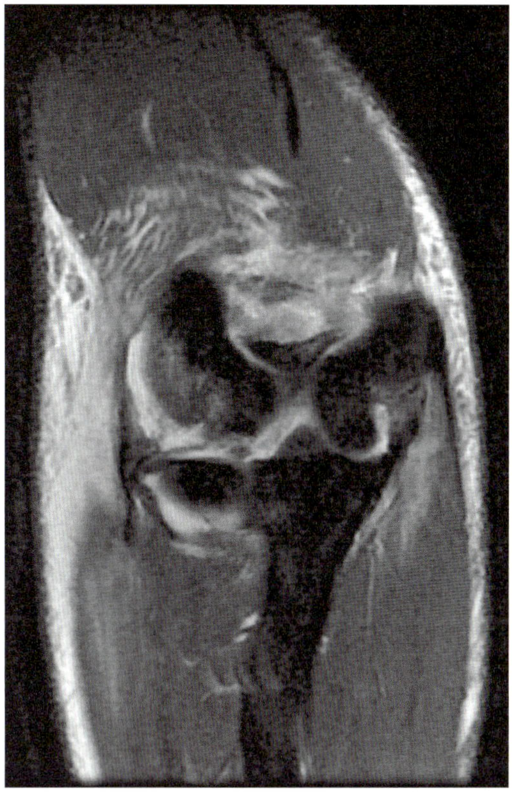

Fig. 21.5 Coronal MRI showing disruption of the LCL complex from the lateral epicondyle to the radius

21.7 Treatment

21.7.1 Nonoperative Management

In more limited instability cases, a compressive sleeve and strengthening of the lateral musculature may be effective. This treatment may be supplemented by topical nonsteroidal anti-inflammatory drugs (NSAIDs) and physiotherapy treatments that allow the athlete to return to sport. Although an attractive option, we were unable to uncover reports of ligament regeneration utilizing biologic supplementation.

21.7.2 Operative Management

The most important is identifying the patients who would benefit from surgery. These include those that are symptomatic with pain, signs of instability, or restrictions in their daily lifestyle [28]. Described are several techniques that have reported success in treating patients.

21.7.2.1 Arthroscopic Repair

Arthroscopic repair is performed in the prone position with the arm stabilized on a bolster. The portals used for accessing the joint include the proximal anteromedial and proximal anterolateral portals for the anterior compartment and the posterior central and posterolateral portals for the posterior compartment.

For an acute ligament rupture, the anterior compartment is accessed first, and a diagnostic arthroscopy is performed. Any hematoma can be evacuated at this time with an arthroscopic shaver. Upon complete anterior evaluation, the arthroscope is placed into the posterior compartment for further diagnostic purposes. At this point in the procedure, it is noted that in an elbow with LCL instability, the arthroscope is able to be placed down the posterolateral gutter across the ulnohumeral articulation into the medial gutter. This is called the "drive-through sign of the elbow." This is only possible in an unstable elbow, and once the complex is repaired, this should no longer be possible.

Continuing down the lateral gutter, one can evaluate the LCL complex and capsule. Visualization is important in this area as the avulsed ligament is often displaced into the radiocapitellar or ulnohumeral joints. Upon viewing of the posterior aspect of the lateral condyle, the normal origin of the LCL complex is noted to be vacant, with evidence of trauma.

The normal origin can be prepared with a soft tissue shaver and an anchor inserted via a straight lateral portal (Fig. 21.6). The sutures can be retrieved out of a clear cannula in the soft spot. Each suture (authors prefer double-loaded anchors) is retrieved using a retrograde retriever placed percutaneously through the ligament from anterior to posterior, creating horizontal mattress sutures (Fig. 21.7). One of the portals can be slightly extended and the sutures retrieved from beneath the anconeus and out the portal. The elbow can be extended to 30° extension and the sutures tied sequentially from anterior and distal to proximal and posterior. While the sutures are tensioned, an adequate repair can be confirmed as the arthroscope should be pushed from the lateral gutter during tensioning (Fig. 21.8). The arthroscope is then placed back into the anterior compartment to confirm restoration of the annular ligament, making this an acceptable repair.

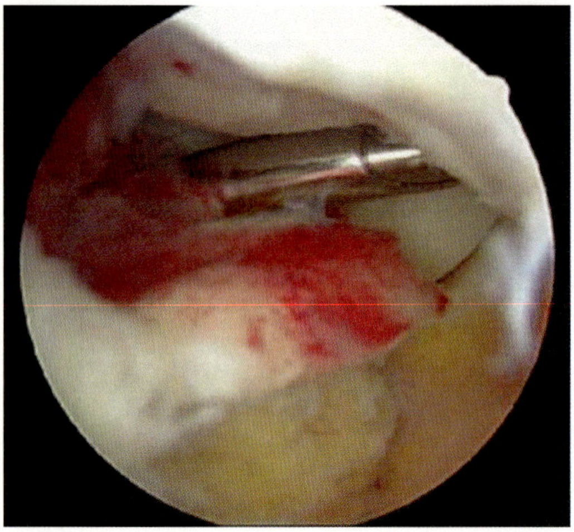

Fig. 21.6 Lateral condyle after preparation with shaver and awl being used for placement of suture anchors

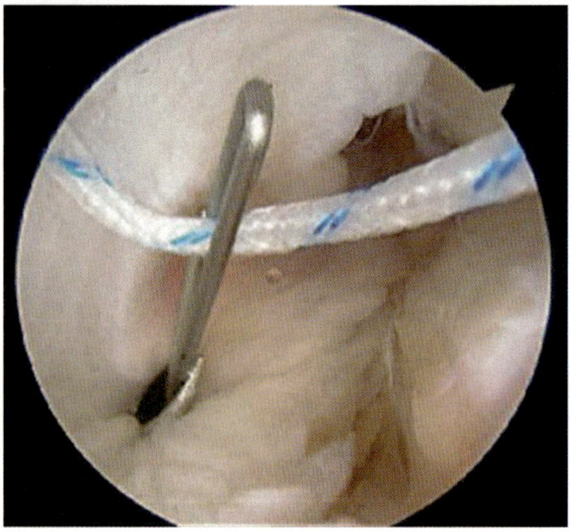

Fig. 21.7 Arthroscopic view of percutaneous retrieval of suture

For patients with chronic ligamentous injury, arthroscopy can still be used to correct the instability. In these cases, absorbable sutures are used to horizontally plicate the ligament complex. Two anchors are normally used, with one at the normal attachment site on the humerus and a

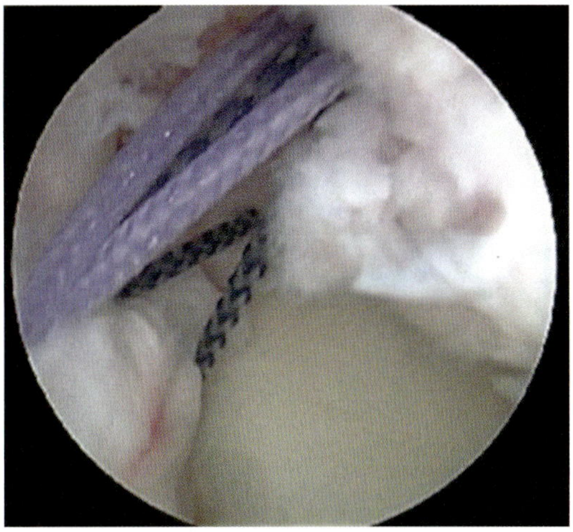

Fig. 21.8 View down the lateral gutter after the sutures have been placed through the LCL complex

second one more proximally. As in the acute repair, the sutures are retrieved using a retrograde retriever, but rather than mattress sutures, one limb is retrieved around the plicated ligament complex and used to shift this complex proximally back to the humerus.

Savoie et al.'s paper on arthroscopic repair found statistically significant improvements with combined objective scores (Andrews-Carson score) and subjective scores [25]. Smith et al. found all 20 patients had satisfactory results after arthroscopic repair of their LCL complex [22]. Spahn et al. reported using arthroscopic electrothermal shrinkage of chronic PLRI, and in 21 patients no complications were seen and all patients reported moderate to good results [29].

21.7.2.2 Open Repair

The practice for open techniques starts with the posterolateral approach to the elbow. The anconeus muscle is split and retracted anteriorly. If there is sufficient tissue to allow for repair, plication can be performed with ligaments repaired back to the humerus as described in the arthroscopic section.

For inadequate tissue or those undergoing revision procedures, palmaris autograft or gracilis allograft can be used. First, identification of the supinator crest of the ulna is dissected free, and the insertion site is identified. A 4 mm bone tunnel is then drilled into the supinator crest to recreate the ulnar attachment of the LCL complex. A small 4.5 or 5 mm interference screw is used to lock the midportion of the graft into place. The two free ends are brought back proximally bringing one end under the annular ligament and one over the ligament. These are then attached to the posterior aspect of the lateral epicondyle (Fig. 21.9). Upon ranging the elbow, the graft should tighten with flexion and be slightly lax in extension.

O'Driscoll et al.'s original patient cohort of five patients all had resolution of their feelings of instability [20]. Sanchez-Sotelo et al. presented 45 patients, 12 with direct repair and 33 with reconstruction, with stability being achieved in 89 % of patients after one operation and 73 % reporting excellent results [30]. Daluiski et al. reported on a cohort of 41 patients undergoing open direct repair for either acute or chronic PLRI. The final mean follow-up Mayo Elbow Performance Scores were 90 (65–100) and 89 (65–100), respectively [28]. Kim et al. discussed 19 patients undergoing acute open repair with 18 cases reporting excellent to good results, and all patients demonstrating a negative lateral pivot shift test at final follow-up [31]. Olsen et al.'s group of 18 patients treated with triceps tendon autograft had 17 patients satisfied with their outcome and 15 returning to normal level of activity [32]. Baghdadi et al. reported on revision allograft reconstructions of the LCL complex with 8 of 11 elbows having restored elbow stability [33]. Cohen reported on 16 elbows with chronic posterolateral instability using an allograft repair and showed that all had resolution of symptoms at follow-up, with full motion returning at 3–4 months [23].

21.8 Postoperative Care

Upon completion of surgery, patients are placed in either a splint or hinged elbow brace at 30° of extension; this relaxes the tension on the repair. Upon successful splinting/bracing, fluoroscopy is obtained to confirm the joint that has been reduced. If not, additional flexion may be added to reduce the joint.

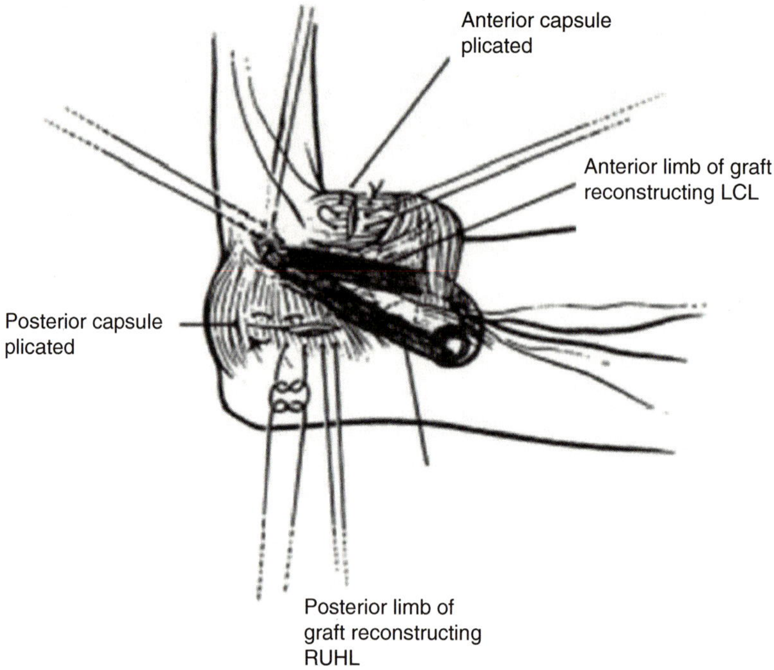

Fig. 21.9 Diagram representing the use of grafts for repair of the LCL complex

Pitfalls

1. Delay in diagnosis due to unfamiliarity with this injury continues despite increasing knowledge of the anatomy and pathology.
2. Physical examination techniques remain elusive, and imaging is often inadequate.
3. The lack of familiarity with the actual ligamentous anatomy, which is often not illustrated correctly in many textbooks, making surgical management somewhat difficult, with some reports showing continuing instability postoperatively [33].
4. Operating on patients with prior surgeries or signs of radiocapitellar arthrosis, who tend to have poorer outcomes [4].

Pearls

1. Listen carefully to the entire history to elucidate the mechanism of injury.
2. Learn how to evaluate the instability on physical examination.
3. Perform cadaveric dissections to truly learn the anatomy; it will facilitate better physical examination techniques as well as teach how to properly restore the three ligaments of the RUHL complex in order to improve the surgical outcome.
4. In athletes, rehabilitation must advance according to soft tissue healing and conclude with high velocity, upper extremity plyometric training before a return to sport is allowed.

The patient returns to clinic several days after surgery, wounds are evaluated, and the elbow is placed in a hinged brace that allows a limited arc of movement. At this point, the patient is instructed in shoulder, wrist, and hand exercises as long as they do not cause elbow pain.

The patient will follow up on 2-week intervals where motion is increased through the brace as swelling and pain allows. Physical therapy begins around 6–8 weeks postoperatively, with full range of motion of the elbow ideally obtained by 8 weeks. Patients must be able to perform the exercises pain-free out of the brace before being allowed to permanently cease of wearing the brace.

21.9 Complications and Pitfalls

The primary complication is recurrence of instability, followed only by postoperative stiffness. Other complications following repair or revision include wound complications necessitating repeat soft tissue surgery, neuritis or nerve transection during surgery, and development of arthritis [28].

21.10 Summary

Lateral collateral ligament complex injuries and posterolateral rotatory instability are conditions that can cause athletes and patients great distress. It can cause acute symptoms affecting play and daily life and can lead to long-term consequences to the elbow joint. It is important for treating physicians to be able to appropriately identify this condition and to deliver patients adequate treatment. Upon successful treatment, patients are provided symptomatic relief and are able to return to sport.

References

1. O'Drisoll SW, Bell DF, Morrey BF. Posterolateral rotatory instability of the elbow. J Bone Joint Surg. 1991;73:440–6.
2. Singleton SB, Conway JE. PLRI: posterolateral rotatory instability of the elbow. Clin Sports Med. 2004;23:629–42.
3. Thornton R, Riley GM, Steinbach LS. Magnetic resonance imaging of sports injuries of the elbow. Top Magn Reson Imaging. 2003;14:69–86.
4. Anakwenze OA, Kancheria VK, Iyengar J, et al. Posterolateral rotatory instability of the elbow. Am J Sports Med. 2014;42:485–91.
5. Reichel LM, Milam GS, Sitton SE, et al. Elbow lateral collateral ligament injuries. J Hand Surg. 2013;38A:184–201.
6. Seki A, Olsen BS, Jensen ST, et al. Functional anatomy of the lateral collateral ligament of the elbow: configuration of Y and its role. J Shoulder Elbow Surg. 2003;11:53–9.
7. Alcid JG, Ahmad CS, Lee TQ. Elbow anatomy and structural biomechanics. Clin Sports Med. 2004;23: 503–17.
8. Bryce CD, Armstrong AD. Anatomy and biomechanics of the elbow. Orthop Clin N Am. 2008;39:141–54.
9. Zoner CS, Buck FM, Cardoso FN, et al. Detailed MRI – anatomic study of the lateral epicondyle of the elbow and its tendinous and ligamentous attachments in cadavers. Am J Roentgenol. 2010;195:629–36.
10. Imatani J, Ogura T, Morito Y. Anatomic and histologic studies of lateral collateral ligament complex of the elbow joint. J Should Elb Surg. 1999;8:625–7.
11. Dewan AK, Chhabra AB, Khanna AJ, et al. MRI of the elbow: techniques and spectrum of disease. J Bone Joint Surg. 2013;95:1–13.
12. Capo JT, Collins C, Beutel BG, et al. Three-dimensional analysis of elbow soft tissue footprints and anatomy. J Shoulder Elbow Surg. 2014;23: 1618–23.
13. Berg EE, DeHoll D. The lateral elbow ligaments: a correlative radiographic study. Am J Sports Med. 1999;27:796–800.
14. Dunning CE, Zarzour ZDS, Patterson SD, et al. Ligamentous stabilizers against posterolateral rotatory instability of the elbow. J Bone Joint Surg. 2001;83:1823–8.
15. Arvind CHV, Hargreaves HG. Tabletop relocation test: a new clinical test for posterolateral rotatory instability of the elbow. J Shoulder Elbow Surg. 2006;15:707–8.

16. McGuire DT, Bain GI. Management of dislocations of the elbow in the athlete. Sports Med Arthrosc Rev. 2014;22:188–93.
17. McCabe MP, Savoie FH. Simple elbow dislocations: evaluation, management, and outcomes. Phys Sportsmed. 2012;40:62–71.
18. McKee MD, Schemitsch EH, Sala MJ, et al. The pathoanatomy of lateral ligamentous disruption in complex elbow instability. J Shoulder Elbow Surg. 2003;12:391–6.
19. Beltran LS, Bencardino JT, Beltran J. Imaging of sports ligamentous injuries of the elbow. Semin Musculoskelet Radiol. 2013;17:455–65.
20. O'Driscoll SW. Classification and evaluation of recurrent instability of the elbow. Clin Orthop Relat Res. 2000;370:34–43.
21. Cheung EV. Chronic lateral elbow instability. Orthop Clin N Am. 2008;39:221–8.
22. Smith JP, Savoie FH, Field LD. Posterolateral rotatory instability of the elbow. Clin Sports Med. 2001;20:47–58.
23. Cohen MS. Lateral collateral ligament instability of the elbow. Hand Clin. 2008;24:69–77.
24. Husarik DB, Saupe N, Pfirrmann CWA. Ligaments and plicae of the elbow: normal MR imaging variability in 60 asymptomatic subjects. Radiology. 2010;257:185–94.
25. Savoie FH, O'Brien MJ, Field LD, et al. Arthroscopic and open radial ulnohumeral ligament reconstruction for posterolateral rotatory instability of the elbow. Clin Sports Med. 2010;29:611–8.
26. Potter HG, Schachar J, Jawetz S. Imaging of the elbow. Oper Tech Orthop. 2009;19:199–208.
27. Wenzke DR. MR imaging of the elbow in the injured athlete. Radiol Clin North Am. 2013;51:195–213.
28. Daluiski A, Schrumpf MA, Schreiber JJ, et al. Direct repair for managing acute and chronic lateral ulnar collateral ligament disruptions. J Hand Surg. 2014;39:1125–9.
29. Spahn G, Kirschbaum S, Klinger HM, et al. Arthroscopic electrothermal shrinkage of chronic posterolateral elbow instability. Acta Orthop. 2006;77:285–9.
30. Sanchez-Sotelo J, Morrey BF, O'Driscoll SW. Long-term outcome of ligamentous reconstruction for posterolateral rotatory instability of the elbow. 18th open meeting, American shoulder and elbow surgeons. Dallas; 16 Feb 2002.
31. Kim BS, Park KH, Song HS, et al. Ligamentous repair of acute lateral collateral ligament rupture of the elbow. J Shoulder Elbow Surg. 2013;22:1469–73.
32. Olsen BS, Sojbjerg JO. The treatment of recurrent posterolateral instability of the elbow. J Bone Joint Surg [Br]. 2003;85-B:342–6.
33. Baghdadi YMK, Morrey BF, O'Driscoll SW, et al. Revision allograft reconstruction of the lateral collateral ligament complex in elbows with previous failed reconstruction and persistent posterolateral rotatory instability. Clin Orthop Relat Res. 2014;473:2061–7.

Radial Head Fractures

22

Bertram The and Denise Eygendaal

22.1 Introduction and Epidemiology

It is estimated that radial head fractures constitute 3 % of all fractures [9], and approximately 33 % of elbow fractures involve the radial head [24], making them the most common elbow fracture in adults. The mean age of patients is 43 years, with 60 % being female [15].

22.1.1 Anatomy and Biomechanics

The elbow consists of three articulations: the ulnohumeral joint allows for flexion and extension of the elbow, whereas the radiocapitellar joint and proximal radioulnar joint, together with the distal radioulnar joint, allow for forearm rotation. The radial head is therefore a key structure during pronation-supination movements. The radial head is elliptical with the articulating dish located eccentrically with respect to the neck [24]. It articulates with the lesser sigmoid notch of the proximal ulna during rotational movements. The articular zone comprises a 250° arc, leaving a non-articular zone of 110°. The latter ranges from 65° in the anterolateral quadrant to 45° in the posterolateral quadrant, measured with the forearm in neutral rotation [5, 12, 25].

The radial head translates an average of 2.1 mm in the AP direction and 1.6 mm in the mediolateral direction during forearm rotation [11].

While the medial collateral ligament provides valgus stability, the radial head is a secondary stabilizer resisting valgus stress, thus becoming more important when ligamentous injury is present [24], in addition to resisting axial and posterolateral rotational forces.

When discussing the treatment of radial head fractures, it is imperative to consider the role of the lateral collateral ligament complex, which is in an intimate relationship with the radial head. This complex consists of the lateral ulnar collateral ligament, the radial collateral ligament, as well as the annular ligament and resists varus and posterolateral instability. It is a known structure at risk for associated injury in displaced radial head fractures, especially when a concommitant dislocation is present. And even when it is uninjured, it is a key structure to bear in mind when approaching the radial head during surgery.

22.2 Injury Patterns and Classifications

Mason classified radial head fractures as nondisplaced, displaced, and displaced and comminuted [18]. Broberg and Morrey later modified this

B. The • D. Eygendaal (✉)
Upper Limb Unit, Amphia Hospital Breda, Breda, The Netherlands

Department of Orthopedic Surgery, Academic Medical Centre, Amsterdam, The Netherlands
e-mail: denise@eygendaal.nl

L.A. Pederzini et al. (eds.), *Elbow and Sport*, DOI 10.1007/978-3-662-48742-6_22

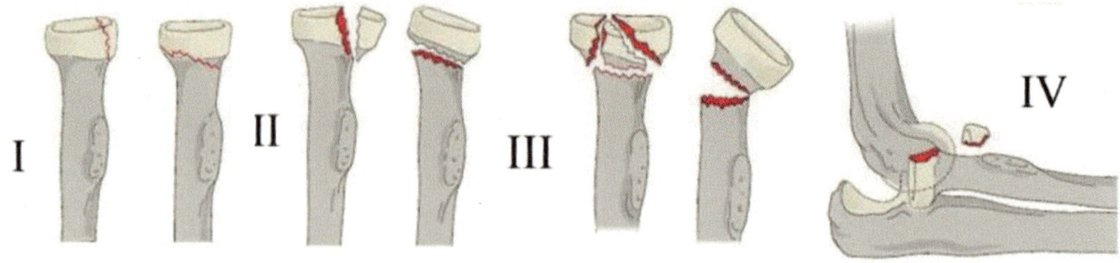

Fig. 22.1 Mason classified radial head fractures as nondisplaced, displaced, and displaced and comminuted [18]. Johnston added a fourth type, which entails all radial head fractures in concomitance with an elbow dislocation

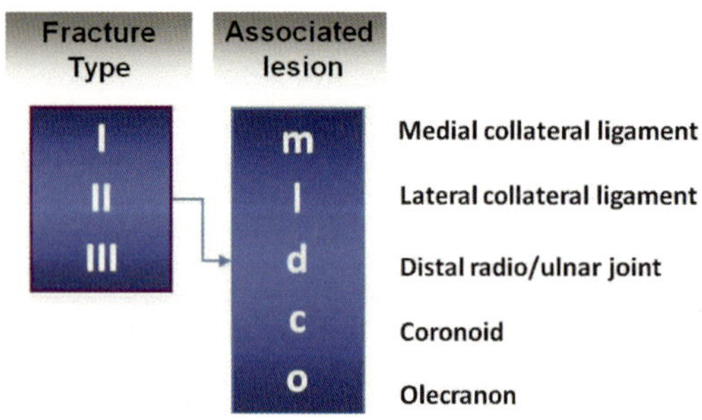

Fig. 22.2 Van Riet and coworkers have proposed a more detailed classification which classifies the associated injuries as well

classification, taking into account parameters of displacement (using a threshold of 2 mm) and size (more or <30 % of the articular surface) [2]. Although an earlier report casted some doubts on the reliability of the Mason classification [20], a more recent report showed satisfactory reliability, outperforming the AO classification [19].

Johnston added a fourth type, which entails all radial head fractures in concomitance with an elbow dislocation (Fig. 22.1). Hotchkiss added treatment recommendations to the aforementioned criteria. Type 1 fractures had <2 mm displacement and no mechanical block during rotational movements and were treated conservatively. Type 2 fractures showed more than 2 mm displacement or a mechanical block and were treated with open reduction and internal fixation. Type 3 fractures were severely comminuted with a mechanical block and were only amenable to treatment with radial head replacement. Van Riet and coworkers have proposed a classification which classifies the associated injuries as well (Fig. 22.2).

22.2.1 Isolated Radial Head Fractures

Nondisplaced radial head fractures are amenable to conservative treatment. They will generally prove to be stable enough to allow for early mobilization. They do not give rise to mechanical blocks or residual locking symptoms and will, almost without exception, lead to bony healing within 6 weeks after trauma. Although seemingly trivial injuries, they usually do give rise to a prolonged period of lateral elbow pain, as well as a slight (but sometimes permanent) extension deficit. This might be indicative of an underappreciation of the true severity of any trauma resulting in a radial head fracture, and the patient is better off being given a heads up in advance on the potentially deceptive nature of this seemingly innocuous type of fracture. The long-term results of conservative treatment of undisplaced fractures are, in general, good. It is mostly the displaced partial articular (Mason type 2) fractures that lead to debates whether conservative or operative treatment should be recommended. A commonly used criterium for operative intervention, when considering the appearance of the fracture fragment, is a displacement of more than 2 mm and a size of the fragment entailing more than 30 % of the articular surface. This is also reflected in the classifications as earlier described. There is some evidence that a more conservative approach might be justified [26], and some surgeons only resort to surgical intervention in case of a mechanical block or other absolute indications for surgery. When opting for operative treatment, it can be noted that the fracture fragment is usually located within the anterolateral quadrant of

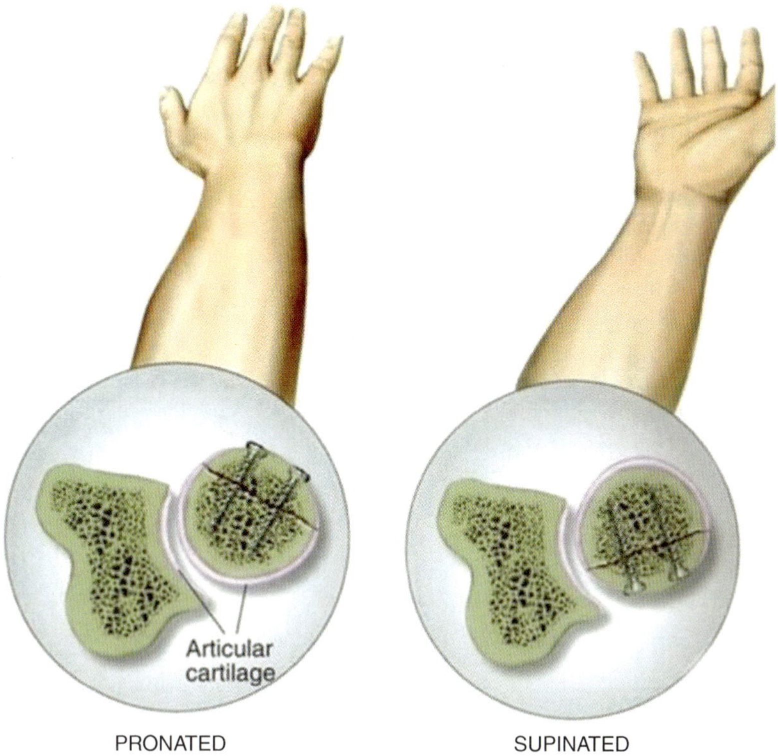

Fig. 22.3 The fracture fragment is usually located within the anterolateral quadrant of the radial head with the forearm in neutral. This corresponds well to the non-articular part of the rim which allows for placement of screws or other fixation devices as desired without compromising the true articular surface

the radial head with the forearm in neutral. This corresponds well to the non-articular part of the rim which allows for placement of screws or other fixation devices as desired without compromising the true articular surface (Fig. 22.3). It should be borne in mind, however, that this also means that, when inadvertently penetrating the overlying cortex, the other end of the screw always ends up damaging the articular surface.

Complete articular fractures with displacement are candidates for surgical intervention and will usually be treated with ORIF or, if not amenable to reconstruction, prosthetic replacement. When the fracture consists of three large fragments, it is usually feasible to reconstruct the articular surface in a satisfactory manner. But even in more comminuted patterns, it might be worthwhile trying to retain the patient's own joint, when the patient is young and active. If reconstruction is not deemed a viable option, the most common alternative is prosthetic replacement of the radial head.

22.2.2 Associated Injuries

Certain radiographic patterns of fracture may be predictive of the presence of other fractures of the elbow or concomitant ligament injuries, thus representing a complex injury pattern. In a series of 121 Mason type 2 fractures, the presence of a fracture fragment that lacked cortical contact with the rest of the proximal radius was associated with such concomitant lesions in 91 % of cases, while this was 33 % when cortical contact remained [23].

The interobserver agreement of determining the lack or presence of cortical contact using AP and lateral x-rays was reported to be moderate [3]. Future studies may clarify the potential added value of CT scans for this particular purpose.

Another study confirmed in a series of 18 patients who were clinically suspected for longitudinal forearm injury that no lesion of the interosseous membrane was present in Mason 1 radial head fractures, as confirmed by MRI. Both Mason 2 and 3 classified radial head fractures were associated with partial or complete tearing of the interosseous membrane in this small series of clinically suspect patients. It was also noted that a substantial part of patients, even those with an intact interosseous membrane, showed edema in the pronator quadratus muscle. This finding correlated with distal forearm pain.

22.2.3 Elbow Dislocations with Radial Head Fracture

Elbow dislocations with a concommitant radial head fracture are typically part of the terrible triad, in which a coronoid fracture and injury of the lateral ulnar collateral ligament are also present. The negative connotation with this injury, as reflected in its given name, is a remnant of the historically poor results originally obtained when treating these patients. Modern insight in the key elements of this injury and advances in the surgical treatment have led to reproducible and generally good results [22]. It might still be an "unhappy" triad, but calling it "terrible" does not seem to be entirely appropriate these days. Conservative treatment is the exception to the rule in this injury pattern. Prerequisites are a radial head fracture and coronoid fracture type that are both fit for conservative treatment, as well as an elbow which is stable from full flexion to at least 45° of flexion. A cast with the elbow in 90° of flexion and full pronation is applied for the first 10 days, followed by dynamic bracing with a progressively more lenient extension block or a removable splint in 30° of extension. Keeping the forearm in pronation during the first weeks unloads the lateral ulnar collateral ligament, as in pronation the radial head is firmly reduced against the capitellum and creates the best chance of healing of this structure without attenuation.

The mainstay of treating the unhappy triad remains surgical intervention. Preoperative imaging, including a CT scan with 3D reconstruction, is helpful in making a tailor-made plan for the individual patient. When performing the surgery, the injuries are assessed from outside-in, while treatment advances from inside-out. This means that the injury to the lateral ulnar collateral ligament is identified first. It is usually avulsed from the proximal (humeral) attachment. Next, the radial head fracture is assessed. If it is deemed to be reconstructible, reconstruction is first delayed until the coronoid fracture has been addressed.

If the decision is made to replace the radial head by a prosthesis, the resection is done next (but no prosthesis is implanted yet) to enhance visualization of the coronoid fragment. Then, starting from the innermost injury, the stepwise treatment is initiated and the coronoid injury is addressed. If it is a mere flake fragment, it might be left untouched. Preoperative imaging might however underappreciate the true size of the coronoid fragment, and, if feasible, any substantial fragment should be reduced and fixed with either screws, transosseous sutures, or suture anchors. Next, the radial head is either fixed or replaced. Finally the lateral ulnar collateral ligament is reattached to its origin. Postoperative rehabilitation is dictated by the stability of the radial head (prosthesis or osteosynthesis) and the quality of the fixation of the coronoid. In general we apply a plaster for 10 days, replace the plaster by a removable cast, and start mobilization against gravity by a specialized physiotherapist. Axial loading is forbidden for 3–4 months as is forceful lifting in supination.

22.3 Presentation and Clinical Exam

Taking a careful history and taking into account the mechanism of injury may lead to important clues to the severity of injury and potential associated injuries. Although some patients are perfectly able to point out the lateral side of the elbow to be involved in the injury, others are not. A careful examination of the elbow will usually reveal tenderness at the lateral side. Both flexion and extension are usually limited as a consequence of the resulting hemarthrosis. Rotational movements may elicit pain or even a mechanical block.

The latter is regarded a strong indication for surgical treatment.

Even after identifying the radial head as the potential site of injury, the remainder of osseous and ligamentous structures should be assessed as well. A concomitant examination of the entire upper extremity is needed to rule out concommitant injury either proximal or distal to the elbow, such as an Essex-Lopresti forearm dissociation.

22.4 Imaging

Conventional x-rays are the mainstay of confirming the diagnosis of a radial head fracture. In the undisplaced fracture type (Mason 1), the only radiographic clue might be a positive fat pad sign. The anterior fat pad is, especially in younger patients, sometimes also visible in the uninjured elbow, but a visible posterior fat pad is highly suggestive of intra-articular fluid or hemarthrosis.

Displaced or comminuted radial head fractures are usually readily visible, although the exact amount of displacement, the percentage of damaged articular surface, and severity of comminution can be difficult to establish.

When relying on these criteria for determining the definitive treatment, a CT scan may be helpful. Evidence suggests that the addition of 3D CT images can lead to improvement of reliability of classifying radial head fractures according to the Broberg and Morrey modification of the Mason classification. Moreover, it seems to lead to a higher sensitivity to detect radial neck fracture and comminution, articular gaps, step off of at least 2 mm, and impaction of the articular surface. The amount of displacement is often overestimated at standard radiographs, while the comminution is often underestimated [13].

22.5 Treatment Options, Complications, and Outcome

22.5.1 Conservative Treatment

A Cochrane review published in 2014 found two randomized controlled trials comparing aspiration versus no aspiration for treating radial head fractures in adults [10]. The two trials included 126 participants, but results were provided for 108 patients only. One trial included Mason 1, 2, and 3 fractures as well as a few cases with hemarthrosis with clinical suspicion of a fracture, but, besides a positive fat pad sign, no clear radiological sign of fracture after trauma [14]. The other trial included Mason types 1 and 2 fractures only [7]. All cases were treated conservatively. The substantial risk of bias in both studies led the authors of the Cochrane review to downgrade the level of evidence to "very low quality", concluding that there is insufficient evidence to determine the effectiveness of joint aspiration for the initial treatment of radial head fractures in terms of function, pain, and range of motion or to determine the safety of the procedure.

One paper reported a 92 % satisfaction rate in a conservatively treated cohort at a mean follow-up duration of 10 years [8]. This comprised only of skeletally mature patients who sustained an isolated injury to the head or neck, classified as a Mason type 1 or 2 fracture. Only 2 patients out of this cohort of 100 patients needed secondary surgery: the first case was an ORIF due to a persistent mechanical block at 10 days post injury (Mason type 2), and the second case was a radial head excision at 8 years post injury due to persistent pain and clicking (Mason type 1). They noted a correlation between the amount of displacement of the fracture – varying from 0 to 5 mm in their series – and a higher DASH score, implicating more disability. Although not statistically significant at a p value of 0.07, they reported a potential cutoff value of 4 mm, where displacement of > = 4 mm resulted in a mean DASH score of 13.7, whereas less displacement resulted in a mean DASH score of 5.2. Other negative predictors of outcome (i.e., a higher DASH score) were age, the presence of comorbidity, socioeconomic deprivation, and the involvement in compensation proceedings.

No prospective, randomized study to compare conservative treatment versus open reduction and internal fixation of stable, but displaced (Mason type 2) fractures has been published yet.

Future studies are still needed to clarify issues in this ongoing discussion [4].

22.5.2 Surgery: ORIF, Resection, Arthroscopy, and Arthroplasty

22.5.2.1 Approach

The aim of the surgical approach is to provide adequate and preferably extensile exposure of the radial head with a safe distance to the main neurovascular structures at all times and safe handling of the ligaments stabilizing the joint. It should allow for early mobilization of the elbow joint and minimize the chances of joint contracture [21].

With better understanding of the importance of the lateral ulnar collateral ligament in preventing posterolateral rotatory instability, the traditional Kocher approach has been modified to perform a slightly more anterior capsulotomy after anterior mobilization of the extensor carpi ulnaris, keeping the anconeus muscle on the posterior side.

The Kaplan approach is slightly more anteriorly oriented as it uses an intermuscular plane between the anterior border of the extensor digitorum communis (EDC) and the extensor carpi radialis longus (ECRL). The interval can be identified by locating the vessels, penetrating the fascia along the anterior margin of the EDC aponeurosis [16].

Dissecting deep to the ECRL, the extensor carpi radialis brevis (ECRB) is encountered. The deepest muscular layer is formed by the supinator muscle, which has an intimate relationship with the posterior interosseous nerve (PIN).

Straying too much to the anterior aspect is therefore undesirable as it would endanger the posterior interosseous nerve, which is known to cross from the anterior side of the most proximal part of the radius to the posterior side more distally. It has been reported that a safe zone of at least 38 mm (with a mean of 52 mm) can be used (measured as the distance from the radiocapitellar joint to the point where the nerve crosses the lateral midline) when approaching the radius from lateral, assuming the forearm is in a fully pronated position. This safe zone decreases to 22 mm (with a mean of 33 mm) in a fully supinated position [6].

Arthroscopic fixation of radial head fractures is a viable alternative; this technique facilitates anatomic reduction of the joint surface but is technically more demanding.

22.5.2.2 Fragment or Radial Head Excision

Excision of small fragments is indicated when the fragments are implicated in a mechanical block and are not amenable to fixation. It has been suggested that excising fragments that are larger than 25 % of the radial head should be avoided, since it might lead to symptomatic instability or painful clicking [1, 17]. This may in turn necessitate a complete radial head excision or a radial head arthroplasty.

Radial head excision can primarily be considered when treating severely comminuted fractures with a stable elbow. Candidates are especially the lower-demand patients or those prone to infectious problems.

22.5.2.3 Arthroplasty

Varying implants to replace the radial head are based on axisymmetric designs, where the artificial head is rotationally symmetric around the stem, which does not reflect the human anatomy as the radial is elliptical in shape. In an attempt to mimic the native anatomy more closely, other designs have been developed. In theory, this may lead to kinematics resembling the normal situation, resulting in better clinical outcome such as relief of pain during movement, minimization of abnormal stress patterns on the capitellar cartilage layer, and better implant survival in the longer term. However a study comparing native kinematics to kinematics after implanting an axisymmetric radial head, a population-based, and a patient-specific design using reverse engineering failed to reveal substantial differences [24]. It was suggested that other factors, such as ligamentous integrity (e.g., the annular ligament), might be of greater importance than implant shape, when considering kinematic changes after radial head replacement. Implants are available in a monopolar and bipolar design; for acute pathology, with a normal alignment of the proximal radius, a monopolar design is preferred. In long-standing pathology, for example, after radial head resection in the past, a bipolar prosthesis is indicated in case of a malalignment of the proximal radius in relation to the capitellum.

In all cases, a modular implant is mandatory because of the great interindividual variation of the anatomy of the proximal radius.

References

1. Beingessner DM, Dunning CE, Gordon KD, Johnson JA, King GJ. The effect of radial head fracture size on elbow kinematics and stability. J Orthop Res. 2005;23(1):210–7. PubMed.
2. Broberg MA, Morrey BF. Results of treatment of fracture-dislocations of the elbow. Clin Orthop Relat Res. 1987;216:109–19. PubMed.
3. Bruinsma WE, Guitton T, Ring D. Science of variation group. Radiographic loss of contact between radial head fracture fragments is moderately reliable. Clin Orthop Relat Res. 2014;472(7):2113–9. doi:10.1007/s11999-014-3592-z. PubMed PMID: 24711128, PubMed Central PMCID: PMC4048410.
4. Bruinsma W, Kodde I, de Muinck Keizer RJ, Kloen P, Lindenhovius AL, Vroemen JP, Haverlag R, van den Bekerom MP, Bolhuis HW, Bullens PH, Meylaerts SA, van der Zwaal P, Steller PE, Hageman M, Ring DC, den Hartog D, Hammacher ER, King GJ, Athwal GS, Faber KJ, Drosdowech D, Grewal R, Goslings JC, Schep NW, Eygendaal D. A randomized controlled trial of nonoperative treatment versus open reduction and internal fixation for stable, displaced, partial articular fractures of the radial head: the RAMBO trial. BMC Musculoskelet Disord. 2014;15:147. doi:10.1186/1471-2474-15-147. PubMed PMID: 24885637; PubMed Central PMCID: PMC4109703.
5. Caputo AE, Mazzocca AD, Santoro VM. The nonarticulating portion of the radial head: anatomic and clinical correlations for internal fixation. J Hand Surg Am. 1998;23(6):1082–90. PubMed.
6. Diliberti T, Botte MJ, Abrams RA. Anatomical considerations regarding the posterior interosseous nerve during posterolateral approaches to the proximal part of the radius. J Bone Joint Surg Am. 2000;82(6):809–13. PubMed.
7. Dooley JF, Angus PD. The importance of elbow aspiration when treating radial head fractures. Arch Emerg Med. 1991;8(2):117–21. PubMed PMID: 1888405, PubMed Central PMCID: PMC1285752.
8. Duckworth AD, Wickramasinghe NR, Clement ND, Court-Brown CM, McQueen MM. Long-term outcomes of isolated stable radial head fractures. J Bone Joint Surg Am. 2014;96(20):1716–23. doi:10.2106/JBJS.M.01354. PubMed.
9. Duckworth AD, Clement ND, Jenkins PJ, Aitken SA, Court-Brown CM, McQueen MM. The epidemiology of radial head and neck fractures. J Hand Surg Am. 2012;37(1):112–9. doi:10.1016/j.jhsa.2011.09.034. Epub 2011 Nov 25. PubMed.
10. Foocharoen T, Foocharoen C, Laopaiboon M, Tiamklang T. Aspiration of the elbow joint for treating radial head fractures. Cochrane Database Syst Rev. 2014;11:CD009949. doi:10.1002/14651858.CD009949.pub2. PubMed.
11. Galik K, Baratz ME, Butler AL, Dougherty J, Cohen MS, Miller MC. The effect of the annular ligament on kinematics of the radial head. J Hand Surg Am. 2007;32(8):1218–24. PubMed.
12. Giannicola G, Manauzzi E, Sacchetti FM, Greco A, Bullitta G, Vestri A, Cinotti G. Anatomical variations of the proximal radius and their effects on osteosynthesis. J Hand Surg Am. 2012;37(5):1015–23. doi:10.1016/j.jhsa.2012.02.005. Epub 2012 Mar 28. PubMed.
13. Guitton TG, Brouwer K, Lindenhovius AL, Dyer G, Zurakowski D, Mudgal CS, Ring DC. Diagnostic accuracy of two-dimensional and three-dimensional imaging and modeling of radial head fractures. J Hand Microsurg. 2014;6(1):13–7. doi:10.1007/s12593-013-0107-1. PubMed PMID: 24876684, PubMed Central PMCID: PMC4037434, Epub 2013 Nov 12.
14. Holdsworth BJ, Clement DA, Rothwell PN. Fractures of the radial head–the benefit of aspiration: a prospective controlled trial. Injury. 1987;18(1):44–7. PubMed.
15. Kaas L, van Riet RP, Vroemen JP, Eygendaal D. The epidemiology of radial head fractures. J Shoulder Elbow Surg. 2010;19(4):520–3. doi:10.1016/j.jse.2009.10.015. Epub 2010 Feb 10. PubMed.
16. Kaplan EB. Surgical approach to the proximal end of the radius and its use in fractures of the head and neck of the radius. J Bone Joint Surg. 1941;23(1):86–92.
17. King GJ, Evans DC, Kellam JF. Open reduction and internal fixation of radial head fractures. J Orthop Trauma. 1991;5(1):21–8. PubMed.
18. Mason ML. Some observations on fractures of the head of the radius with a review of one hundred cases. Br J Surg. 1954;42(172):123–32. PubMed.
19. Matsunaga FT, Tamaoki MJ, Cordeiro EF, Uehara A, Ikawa MH, Matsumoto MH, dos Santos JB, Belloti JC. Are classifications of proximal radius fractures reproducible? BMC Musculoskelet Disord. 2009;10:120. doi:10.1186/1471-2474-10-120. PubMed PMID: 19793401; PubMed Central PMCID: PMC2761854.
20. Morgan SJ, Groshen SL, Itamura JM, Shankwiler J, Brien WW, Kuschner SH. Reliability evaluation of classifying radial head fractures by the system of Mason. Bull Hosp Jt Dis. 1997;56(2):95–8. PubMed.
21. Patterson SD, Bain GI, Mehta JA. Surgical approaches to the elbow. Clin Orthop Relat Res. 2000;370:19–33. Review. PubMed.
22. Pugh DM, Wild LM, Schemitsch EH, King GJ, McKee MD. Standard surgical protocol to treat elbow dislocations with radial head and coronoid fractures. J Bone Joint Surg Am. 2004;86-A(6):1122–30. PubMed.
23. Rineer CA, Guitton TG, Ring D. Radial head fractures: loss of cortical contact is associated with concomitant fracture or dislocation. J Shoulder Elbow Surg. 2010;19(1):21–5. doi:10.1016/j.jse.2009.05.015. Epub. PubMed.

24. Shannon HL, Deluce SR, Giles JW, Johnson JA, King GJ. The effect of radial head implant shape on radiocapitellar kinematics during in vitro forearm rotation. J Shoulder Elbow Surg. 2014;S1058–2746(14):00518–7. doi:10.1016/j.jse.2014.09.019.
25. Smith GR, Hotchkiss RN. Radial head and neck fractures: anatomic guidelines for proper placement of internal fixation. J Shoulder Elbow Surg. 1996;5(2 Pt 1):113–7. PubMed.
26. Yoon A, King GJ, Grewal R. Is ORIF superior to nonoperative treatment in isolated displaced partial articular fractures of the radial head? Clin Orthop Relat Res. 2014;472(7):2105–12. doi:10.1007/s11999-014-3541-x. PubMed PMID: 24577616, PubMed Central PMCID: PMC4048435.

Capitellar and Trochlear Fractures 23

R. Rotini, M. Cavaciocchi, G. Bettelli,
and A. Marinelli

23.1 In Which Sports and Why?

A coronal shear fracture of the capitellum and trochlea can result from a low-energy trauma (typically in patients with poor bone quality) or from a high-energy trauma (as in sportsmen with good bone quality).

We cannot define a sport-specific correlation for this kind of lesions, because the proposed mechanisms of injury (a direct trauma on the elbow or, more commonly, an axial load transmitted to the capitellum by the radial head caused by a fall on the outstretched hand with the elbow partially flexed and the forearm partially pronated) can be found in several sports. Basing on our experience, coronal shear fractures of the distal humerus are more frequent in patients practicing basketball, cycling, ski, snowboard, skating, rugby, and motocross.

23.2 Introduction

Coronal shear fractures of the distal humerus can involve the capitellum, the trochlea, or a combination of both. Capitellar fractures are uncommon, representing only 1 % of all elbow fractures, basing on Morrey data [1]. In our experience, the incidence of isolated capitulum fractures has been progressively increasing over the last years. Isolated trochlear fractures, on the other hand, still remain very rare.

These fractures are generally considered to be more common in female athletes because of their increased elbow carrying angle determining a greater contact force on the capitellum and the lateral column during a fall with the extended elbow.

Different names have been proposed over the last 30 years for this type of fractures (Table 23.1). The evolution of the names reflects the progressive improvement of their understanding.

Initially they were defined as "isolated fractures of the capitellum" and were classified according to Broberg and Morrey in three types [1]: Type I fracture, also called "Hahn-Steinthal fractures," that consists of a single and large hemispherical osseous fragment involving the entire capitellum with a good subchondral bone, Type II also called "Kocher-Lorenz" which consists of an osteochondral fracture with minimal

Table 23.1 Capitellar and trochlear fractures: different names proposed over the last 30 years

Fractures of the capitellum	Bryan et al. (1985)
Coronal shear fractures	McKee et al. [2]
Articular fractures of the distal humerus	Ring et al. [3]
Predominantly articular fractures	Davies et al. [6]
Capitellar and trochlea fractures	Dubberley et al. [5]
Apparent capitellar fractures	Ring [4]

R. Rotini (✉) • M. Cavaciocchi • G. Bettelli
A. Marinelli
Shoulder and Elbow Unit, Istituto
Ortopedico Rizzoli, Bologna, Italy
e-mail: roberto.rotini@ior.it

L.A. Pederzini et al. (eds.), *Elbow and Sport*, DOI 10.1007/978-3-662-48742-6_23

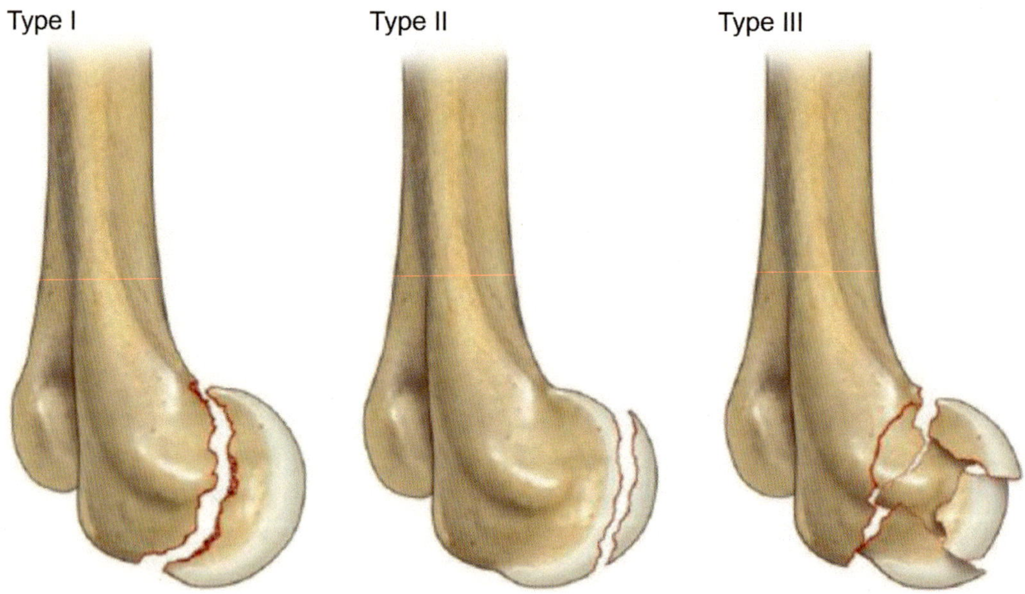

Fig. 23.1 Classification of capitellar fractures according to Broberg and Morrey in three types [1]: Type I, single and large hemispherical osseous fragment involving the entire capitellum with a good subchondral bone. Type II, osteochondral fracture with minimal subchondral bone. Type III, comminuted or compression fracture of the capitellum

subchondral bone, and Type III consisting of a comminuted or compression fracture of the capitellum (Fig. 23.1).

Afterward, as also the trochlea was sometimes involved, a fourth type was added to the previous classification [2] and named "coronal shear fractures."

Some years later Ring [3] defined generically all these types of fractures "articular fractures of the distal humerus." He noted in fact that these lesions are often not only coronal shear fractures of the capitellum and the trochlea, but they more frequently involve or extend to the lateral epicondyle, the lateral column, the posterior part of the trochlea, and the medial epicondyle, as well as in a subsequent progression of severity caused by the energy and the mechanism of trauma.

To emphasize the important concept that isolated capitellar fractures, as seen on plain X-rays, are uncommon, and very often they present an involvement of the lateral portion of the trochlea at least, Ring proposed the name of "apparent capitellar fracture" [4].

Later Dubberley proposed the name of "capitellar and trochlea fractures" [5] and a new classification system based on the extension of the fracture on the coronal plane, the presence of fragmentation, and posterior comminution as prognostic factors (Figs. 23.2 and 23.3).

The Dubberley and AO/ASIF classifications are currently widely accepted.

According to the AO/ASIF classification, these fractures are grouped as 13 – B3 (distal part of the humerus, partial articular, on the frontal plane), with B3.1 indicating capitellar fractures, B3.2 trochlear fractures, and B3.3 capitellar and trochlear fractures [7].

Recent evidences support the idea that isolated fractures of the capitellum are rare: a portion of the trochlea (the lateral) is involved in almost 80 % of the cases [3, 5, 8, 9]. Lateral collateral ligament injuries are associated up to 40 % of cases, and radial head fracture is reported from 10 to 30 % of cases [5, 10].

23.3 History and Physical Examination

If an athlete presents with elbow pain, joint effusion, and flexion impairment after a direct or indirect trauma, a thorough investigation is mandatory to exclude an articular fracture.

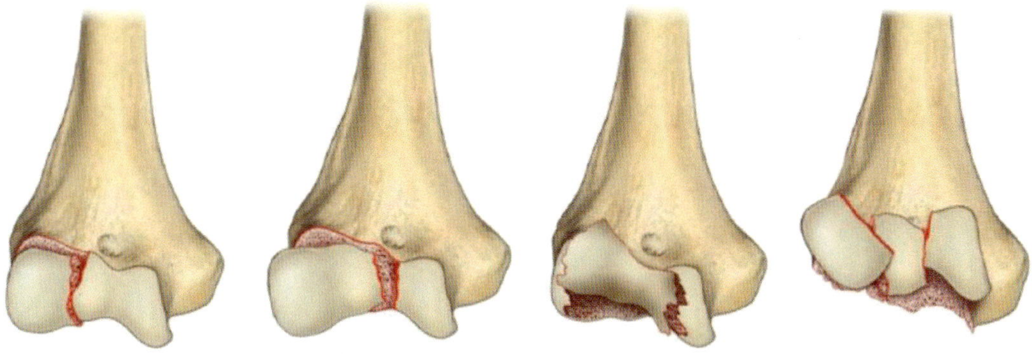

Fig. 23.2 Dubberley proposed the name of "capitellar and trochlea fractures" [5] and a new classification system based on the extension of the fracture on the coronal plane, the presence of fragmentation 78, and posterior comminution as prognostic factors

On plain X-ray, mostly in the anteroposterior views, these types of fracture can be difficult to identify. Capitellar fractures extending to the trochlea may be detected by a pathognomonic radiographic feature visible on the lateral view and called "double-arc sign." It is formed by the subchondral bone of the capitellum and the lateral trochlear ridge, typically rotated and displaced in a proximal direction.

CT scan is essential for a correct comprehension of the fracture pattern and thus for the surgical planning. It allows to correctly identify the degree of involvement of the capitellum and the trochlea, the columns, the posterior trochlea, and also the presence of posterior impaction or comminution which affect surgical fixation, rehabilitation, and prognosis. Moreover CT scan can clearly show possible associated lesions, like radial head or proximal ulnar fractures.

23.4 Treatment Options (Evidence Based)

Several methods have been described for the treatment of capitellum and trochlea fracture, including conservative treatment, simple excision, open reduction and internal fixation (ORIF), arthroscopic reduction and internal fixation (ARIF), and elbow replacement (total elbow arthroplasty or distal humeral hemiarthroplasty).

Nowadays it is well known that conservative treatment of displaced capitellar and trochlear fractures leads invariably to poor results (Fig. 23.4).

If the severity of the comminution of the capitellum precludes any attempt of ORIF, fragment excision performed either with open technique or arthroscopically can be a reasonable salvage option.

In this situation it is important to remember that the capitellum does not contribute significantly to the ulnohumeral joint stability when all the other stabilizers are intact. On the contrary, the whole trochlea articular surface is necessary for a normal elbow kinematics, even when all the other stabilizers are intact [11].

However, thanks to the great improvement in surgical approaches and fixation techniques, nowadays, it is possible to perform ORIF in the majority of cases.

The first option is fixation with screws. If the fragments are too small, or the subchondral bone is not thick enough to accept one or more screws, resorbable pins can be used.

If posterior comminution is present (Dubberley/AO type B fractures), every single case should be carefully evaluated intraoperatively. It is therefore necessary to have different fixation devices available in theater, in addition to the screws, such as Kirschner wires, resorbable pins, anatomical plates, bone graft, external fixator, and prosthesis.

The prosthetic replacement, by total elbow arthroplasty or distal humerus hemiarthroplasty,

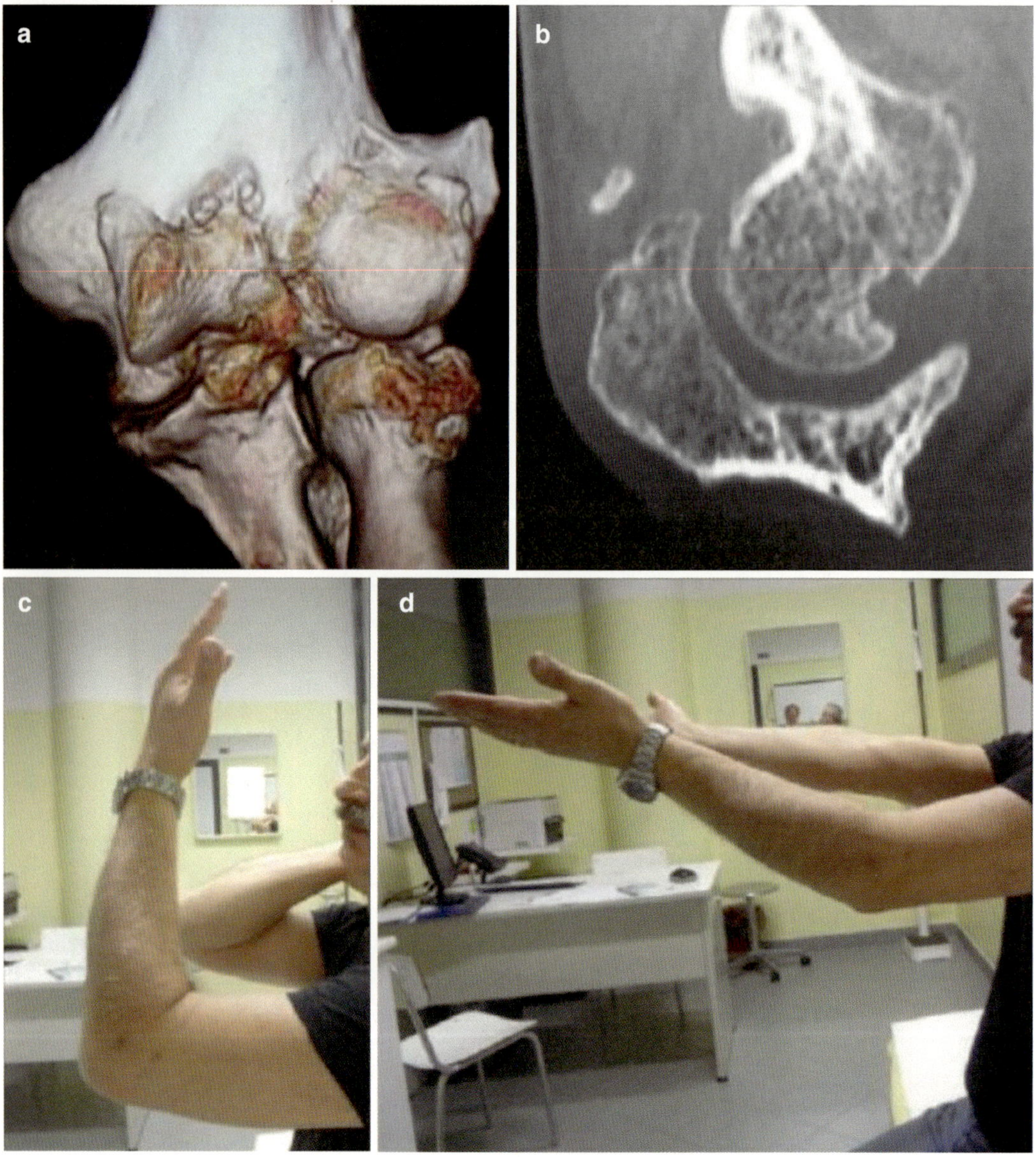

Fig. 23.3 Conservative treatment of displaced capitellar and trochlear fractures leads invariably to poor results. Clinical case: (**a**, **b**) Pre-operative CT Scan, (**c**, **d**) clinical result with flexion and extension limitation

is not indicated for young patients and athletes and its indications and results will not be discussed in this chapter.

23.4.1 Surgical Technique

If olecranon osteotomy is not indicated, our preferred approach is a lateral skin incision, centered over the lateral epicondyle and extended from the anterior aspect of the lateral column to approximatively 2 cm distal to the radial head.

Proximally the distal and anterior part of the lateral column is exposed, while distally the Kocher interval is developed, preserving the LUCL. With the elbow flexed, it is possible to have a good exposure of the capitellum and the lateral part of the trochlea by placing a large and blunt Hohmann retractor beneath the anterior capsule and the brachialis muscle, just over the medial column.

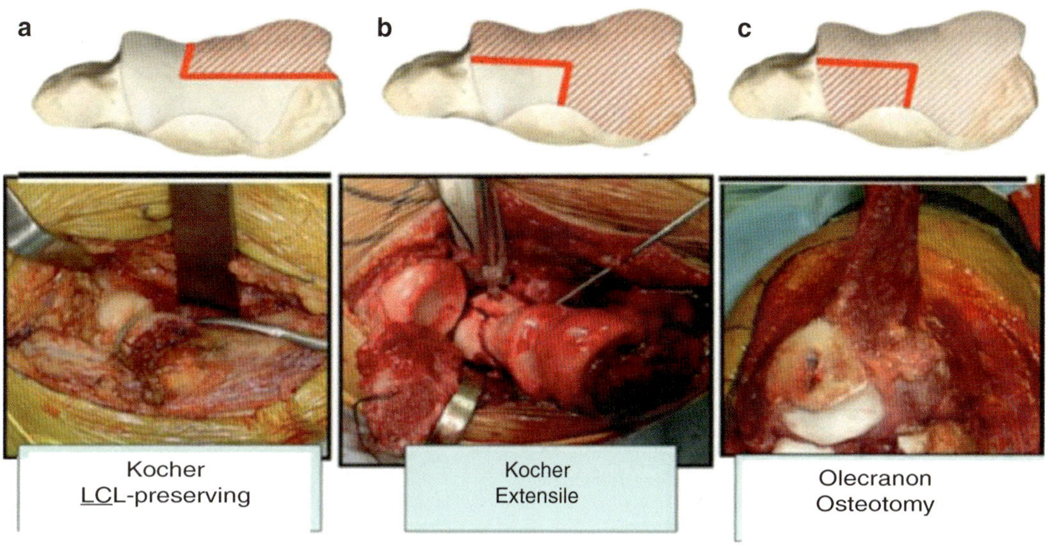

Fig. 23.4 Fractures involving the capitellum and a small part of the trochlea (Type 1 of Dubberley classification) can be treated through a Kocher approach preserving the lateral collateral ligament (**a**). With greater involvement of the trochlea, with or without fragmentation (Type 2 and 3 of Dubberley classification), the extensile posterolateral approach described by Morrey is necessary (**b**). When the posterior trochlea and the medial epicondyle are involved, a trans-olecranic approach is recommended (**c**)

If a bigger part of the anterior trochlea is involved, an extensive lateral exposure with elbow subluxation is indicated. If also the posterior trochlea and/or the medial epicondyle are involved, then olecranon osteotomy is necessary.

Regardless of the chosen approach, the articular fragments are carefully reduced and temporarily fixed with Kirschner wires placed along the fracture margin in order to avoid interference with subsequent placement of the screws; if the fragments don't reduce, the posteroinferior aspects of the distal lateral column and trochlea should be inspected for impaction and comminution. Definitive fixation of the capitellar and trochlear fragments is then achieved with screws, ideally at least two with divergent directions.

The direction of insertion of the screws can be decided based on the fracture pattern and on the surgeon preference: with out-in direction (from posterior to anterior), using partially threaded cancellous screws or with in-out direction (from anterior to posterior) using cannulated, headless, variable thread pitch screws (metallic or resorbable) buried beneath the articular surface.

Table 23.2 Advantages and disadvantages of two different techniques for screws insertion (out-in or in-out direction)

Screws out-in direction
Advantages
No cartilage damage to insert the screws
Screws easy to remove if avascular necrosis occurs
Cheaper screws can be used
Disadvantages
Not useful in very thin fragments
Less precision in screw insertion
Bigger posterior soft tissue detachment
Screws in-out direction
Advantages
More precise entry point to fix the fracture
More fixation strength in thin fragments
Disadvantages
Possible difficulties in screw's removal
A little damage is produced on the cartilage

We prefer the in-out technique to obtain a stronger and more accurate fixation, preserving the posterior vascular support that is the main blood supply for the lateral column and the capitellum. The specific advantages and disadvantages of in-out and out-in technique are summarized in Table 23.2.

In complex fractures supplemental fixation as resorbable pins, mini-fragment screws, or plates may be needed. If the lateral column is also involved, a short precontoured buttress plate is recommended.

The role of the arthroscopic technique in the management of this type of fractures likely will increase in the future. Until now only very few cases have been reported [12–14]. The accepted indications are Type 1A or 2A of Dubberley classification.

The difficulties in the management of posterior comminution, the frequently associated lateral column fractures and lateral collateral ligament injuries, still limit the indications for arthroscopic treatment.

23.4.2 Postoperative Treatment

After surgery the elbow is immobilized in a lightweight, removable thermoplastic orthosis, with the elbow at 90° of flexion. Based on the intraoperative assessment of the quality of the fixation, the rehabilitation program is then established. In the majority of cases, active auto-assisted motion can be encouraged on the first postoperative day.

After 3–4 weeks the use of the thermoplastic orthosis is progressively discontinued and a formal physiotherapy program can be started.

A splinting daily program with a mobilization brace [15] can be used in case of stiffness after 4 weeks.

Pearls of Treatment

1. *Recognizing the specific type of injury*

   These types of injuries present a wide spectrum of fracture patterns ranging from relatively simple lesions that involve only the capitellum, with good subchondral bone, to very complex fractures with extensive fragmentation and comminution.

   On a plain X-ray, the true extent of the injury, like posterior comminution and trochlear involvement, can be easily underestimated.

   A good quality CT scan study with two- and three-dimensional reconstructions is usually recommended for the preoperative planning.

   In almost 80 % of the cases, the capitellar fracture extends medially to involve a part of the trochlea [3, 5, 8, 9], in up to 40 % of the cases the lateral collateral ligament is injured, and a radial head fracture is present in almost 10–30 % of the cases [5, 10].

   More complex fracture patterns nearly always involve a fracture of the lateral epicondyle. Understanding the fracture complexity is fundamental to plan the right approach and the surgical instruments that need to be available in the operating room.

2. *Choosing the right approach*

   The strategic choice of the right approach can be the key element for a successful treatment:

   - Fractures involving the capitellum and a small part of the trochlea (Type 1 of Dubberley classification) can be treated through a Kocher approach preserving the lateral collateral ligament (Fig. 23.4a). The fixation technique can be performed with out-in or in-out direction using cannulated, headless, variable thread pitch screws (Table 23.2).
   - In more complex fractures with greater involvement of the trochlea, with or without fragmentation (Type 2 and 3 of Dubberley classification), the extensile posterolateral approach described by Morrey is necessary (Fig. 23.4b). It consists in performing a proximal column procedure with the detachment of the common extensor tendon, the lateral collateral ligament, and the capsule. Moreover the triceps is detached from the posterior humerus, and, if needed, the anconeus is detached from the ulna. After that, it is possible to subluxate the elbow with a stress

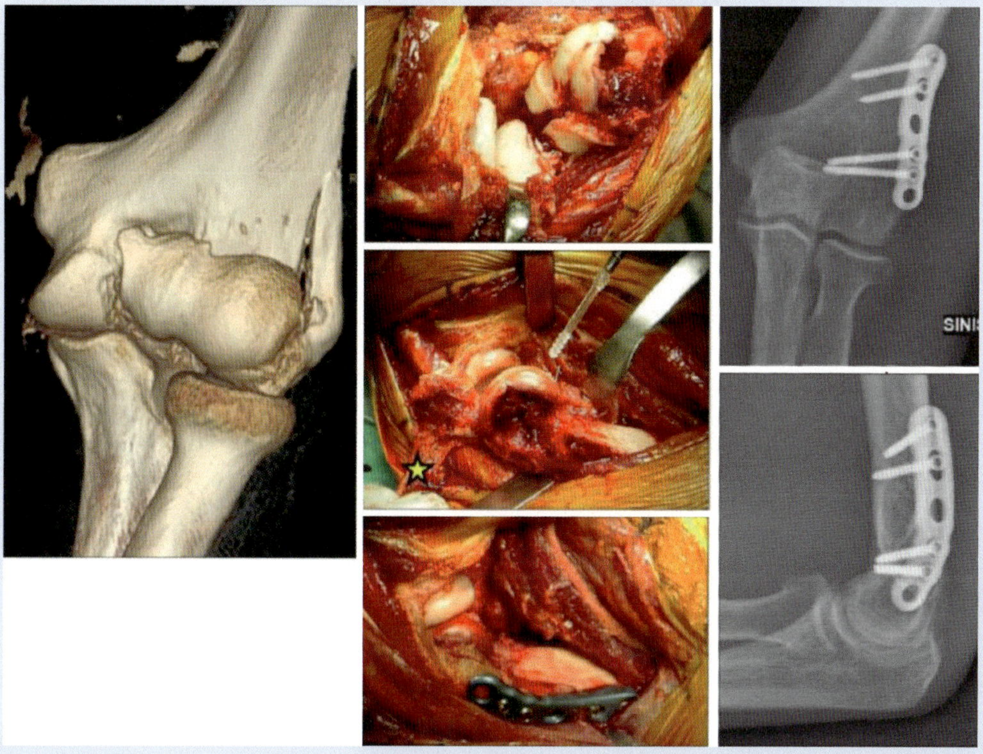

Fig. 23.5 In case of fracture of the lateral epicondyle, it is possible to take advantage of this fracture preserving the lateral collateral ligament

maneuver in varus, flexion, and supination, in order to expose the anterior articular surface of the distal humerus.

- In the same way, in case of fracture of the lateral epicondyle, it is possible to take advantage of this fracture preserving the lateral collateral ligament (Fig. 23.5).
- When the posterior trochlea and the medial epic.5eve a better exposure and an adequate fixation (Fig. 23.4c).
- In case of associated olecranon fractures, it is possible to take advantage of the fracture for the approach.

3. *Trying fixation in every possible case*

In these types of fractures, the percentage of clinically significant avascular necrosis is less common than expected, also in cases of severe comminution or when the fracture reconstruction is made on the back table. So we believe it is important to primarily attempt to perform a good fragment fixation in every possible case, considering fragment removal or prosthetic replacement only in very selected cases.

4. *Considering the use of resorbable screws and pins*

The use of resorbable screws and pins with anterior to posterior direction can avoid further surgery to remove the implants, as it happens, for example, in case of avascular necrosis causing hardware protrusion.

It is important to consider that in some cases, screw removal can be difficult, especially when they are inserted with a dislocated elbow or through a trans-olecranic approach. In these cases the exposure needed for hardware removal can be very aggressive and thus resorbable screws are an appealing option. The specific advantages and disadvantages of resorbable or metallic screws are summarized in Table 23.3.

The time of resorption depends on many variables, like materials, processing techniques, size and shape of the screws, type of bone, and mechanical stress received. However, the companies report a mean time of resorption of 3–5 years.

5. *Using superior and medial border of the capitellum as reliable reference points*

   In some cases difficulties are encountered in achieving anatomical reduction of the fragment because of the impaction causing a plastic deformation of the posterior part of the capitellum and/or trochlea. Such posterior impaction is not easily detectable on plain X-rays or on the surgical field. In these cases the inferior and lateral part of the posterior capitellum are the most deformed parts, and the inferior aspect of capitellum should not be used as a reference for final reduction. On the contrary the superior and medial margin of the capitellar fragment should be used as reference.

Table 23.3 Advantages and disadvantages of two different kind of screws (resorbable and metallic)

Resorbable screws
Advantages
No removal
Lower image distortion (CT scan or MRI)
Disadvantages
More expensive (at least three times)
Possible local inflammatory reaction
Require precise and accurate technique
In osteoporotic bone less compression strength
Metallic screws
Advantages
Cheaper
More mechanical compression strength, mostly in weak bone
Easier surgical technique
No risk of local inflammatory reaction
Disadvantages
Possible need of removal
Metal artifact on CT scan or MRI

23.5 Results After Treatment

The rarity of these fractures makes prospective or randomized studies extremely difficult to perform. Until now all the few studies reported in the literature are therefore retrospective case series (level IV evidence).

In our experience, and according to the published data, positive results can be achieved in the majority of patients treated with ORIF by means of current surgical techniques and fixation devices [2, 3, 5, 8–10]. In particular for simplest fractures involving only the capitellum or a limited part of the trochlea, without posterior comminution, the overall reported outcomes are good to excellent. On the other hand, a greater extension of the fracture to the trochlea, multiple fragments, and posterior comminution are well-recognized negative prognostic factors. In the presence of such negative predictive factors, complications are frequently reported and outcomes are relatively poor, even for high-volume surgeons/centers (Table 23.4). Reoperation rate is still high (10/21 Ring et al. [3] – 12/28; Dubberley et al. [5] – 18/27; Guitton et al. [9]) and is mainly due to the need for contracture release and hardware removal (it would be better to write down percentage/rate, instead of case number if possible).

Mild to moderate post-traumatic osteoarthritis may be anticipated at midterm follow-up, especially in complex cases.

On the opposite, despite the size of the fragments, the displacement, the possible presence of posterior metaphyseal comminution, and the limited soft tissue attachments, avascular necrosis is rare and usually poorly symptomatic.

In conclusion the improved understanding of these fractures has led to greater efficacy of treatment compared to the past years. Nevertheless, complex cases are still challenging and complication rate is still high.

References

1. Bryan R, Morrey B. Fractures of the distal humerus. In: Morrey B, editor. The elbow and its disorders. Philadelphia: WB Saunders; 1985. p. 325–33.
2. McKee MD, Jupiter JB, Bamberger HB. Coronal shear fractures of the distal end of the humerus. J Bone Joint Surg Am. 1996;78(1):49–54.
3. Ring D, Jupiter JB, Gulotta L. Articular fractures of the distal part of the humerus. J Bone Joint Surg Am. 2003;85-A(2):232–8.
4. Ring D. Apparent capitellar fractures. Hand Clin. 2007;23(4):471–9.
5. Dubberley JH, Faber KJ, Macdermid JC, Patterson SD, King GJ. Outcome after open reduction and internal fixation of capitellar and trochlear fractures. J Bone Joint Surg Am. 2006;88(1):46–54.
6. Davies MB, Stanley D. A clinically applicable fracture classification for distal humeral fractures. J Should Elb Surg. 2006;15(5):602–8.
7. Bandi W, Muller ME. Arbeitsgemeinschaft fur Osteosynthesefragen. Manual of internal fixation: techniques recommended by the AO-Group. Berlin: Springer; 1979.
8. Watts AC, Morris A, Robinson CM. Fractures of the distal humeral articular surface. J Bone Joint Surg (Br). 2007;89(4):510–5.
9. Guitton TG, Doornberg JN, Raaymakers EL, Ring D, Kloen P. Fractures of the capitellum and trochlea. J Bone Joint Surg Am. 2009;91(2):390–7.
10. Mighell M, Virani NA, Shannon R, Echols Jr EL, Badman BL, Keating CJ. Large coronal shear fractures of the capitellum and trochlea treated with headless compression screws. J Should Elb Surg. 2010;19(1): 38–45.
11. Sabo MT, Fay K, McDonald CP, Ferreira LM, Johnson JA, King GJ. Effect of coronal shear fractures of the distal humerus on elbow kinematics and stability. J Should Elb Surg. 2010;19(5):670–80. doi:10.1016/j.jse.2010.02.002. Epub 2010 Apr 24.
12. Hardy P, Menguy F, Guillot S. Arthroscopic treatment of capitellum fracture of the humerus. Arthroscopy. 2002;18(4):422–6.
13. Mitani M, Nabeshima Y, Ozaki A, Mori H, Issei N, Fujii H, Fujioka H, Doita M. Arthroscopic reduction and percutaneous cannulated screw fixation of a capitellar fracture of the humerus: a case report. J Should Elb Surg. 2009;18(2):e6–9.
14. Kuriyama K, Kawanishi Y, Yamamoto K. Arthroscopic-assisted reduction and percutaneous fixation for coronal shear fractures of the distal humerus: report of two cases. J Hand Surg [Am]. 2010;35(9):1506–9.
15. Marinelli A, Bettelli G, Guerra E, Nigrisoli M, Rotini R. Mobilization brace in post-traumatic elbow stiffness. Musculoskelet Surg. 2010;94 Suppl 1:S37–45.

Index

L.A. Pederzini et al. (eds.), *Elbow and Sport*, DOI 10.1007/978-3-662-48742-6

Printed by Printforce, the Netherlands